THE BIOLOGY AND IDENTIFICATION
OF THE COCCIDIA (APICOMPLEXA)
OF MARSUPIALS OF THE WORLD

THE BIOLOGY AND IDENTIFICATION OF THE COCCIDIA (APICOMPLEXA) OF MARSUPIALS OF THE WORLD

DONALD W. DUSZYNSKI

Professor Emeritus of Biology, The University of New Mexico
Albuquerque, NM, USA

AMSTERDAM • BOSTON • HEIDELBERG • LONDON
NEW YORK • OXFORD • PARIS • SAN DIEGO
SAN FRANCISCO • SINGAPORE • SYDNEY • TOKYO
Academic Press is an imprint of Elsevier

Academic Press is an imprint of Elsevier
125 London Wall, London EC2Y 5AS, UK
525 B Street, Suite 1800, San Diego, CA 92101-4495, USA
225 Wyman Street, Waltham, MA 02451, USA
The Boulevard, Langford Lane, Kidlington, Oxford OX5 1GB, UK

Library of Congress Cataloging-in-Publication Data
A catalog record for this book is available from the Library of Congress

British Library Cataloging-in-Publication Data
A catalog record for this book is available from the British Library

ISBN: 978-0-12-802709-7

For information on all Academic Press publications
visit our website at http://store.elsevier.com/

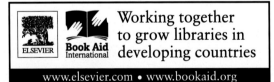

Working together
to grow libraries in
developing countries

www.elsevier.com • www.bookaid.org

Publisher: Janice Audet
Acquisition Editor: Linda Versteeg-buschman
Editorial Project Manager: Halima Williams
Production Project Manager: Julia Haynes
Designer: Mark Rogers

Typeset by TNQ Books and Journals
www.tnq.co.in

Printed and bound in the United States of America

Dedication

This book is dedicated to the *Spirit of International Cooperation* of my colleagues who work on marsupials and their protist parasites, both in Australia and in the Americas.

Australia. About 20 years ago, when I first began trying to archive every known reprint on the coccidia of vertebrates, Dr Mick O'Callaghan (now retired), Central Veterinary Laboratories, Department of Agriculture, Adelaide, South Australia, sent me the negatives of many of the *Eimeria* species that he and his colleagues had described from a variety of macropodid hosts. Many of these had never been published, and I am fortunate to be able to share these new images (photomicrographs) of previously described *Eimeria* species in this book. Professor Peter O'Donoghue, Department of Microbiology and Parasitology, University of Queensland, Brisbane, offered me access to his professional library and helped me retrieve some of the very early reprints that were unavailable to me. Professor Ian Beveridge, Faculty of Veterinary Science, University of Melbourne, NSW, sent me original reprints of several of his papers that I only had as badly printed copies. It's much easier to extract images from the original glossy reprint. He also sent me a spread sheet of all the *Klossiella* species he had worked on, to ensure I didn't miss any of the descriptions. Dr Ian Barker, Institute of Medical and Veterinary Science, Adelaide, South Australia, immediately volunteered to help me in every way he could when he learned that I was writing this book, offering anything of his that I needed, from plates used in his previous papers to any negatives he possessed in his files. These guys have been friends for decades, and they always are eager to help colleagues solve problems. I need to mention two other Australian parasitologists: Dr Una Ryan, Division of Veterinary and Biomedical Sciences, Murdoch University, Western Australia, and Dr Michelle Power, Department of Biological Sciences, Macquarie University, Sydney, NSW. I have known and admired Una for a long time, and she has helped me in other publications to understand the current molecular literature on *Cryptosporidium*. I had the great opportunity, a few years ago, to meet Michelle only once, when she was visiting Dr Robert Miller's laboratory in Biology at the University of New Mexico. I'm sure I bored her to tears with my diatribe about the many, seemingly insoluble, problems we face working with the coccidia. I think these two young scientists are doing some of the most interesting, insightful, and careful work in molecular parasitology today. They are developing protocols to better help us understand the genetic diversity of *Cryptosporidium* species that have so few structural details of their oocysts that they are impossible to distinguish morphologically. Their work has many applications to other coccidian groups, especially *Sarcocystis* species, in which the exogenous sporocysts are all nearly identical, and the protocols to be able to distinguish cryptic *Eimeria* species that may have very similar-looking sporulated oocysts in sometimes distantly related hosts. I feel truly honored to know all of these people.

The Americas. There are three individuals I want to thank and make special reference to. In Brazil, Dr Ralph Lainson, Departamento de Parasitologia, Instituto Evandro Chagas, Belém, has been a friend and colleague ever since Steve Upton and I visited him in the Belém hospital (his appendix ruptured a day or two before we arrived to visit his laboratory!), and he always has been eager to cooperate with reprint requests and permission to use his drawings and photomicrographs in our various research endeavors. In Costa Rica, Professor Misael Chinchilla, Research Department, Universidad de Ciencias Médicas (UCIMED), San José, Costa Rica, was kind enough to include me in the work he was doing with Dr Idalia Vanlerio, also at UCIMED, involving one of the eimerians cited in this book, *Eimeria marmosopos*. Their landmark experimental work with this apicomplexan established the first *complete* endogenous life cycle known for any of the 56 *Eimeria* and 1 *Isospora* species described to date from marsupials. Finally, in the USA, when I was struggling to locate some of the very ancient literature on *Sarcocystis* species, Dr J.P. Dubey, United States Department of Agriculture, Agricultural Research Service, Parasite Biology, Epidemiology, and Systematics Laboratory, Beltsville, Maryland, was kind enough to help locate several older publications for me and, in addition, he sent me a Word.doc copy of his soon-to-be-published revision of *Sarcocystosis of Animals and Man*.

If the rest of the world's humans could be this welcoming and willing to understand and cooperate in helping others to solve their problems, it'd be a better planet on which to live. Everyone should be a parasitologist!

Contents

5. Order Peramelemorphia—Eimeriidae   87

6. Adeleidae in Marsupials   93

7. Sarcocystidae: Sarcocystinae (*Sarcocystis*) in Marsupials   105

11. Discussion, Summary, and Conclusions   175

Preface and Acknowledgments

When I was in graduate school at Colorado State University, working on coccidia in Bill Marquardt's laboratory (1966–1970), the "Bible on Coccidia" at that time was László Pellérdy's *Coccidia and Coccidiosis* (1965). Our library had only one copy, and there was constant competition among Bill's graduate students to see who could check it out, and keep it for the longest period of time. I don't know why I remember that.

Long after being hired (1970) at the University of New Mexico, progressing through the ranks, serving a decade as chairman of Biology, hiring 18 faculty members, and having the good fortune to be surrounded by a cohort of my marvelous graduate students, I was reinvigorated (1991) to get back into my research on the coccidia, and to a make a meaningful contribution to coccidian biology, taxonomy, and systematics. Fortunately, instead of Murphy (aka Murphy's Law), Serendipity intervened (my friend Terry Yates defined serendipity this way: "Even a blind hog gets an acorn every now and then!"). In 1992–1993, the National Science Foundation (NSF) announced the first call for its new initiative, Partnerships for Establishing Expertise in Taxonomy (PEET), to support research that targeted groups of poorly known organisms. The coccidia certainly passed that test. NSF designed PEET "to encourage the training of new generations of taxonomists and to translate current expertise into electronic databases and other formats with broad accessibility to the scientific community." Three major elements were required to submit a proposal in the first PEET Special Competition: (1) Monographic research; (2) Training students in taxonomic method; and (3) Computer infrastructure. We had all those pieces in place at University of New Mexico (UNM), so I submitted a proposal, and in 1995, I was honored to be in the first cohort of PEET recipients to begin work on "The Coccidia of the World (DBS/DEB-9521687)." Professor Pellédy's "Bible" had an obvious influence on that title. My colleague from Kansas State University (and former graduate student), Dr Steve Upton, was my co-PI. Together, Steve and I were able to visit many of the labs doing research at the time on coccidian taxonomy and systematics (Australia, Brazil, France, Hungary, Russia, others), and set up our network for cooperative interactions for the future. The Coccidia of the World online database, which many who may read this book have used (http://biology.unm.edu/coccidia/home.html), was one outcome of the PEET award (sadly, without current funding—although still useful to many—it is now out of date, and is in desperate need of someone to take over its upgrade and management). A good number of high school, undergraduate, and graduate students benefited from this PEET initiative that, in different ways, helped focus their careers in biology and/or parasitology. And our revisionary monographic work since 1998 resulted from the foundation of historic reference materials that we acquired and archived over the years, including marmotine squirrels (Wilber et al., 1998); primates and tree shrews (Duszynski et al., 1999); insectivores (Duszynski and Upton, 2000); *Eimeria* and *Cryptosporidium* in wild mammals (Duszynski and Upton, 2001), bats (Duszynski, 2002); amphibians (Duszynski et al., 2007); snakes (Duszynski and Upton, 2009), rabbits (Duszynski and Couch, 2013); turtles (Duszynski and Morrow, 2014); and this treatise on coccidia species known from marsupials.

We all stand on the shoulders of others. I am most grateful to the following friends and colleagues, without whose acquaintance, friendship, and support this book would not have been completed. I thank Lee Couch, friend and wife, Department of Biology, The UNM, for her help scanning, adjusting, and archiving all the line drawings and photomicrographs used in the species descriptions in this book, and for proofreading and editorial suggestions. Special thanks are due to Dr Norman D. Levine (deceased) who, many years ago after his retirement from the University of Illinois, sent me a preliminary manuscript hand-typed on yellow paper (ca. 1990), of a list of the coccidia then known from marsupials, and he suggested that if I ever got some free time that this would be a good project to undertake. To Dr Rob Miller, colleague, friend, and current Chair of Biology at UNM, who said last year, over a few beers, "Why don't you write your next book on the coccidia of marsupials?" Rob also took, and gave me permission to use, the original koala photo that adorns the cover of this book. Thus, two colleagues and friends, whose professional careers were in different places, at different times, and in quite different areas of biology, gave me the impetus to start this project. Some of the many shoulders I stand on are those of my parasitology colleagues in Australia, and in South, Central, and North America, who work on the coccidian parasites of marsupials. They impressed me so strongly with their willingness to help me in every way, that I dedicate this book to them so they can be individually named and thanked.

Finally, and once again, the steadfast professional staff at Elsevier took my Word.docs and translated that ugly caterpillar into this lovely book. I am especially grateful to Linda Versteegbuschman, Acquisitions Editor; Halima Williams, Editorial Project Manager, Life Sciences; Julia Haynes, Production, Project Manager, Mark Rogers, Designer, and Janice Audet, Publisher.

Donald W. Duszynski
Professor Emeritus of Biology
The University of New Mexico
Albuquerque, NM 87131
February, 2015

Introduction

There have been a number of review articles, monographs, and books on the coccidian parasites of several vertebrate host groups that precede this one; they are listed in the Preface. Like the others, this book is intended to be the most comprehensive discourse, to date, describing the structural and biological knowledge on the coccidian parasites (Apicomplexa) that infect marsupials.

The phylum Apicomplexa Levine, 1970, was created to provide a descriptive name that was better suited to the organisms contained within it than was the long-used Sporozoa Leuckart, 1879. The latter name became unsuitable and unwieldy, because it was a catch-all category for any protist that was not an amoeba, a ciliate, or a flagellate; thus, it contained many organisms that did not have "spores" in their life cycle, as well as many groups, such as the myxo- and microsporidians, that were not closely related to the more traditional sporozoans, such as malaria and intestinal coccidia. Two things about this phylum name bear mentioning. First, it was not possible to create the name for, and classify organisms in, the phylum until after the advent of the transmission electron microscope (TEM). The widespread use of the TEM in the 1950s and 1960s, examining the fine structure of "zoites" belonging to many different protists, revealed a suite of common, shared structures (e.g., polar ring, conoid, rhoptries, etc.) at one

end (now termed anterior) of certain life stages; these structures, in whatever combination, were termed the apical complex. When parasitic protozoologists sought a more unifying and, hopefully, more phylogenetically relevant term, Dr Norman D. Levine, from the University of Illinois, came up with "Apicomplexa." Unfortunately—and this is only my opinion—the name is incorrect because it means, "complex bee," having the prefix, *Api-* (L), a bee. When Levine created the name he should have coined Apical-complexa, with the prefix *Apical-* (L), meaning "the top," or "at the top." No matter; the phylum Apicomplexa is almost universally recognized now as a valid taxon.

Within the Apicomplexa, the class Conoidasida Levine, 1988 (organisms with all organelles of the apical complex present), has two principal lineages: the gregarines and the coccidia. Within the coccidia, the order Eucoccidiorida Léger and Duboscq, 1910, is characterized by organisms in which **merogony**, **gamogony**, and **sporogony** are sequential life cycle stages, and they are found in both invertebrates and vertebrates (Lee et al., 2000; Perkins et al., 2000). There are two suborders in the Eucoccidia: Adeleorina Léger, 1911 and Eimeriorina Léger, 1911. Species within the Eimeriorina differ in two biologically significant ways from those in the Adeleorina: (1) Their macro- and microgametocytes develop independently (i.e., without syzygy); and (2) their microgametocytes usually produce many microgametes versus the small number of microgametes produced by microgametocytes of adeleids (Upton, 2000). Coccidians from these two groups are commonly found in the marsupials that have been examined for them, and are represented by about 86 species that fit taxonomically into seven genera in four families. In the Adeleorina: Klossiellidae Smith and Johnson, 1902, 11 *Klossiella* species; and in the Eimeriorina: Cryptosporidiidae Léger, 1911, 6 *Cryptosporidium* species; Eimeriidae Minchin, 1903, 56 *Eimeria* and 1 *Isospora* species; Sarcocystidae Poche, 1913, 1 *Besnoitia*, 10 *Sarcocystis* species, and *Toxoplasma gondii*.

The taxonomy and identification of coccidian parasites used to be a relatively simple affair based on studying the morphology of oocysts found in the feces. Morphology of sporulated oocysts is still a useful tool, as demonstrated in this book by most of the *Eimeria* and *Isospora* species now known from marsupials. My interest here is not just in taxonomy per se, but simply to derive as robust and reasonable a list of all apicomplexan species that occur naturally in marsupials, and use the gastrointestinal or urinary tracts to discharge their resistant propagules.

However, morphology alone is no longer sufficient to identify many coccidian species, especially those in genera such as *Cryptosporidium* and *Sarcocystis*, which have species with oocysts and sporocysts, respectively, that are very small in size and have an insignificant suite of structural characters. In addition to morphology, identifications now should be supplemented with as much knowledge as can be gleaned from multiple data sets including, but not limited to, location of sporulation (endogenous vs exogenous), length of time needed for exogenous sporulation at a constant temperature, morphology and timing of some or all of the developmental stages in their endogenous cycle, length of prepatent and patent periods, host-specificity via cross-transmission experiments, observations on histological changes, and pathology due to asexual and sexual endogenous development, and others, to clarify the complex taxonomy of these parasites. Amplification of DNA, sequencing of gene fragments, and phylogenetic analysis of those sequences are now sometimes needed to correctly assign a parasite to a group, genus, or even species (e.g., see Merino et al., 2008, 2009, 2010). Thus, there seems a clear need to use molecular tools to ensure accurate species identifications in groups where it is needed most, if we are to truly understand the host–parasite associations of these species and genera.

It needs to be kept in mind, however, that molecular data alone are insufficient for a species description and name, although their use as a valuable tool can help sort out many taxonomic problems. For example, molecular methods helped differentiate between the *Isospora* species with and without Stieda bodies; those with Stieda bodies share a phylogenetic origin with the eimeriid coccidia, while those without Stieda bodies may best be placed in the *Cystoisospora* (Carreno and Barta, 1999). Molecular techniques also have helped resurrect some genera (Modrý et al., 2001), and have allowed proper phylogenetic assignment when only endogenous developmental stages were known (Garner et al., 2006). Tenter et al. (2002) proposed that we need an improved classification system for parasitic protists, and that to build one we need to include molecular data to supplement morphological and biological information. Such combined data sets will enable phylogenetic inferences to be made, which in turn will result in a more stable taxonomy for the coccidia. We seem to slowly be moving in the right direction.

As a quick overview, Chapter 2 presents some basic information about the physical characteristics of marsupials, and recent thoughts on how and when they evolved. Chapters 3, 4, and 5 cover the 56 *Eimeria* and 1 *Isospora* species in the Eimeriidae (Eimeriorina) that have been reported from the three marsupial orders (Didelphimorphia, Diprotodontia, and Peramelemorphia) in which they were found. In Chapter 6, I outline what we know about the 11 *Klossiella* species in the Klossiellidae (Adeleorina) known from marsupials. Along with the Eimeriidae, the other important apicomplexan family is the Sarcocystidae; it has two subfamilies, Sarcocystinae Poche, 1913 (*Sarcocystis*) and Toxoplasmatinae Biocca, 1957 (*Besnoitia, Toxoplasma*, others). These are covered separately in Chapters 7 and 8, respectively. Chapter 9 documents the six *Cryptosporidium* species known to date from marsupials. Chapter 10 entitled *Species Inquirendae*, details all of the apicomplexans that have been mentioned to occur in marsupials, but from which there is not enough clear documentation to label them "species" that really exist in nature. Chapter 11 offers a brief summary of the salient data and ideas presented in the previous chapters, and reiterates some of those topics/issues discussed in previous works, including an overview of where we stand now regarding examining vertebrate hosts for apicomplexans. The formal chapters are followed, in order, by three Tables (11.1. parasite–host; 11.2. host–parasite; 11.3. eimeriid oocyst/sporocyst features), a Glossary and a List of Abbreviations, a complete list of all references cited, and an Index.

Throughout the chapters of this book, I use the standardized abbreviations of Wilber et al. (1998) to describe various oocyst structures: length (L), width (W), and their ratio (L/W), micropyle (M), oocyst residuum (OR), polar granule (PG), sporocyst (SP) L and W and their L/W ratio, Stieda body (SB), substieda body (SSB), parastieda body (PSB), sporocyst residuum (SR), sporozoite (SZ), refractile body (RB), and nucleus (N). Other abbreviations used, as well as definitions of some terms that may be unfamiliar, are **bolded** in the text and are found in the Glossary. All measurements in the chapters are in micrometers (μm) unless indicated otherwise (usually in mm).

Review: Marsupials and Marsupial Evolution

WHAT ARE MARSUPIALS?

Ever since the first Europeans reached Australia, people—especially biologists—became fascinated by the curious animals they found there called marsupials. Immediately intriguing to many was the question of the evolutionary relationships between the living Australian and South American marsupials.

Before I discuss the apicomplexan parasites of marsupials, I think it is useful to have a basic sense of what marsupials are and of how they fit into the web of living things, particularly other mammals. There are three subclasses of **extant** mammals: the most primitive are the **monotremes** or egg-laying mammals (e.g., echidnas (spiny anteaters), duck-billed playtpus), the **metatheria** or marsupials, and the **eutherians** or **placental** mammals. Marsupials can be distinguished from all other mammals by some unique anatomical and physiological characters of reproduction. Most females possess an abdominal pouch; in some it is well developed, in some it consists only of folds of skin around the mammae, while in others, the pouch only develops during the female's reproductive season, and a few, small marsupials have no pouch at all. All marsupials lack a complete placenta, and the female reproductive tract is **bifid**; that is, both the vagina and the uterus are double. In males, the scrotum is in front of the penis (except in one order, the Notoryctemorphia), many have a bifid penis, but they do not possess a **baculum**. There also are skull, jaw, and tooth characteristics (~five upper, four lower incisors, a canine, three premolars, and four molars) to help set marsupials apart from placental mammals (Nowak, 1991). In Australia, and as a group, marsupials exploit many types of habitats; some of them climb (didelphids), hop (kangaroos), dig (bandicoots, wombats), or even swim (the yapok) (Nowak, 1991). Most are herbivores, some are insectivores, but only a few are predators.

In previous classifications of mammals (e.g., Nowak, 1991), all marsupials were placed in a single order, Marsupialia, but molecular and genetic research within the last decade or two has allowed mammalogists to partition them into seven orders within two superorders: **Ameridelphia** (Didelphimorphia, Microbiotheria, Paucituberculata), the American marsupials, and **Australidelphia** (Dasyuromorphia, Diprotodontia, Notoryctemorphia, Peramelemorphia), the Australian marsupials (Wilson and Reeder, 2005). However, the key to marsupial evolutionary history and relationships falls to the monotypic South American order Microbiotheria. Recent molecular work suggests that this primitive "Monito del Monte," *Dromiciops gliroides* Thomas, 1894, from Chile, is the link to a complex, ancient, biogeographic history of marsupials (see below).

The marsupials are not a stagnant lineage, because we know that their number of species continues to increase; some because newer molecular techniques have allowed more critical and detailed comparisons of species limits, allowing cryptic species to be delineated, but most by the discovery of new species, previously undocumented to science. For example, Walker et al. (1975) said that the order Marsupialia contained 9 families, 81 genera, and about 244 species; Nowak (1991) listed 16 families, 78 genera, and 280 species; Wilson and Reeder (1993) recorded 7 orders, 19 families, 83 genera, and 272 species; and Wilson and Reeder (2005) updated their records in 7 orders to 21 families, 92 genera, and 331 species.

MARSUPIAL EVOLUTION

In this section, I want to *briefly* review some of the most recent and, I believe, pertinent literature on who begat whom—as best I can understand it—within the marsupials. Waddell et al. (2001) pointed out that a major effort is being undertaken to sequence an array of mammalian genomes. Only by sequencing multiple genomes, and then analyzing and comparing them, can biologists make use of these sequence differences to understand the evolutionary process from any hypothesized clades that emerge; this progression is called **comparative genomics**. Early in the first decade of this century (2000s), once molecular analyses of various mammalian evolutionary trees began to gain traction, there were many reconstructions and diverse revisions, the aspects of which were sometimes hotly debated (Kriegs et al., 2006). One of the confounding issues was **molecular homoplasies**; that is, shared similar characteristics due to such things as directional mutation pressure, but lacking common ancestry. Then **retroposed elements** were discovered to be useful.

Retroposed elements, or **retroposons**, are repetitive fragments of DNA that are inserted randomly into chromosomes after they have been reverse-transcribed from any RNA. This means there is negligible probability of the same element integrating independently into **orthologous** positions in different species (Kriegs et al., 2006; Nilsson et al., 2010). Thus, the presence or absence of these elements provides a source of information on rare genomic changes that can be an incomparable strategy for molecular systematists to use. Kriegs et al. (2006) emphasized that retroposons are, "…a virtually ambiguity-free approximation of evolutionary history."

Mikkelsen et al. (2007) reported on their genome sequences of *Monodelphis domestica* (Wagner, 1842), the gray, short-tailed opossum, which was the first marsupial species to be completely sequenced. This important research milestone allowed opossum (i.e., marsupial) and eutherian (placental) genomes to be compared for the first time. Their comparison of these genomes revealed a sharp difference in evolutionary innovation between protein-coding and noncoding elements, and allowed them to conclude that metatherian (marsupial) and eutherian lineages diverged from each other sometime between 130 and 180 million years ago (**MYA**), long before the radiation of the extant eutherian clades (~100 MYA) (Mikkelsen et al., 2007). Interestingly, although marsupials seem to have originated in, and then radiated from, North America, only one extant species, *Didelphis virginiana* Kerr, 1792, the Virginia opossum, is now found in North America. All other American marsupial species (93 species) are found in Central and South America, while the majority of marsupials (72%), about 237 species that include the familiar kangaroos, bandicoots, wallabies, koalas, and others, are found in Australia.

Nilsson et al. (2010) pointed out that the evolutionary/phylogenetic relationship between the three **Ameridelphia** and the four **Australidelphia** marsupial orders was unclear and debated intensively ever since the small species, *D. gliroides*, was taxonomically moved from the Didelphimorphia into a new order, Microbiotheria, and into the cohort Australidelphia, which was originally based on ankle joint morphology (Szalay, 1982). The Australidelphia now comprises the four Australian marsupial orders and the South American order Microbiotheria. Nilsson et al. (2010) expanded upon the work of Mikkelsen et al. (2007) using retroposon insertion markers to explore the basal relationships among marsupial orders. Nilsson et al. (2010) found that Australidelphia orders share a single origin with Microbiotheria, as their closest sister group, supporting a clear divergence between South American and Australian marsupials. Their data place the American opossums (Didelphimorphia) as the first branch of the marsupial tree, and placed into a paleobiogeographic context, indicated a single marsupial migration from South America to Australia, which is remarkable, given that South America, Antarctica, and Australia were connected in the South Gondwanan continent for many millennia (Nilsson et al., 2010).

The two recently sequenced marsupial genomes, the South American opossum (*M. domestica*) (Mikkelsen et al., 2007), and the tammar wallaby, *Macropus eugenii* (Desmarest, 1817), along with the identification and use of retroposed elements, allow systematists the unique opportunity to help resolve marsupial and eutherian mammal relationships. The presence of one retroposed element in the orthologous genomic loci of two species signals a common ancestry, while its absence in another species signals a prior divergence (Shedlock and Okada, 2004). No other sequenced mammalian genome has shown as high a percentage of discernible retroposed elements as marsupials (52%) (Mikkelsen et al., 2007). Nilsson et al. (2010) screened the genomes of *M. domestica* and *M. eugenii* for retroposons, and from analysis of ~217,000 retroposon-containing loci, they identified 53 that helped resolve most branches of the marsupial evolutionary tree. They found that *D. gliroides* is only distantly related to Australian marsupials, supporting a single Gondwanan migration of marsupials from South America to Australia. They also found that 10 of the 53 phylogenetically informative markers accumulated in the marsupial genome since they split from the placental mammals ~130 MYA (Lou et al., 2003; Kullberg et al., 2008), and before the earliest divergence of the modern marsupial mammals, 70–80 MYA (Nilsson et al., 2004; Beck, 2008). All 10 were absent in other mammals, significantly confirming the monophyly of marsupials (Waddell et al., 2001). Using the 43 other retroposon markers, they established the first molecular support for the earliest branching of Didelphimorphia, confirming it as the sister group to the remaining six marsupial orders; skull and postcranium morphological data also support Didelphimorphia as the sister group to all marsupials (Horovitz and Sánchez-Villagra, 2003). Another of Nilsson et al. (2010) observations was that 13/53 (25%) of the original markers were present in the Microbiotheria (South America) and in the four Australian orders, but not in either Didelphimorphia or Paucituberculata from the Americas, significantly supporting the monophyly of the Australidelphia (Szalay, 1982). The original 53 markers also significantly supported the monophyly of each of the five multispecies marsupial orders:

Dasyuromorphia, Didelphimorphia, Diprotodontia, Paucituberculata, and Peramelemorphia.

CREATING ZOONOSES

Although Australian marsupials have been geographically isolated from their American cousins for millennia, Power (2010) correctly and importantly pointed out that human influence has seen Australian and American species dispersed to different continents for zoological displays and for the pet trade, particularly in the USA. In Australia, marsupials represent normal and abundant wildlife species and, hence, are naturally present in water catchments across the country. Many marsupials also have adapted to human settlements, such as opossums in urban areas throughout the Americas and Australia, and kangaroos in agricultural areas of Australia. The dispersal of marsupial wildlife species into areas dominated by human activities increases the chance for their interactions with humans and introduced placental mammal species such as cattle, sheep, dogs, and cats. Such interactions at the wildlife, domestic animal, and human interface can and do present risks for pathogen transfer and **zoonoses** that are conducive to emerging disease (Daszak et al., 2000). These interactions also predispose wildlife to parasite species that are atypical in their natural habitats. As we will see in the chapters that follow, this certainly is true of apicomplexan parasites that infect marsupials along with other animals.

Order Didelphimorphia—Eimeriidae

ORDER DIDELPHIMORPHIA GILL, 1872

INTRODUCTION

The Didelphimorphia is the only substantially intact radiation of New World marsupials; it is represented by a single family, Didelphidae, commonly known as opossums. According to Voss and Jansa (2009), didelphids were the first **metatherians** to be encountered by European explorers (Eden, 1555), the first to be described scientifically (Tyson, 1698), and the first to be classified by taxonomists (Linnaeus, 1758). In this chapter, and throughout this book, I use the taxonomic presentation and arrangement provided by Wilson and Reeder (2005) for each of the seven marsupial orders. I have chosen to use their organizational scheme so I can be internally consistent in presenting the apicomplexan parasites known from each marsupial taxon. Wilson and Reeder (2005) recognize 87 **extant** species in 17 genera within the Didelphidae. Although steady advances in didelphid taxonomy were made from the seventeenth through the twentieth centuries, most involved the description of new species. Thus, the arrangement I use for marsupial taxa in this book does not necessarily reflect the evolutionary or phylogenetic relationship of, or within, any marsupial order.

Most didelphids (opossums) have pointed muzzles, well-developed **vibrissae**, prominent eyes, membranous ears, nonspinous **pelage**, and other morphological, cranial, and dental features that unite them. In many respects, they resemble some ancestral marsupials (e.g., *Dromiciops*), as well as certain unspecialized **placental** mammals (e.g., tree shrews). Closer inspection, however, reveals numerous distinctive and some phylogenetically informative details. These are small- to medium-sized mammals. They can vary in head-and-body length from as small as 68 mm at one extreme to about 500 mm at the other, and in weight from about 10 g to more than 3000 g. Most didelphids, however, range in head-and-body length from about 100 to 300 mm and weigh between 20 and 500 g (Voss and Jansa, 2009).

All didelphids have nonspinous fur, which is soft to the touch. A few taxa (e.g., *Caluromys*) have somewhat woolly fur that does not lie flat or exhibit the glossy highlights typically seen in the pelts of many other taxa, but textural differences are hard to define by objective criteria. The only superficial feature of didelphid body pelage that is taxonomically useful is the presence of long, coarse, nonpigmented guard hairs that project conspicuously from under the fur (e.g., in *Didelphis* spp.). Dorsal body pelage of most didelphids is uniformly colored in some shade of brown or gray, but other taxa can be distinctively marked (e.g., *Chironectes*, black transverse scapular stripes/bars on a gray background; *Monodelphis*, with three longitudinal stripes).

Many females that are in the process of, or have produced offspring (**parous** adults), have pouchlike enclosures (**marsupium**, singular; **marsupia**, plural) for nursing young, but these are absent in some didelphids. When present, there seems to be no intraspecific variation in this female reproductive structure, although distinctly different pouch configurations can be recognized among different opossum species. Genera of parous adult females that, apparently, do not have marsupia include *Glironia*, *Gracilinanus*, *Hyladelphys*, *Lestodelphys*, *Marmosa*, *Marmosops*, *Metachirus*, *Monodelphis*, *Thylamys*, and *Tlacuatzin*, while well-developed pouches are found in *Caluromys*, *Chironectes*, *Didelphis*, *Lutreolina*, and *Philander*. The presence or absence of a pouch remains undocumented for many opossums (e.g., *Caluromysiops*). While intraspecifically consistent, the marsupium of some species may consist of deep lateral skin folds that enclose the nursing young and open in the midline; in others, the lateral pockets are joined posteriorly, forming a more extensive enclosure that opens anteriorly (Enders, 1937; Voss and Jansa, 2009), yet in others, the lateral pockets are connected anteriorly, forming a marsupium that opens posteriorly (Krieg, 1924; Oliver, 1976). In all marsupials that possess marsupia, the mammae are contained within it, but the mammae of pouchless taxa are variously distributed (Voss and Jansa, 2009). In most pouchless didelphids, the mammae are confined to a somewhat circular inguinal/abdominal array that occupies the same anatomical position as the pouch in taxa that possess a marsupium. However, a few other pouchless opossums have bilaterally paired mammae that extend anteriorly, well beyond the pouch region. Although most of these anterior teats are not actually located on the upper chest, many mammalogists still refer to them as pectoral or thoracic mammae (e.g., Reig et al., 1987). In addition to bilaterally paired mammae, most didelphids have an unpaired median teat that occupies the ventral midline, approximately in the center of the abdominal-inguinal array (Voss and Jansa, 2009). Mammary counts for didelphids are, therefore, usually odd-numbered, but there are exceptions.

All male opossum species examined to date have a **bifid** penis, although the male genitalia exhibit conspicuous variations in length, shape, urethral grooves, and other details. Unfortunately, these characters of male genitalia have been unstudied in many opossum species.

Although most didelphids have a tail substantially longer than their combined head-and-body length, some taxa are much shorter-tailed. For example, some arboreal species have a tail that may be almost twice as long as their head-and-body length, while some terrestrial forms have a tail that, generally, is less than half of their head-and-body

length. This does not, however, imply that arboreal taxa are always longer-tailed than terrestrial forms.

Linnaeus (1758) described five species of didelphid marsupials, all of which he placed in the genus *Didelphis* (Voss and Jansa, 2009); four of those species are still recognized as valid, but three now reside in different genera (*Philander, Opossum, Murina*). As time advanced and knowledge of new forms increased, new generic names for opossums proliferated, especially during the eighteenth and nineteenth centuries, but without a consistent binomial usage. It was not until Thomas's (1888) catalog of the marsupials in the British Museum of Natural History (Voss and Jansa, 2009) that some context began to take place. He recognized only *Didelphis* and *Chironectes* as genera, while including other taxa as subgenera of *Didelphis*, including *Metachirus, Micoureus,* and *Philander*. As knowledge of didelphid diversity increased in the years following Thomas's classification, Matschie (1916) persisted in referring all nonaquatic opossums to the genus *Didelphis*; he also recognized more subgenera of *Didelphis* than Thomas did, resurrecting old names or describing new ones to suit his needs (according to Voss and Jansa, 2009). Although Cabrera's (1919) classification, among others, rejected Linnaeus's inclusive concept of *Didelphis*, it was influential in establishing modern **binomial** usage, but he made no use of subfamilies, tribes, or other suprageneric categories to indicate relationships among living opossums. Cabrera's (1958) checklist of South American mammals was one of the last attempts to classify extant opossum diversity by traditional (prephylogenetic) criteria, and it remained more-or-less unchallenged until the advent of molecular systematics in the mid-1970s (Voss and Jansa, 2009).

The first classifications of opossum-like marsupials based on an explicitly phylogenetic analysis were by Reig et al. (1985, 1987), and their classification also was the first to incorporate results from molecular and cytogenetic research. Kirsch and Palma (1995) were among the first to incorporate the results of DNA–DNA hybridization experiments into a classification, and McKenna and Bell's (1997) classification followed that of Reig et al. (1985) to some extent. However, no comprehensive phylogenetic synthesis was attempted until Voss and Jansa (2009) summarized more than a decade of morphological and molecular research on the phylogenetic relationships of didelphid marsupials. Their observations, representing diverse functional, morphological, **karyotypic**, and molecular data (some gleaned from the literature, some original sequencing data), provided the basis for a new phylogenetic inference on the didelphids. Using separate parsimony, likelihood, and Bayesian analyses of six data partitions (morphology + karyotypes, five genes), they found highly congruent estimates of didelphid phylogeny, with few examples of conflict among strongly supported nodes.

Of the many genes that have been sequenced to date from one or more didelphid marsupials— including the entire genome of *Monodelphis domestica* (Mikkelsen et al., 2007)—only a few had been sequenced from enough taxa to be useful to Voss and Jansa (2009) for phylogenetic inference; these included: Breast Cancer Activating 1 Gene; Dentin Matrix Protein 1 Gene; Interphotoreceptor Retinoid Binding Protein Gene; Recombination Activating 1 Gene; and the von Willebrand Factor. These five protein-coding nuclear loci were obtained from many species representing almost all the currently recognized genera.

The classification scheme resulting from the analysis of Voss and Jansa (2009) differs somewhat from the one I use in this chapter (Gardner, 2005, in Wilson and Reeder, 2005), but theirs is more phylogenetically accurate. Voss and Jansa (2009) list the Didelphidae with 4

subfamilies (-inae), 4 tribes (-ini), 18 genera, and 97 species:

Didelphidae:
  Glironiinae: *Glironia* (1)
  Caluromyinae: *Caluromys* (3),
  Caluromysiops (1)
  Hyladelphinae: *Hyladelphys* (1)
  Didelphinae:
  Marmosini: *Marmosa* (15), *Monodelphis* (22), *Tlacuatzin* (1)
  Metachirini: *Metachirus* (1)
  Didelphini: *Chironectes* (1), *Didelphis* (6), *Lutreolina* (1), *Philander* (7)
  Thylamyini: *Chacodelphys* (1), *Cryptonanus* (5), *Gracilinanus* (6), *Lestodelphys* (1), *Marmosops* (15), *Thylamys* (9)

Gardner (2005, in Wilson and Reeder, 2005) lists the Didelphidae with only 2 subfamilies, 17 genera, and 87 species; this is the order in which their apicomplexan parasites will be presented below, in those genera from which one or more have been described:

Didelphidae:
  Caluromyinae: *Caluromys* (3), *Caluromysiops* (1), *Glironia* (1)
  Didelphinae: *Chironectes* (1), *Didelphis* (6), *Gracilinanus* (9), *Hyladelphys* (1), *Lestodelphys* (1), *Lutreolina* (1), *Marmosa* (9), *Marmosops* (14), *Metachirus* (1), *Micoureus* (6), *Monodelphis* (18), *Philander* (4), *Thylamys* (10), *Tlacuatzin* (1).

Reiterating what was stated in Chapter 1, in the descriptions of coccidian exogenous stages given below, and throughout the other chapters, I use the standardized abbreviations of Wilber et al. (1998): oocyst length (L), width (W), and their ratio (L/W), micropyle (M), oocyst residuum (OR), polar granule (PG), sporocyst (SP) L and W and their L/W ratio, Stieda body (SB), substieda body (SSB), parastieda body. (PSB), sporocyst residuum (SR), sporozoite (SZ), refractile body (RB), and nucleus (N). All measurements are in micrometers (μm) unless otherwise stated.

SPECIES DESCRIPTIONS

FAMILY DIDELPHIDAE GRAY, 1821 (17 GENERA, 87 SPECIES)

SUBFAMILY CALUROMYINAE KIRSCH, 1977

GENUS CALUROMYS J.A. ALLEN, 1900 (3 SPECIES)

EIMERIA CALUROMYDIS LAINSON AND SHAW, 1989

Type host: *Caluromys philander philander* (L., 1758), Bare-tailed Woolly Opossum.

Type locality: SOUTH AMERICA: Brazil: Pará State, Island of Tocantins.

Other hosts: None to date.

Geographic distribution: SOUTH AMERICA: Brazil.

Description of sporulated oocyst: Oocyst shape: spheroidal to subspheroidal; number of walls: seemingly of a single layer (?); wall characteristics: prominently mammillated outer surface that appears striated in optical section, brownish-yellow, ~3.2 (2.5–4) thick; L×W (n=50): 31.8×31.2 (26–36×25–35); L/W ratio: 1.0; M, OR, PG: all absent. Distinctive features of oocyst: rough, thick, yellow-brown outer wall surface that appears striated and lack of M, OR, and PG.

Description of sporocyst and sporozoites: Sporocyst shape: ovoidal; L×W (n=20): 14.8×9.7 (12.5–16×9–10); L/W ratio: 1.5; SB: inconspicuous at pointed end of sporocyst; SSB: prominent and large; PSB: absent; SR: present; SR characteristics: "bulky," composed of granules and spherules; SZ: sausage-shaped, longer than, and lying lengthwise in, the sporocysts so they are recurved back on themselves (line drawing); RB: not visible. Distinctive features of sporocyst: long SZ with SR that almost completely fills the SP and obscures the SZs.

Prevalence: Found in 2/13 (15%) of the type host.

Sporulation: "Not determined, but within 14 days" (Lainson and Shaw, 1989).

Prepatent and patent periods: Unknown, oocysts were collected from the feces.

Site of infection: Unknown.

Endogenous stages: Unknown.

Cross-transmission: None to date.

Pathology: Unknown.

Materials deposited: A specimen of the "woolly opossum is lodged with the Smithsonian

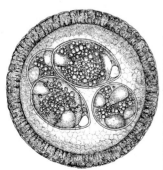 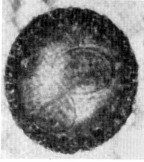 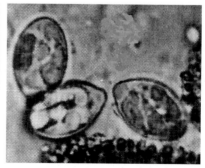

FIGURES 3.1–3.3 **3.1.** Line drawing of the sporulated oocyst of *Eimeria caluromydis*. **3.2.** Photomicrograph of a sporulated oocyst of *E. caluromydis*. **3.3.** Photomicrograph of sporocysts of *E. caluromydis*. All figures slightly modified from Lainson and Shaw, 1989, the *Bulletin du Museum National d'Histoire Naturalle (Paris)*, and with permission from the senior author.

Institution, Washington, D.C., USA." Phototypes are deposited with the Department of Parasitology, the Instituto Evandro Chagas, Belém, Pará, Brazil, and with the Muséum National d'Histoire Naturelle (Laboratoire des Vers), Paris, P-6555.

Remarks: Lainson and Shaw (1989) felt that the remarkably thick, dense, and mammillated wall of this species "effectively distinguished the parasite from the four other *Eimeria* species described from American marsupials, and in addition, the oocysts of *E. gambai* and *E. haberfeldi* are ovoid."

EIMERIA HABERFELDI CARINI, 1937

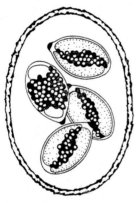

FIGURE 3.4 Line drawing of the sporulated oocyst of *Eimeria haberfeldi* modified from Carini, 1937.

Type host: *Caluromys philander* (L., 1758), Baretailed Woolly Opossum.

Type locality: SOUTH AMERICA: Brazil: near São Paulo.

Other hosts: None to date.

Geographic distribution: SOUTH AMERICA: Brazil.

Description of sporulated oocyst: Oocyst shape: ovoidal or ellipsoidal; number of walls: 1 (line drawing); wall characteristics: rough scabrous outer surface, with radial striations, brownish-yellow, ~2.0 thick; L × W: 30 × 20; L/W ratio: 1.5; M,

OR, PG: all absent. Distinctive features of oocyst: scabrous brown outer wall that appears radially striated in optical section and lack of M, OR, and PG.

Description of sporocyst and sporozoites: Sporocyst shape: ovoidal; L × W: 13 × 8; L/W ratio: 1.6; SB: prominent, at pointed end of sporocyst; SSB, PSB: both absent; SR: present; SR characteristics: "copious" mass of granules and spherules that fill the space between the SZ and sometimes almost fill the SP (line drawing); SZ: sausage- or banana-shaped (line drawing) lying lengthwise in the sporocysts, usually without RB. Distinctive features of sporocyst: massive SR filling much of the space in the SP.

Prevalence: Found in 1/1 of the type host.

Sporulation: In about 6 days (according to Pellérdy, 1974).

Prepatent and patent periods: Unknown, oocysts were collected from the feces.

Site of infection: Carini (1937) said that propagating forms of this eimerian were found "in the first part of the intestine," but Pellérdy (1974) mistranslated that to say the site of infection was the posterior third of the small intestine.

Endogenous stages: Meronts were extremely rare, but Carini (1937) found a few that were spheroidal, 12–15 wide, beneath the host cell nucleus (**HCN**) in the epithelial cells of the villi of the anterior small intestine; each meront contained 9–13 fusiform, slightly curved merozoites. Carini (1937) said that the sexual forms in the tissue sections he examined were numerous. Microgamonts were spheroidal, 20–22 wide, beneath the HCN, each with about 100 microgametes that resemble slightly curved small rods. Macrogametes were found apparently above or below the HCN and were spheroidal with alveolar protoplasm. Carini (1937) said that after fertilization, numerous granules appeared (wall-forming bodies) "which later take part in the formation of the capsule."

Cross-transmission: Carini (1937) was unable to infect two opossums, *Didelphis aurita*, with this species by feeding them drops of slurry containing oocysts. He examined the feces daily for 20 days postinoculation (**PI**) and never saw oocysts.

Pathology: Unknown.

Materials deposited: None.

Etymology: This species was named as a tribute to Professor Walter Haberfeld.

Remarks: This was the first eimerian ever found in a *Caluromys* species (at that time) so Carini (1937) did not see the need to compare it to other forms.

GENUS *DIDELPHIS* L., 1758 (6 SPECIES)

EIMERIA AURITANENSIS TEIXEIRA, RAUTA, ALBUQUERQUE, AND LOPES, 2007

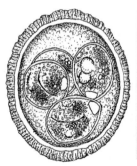 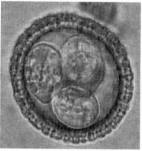

FIGURES 3.5, 3.6 **3.5.** Line drawing of the sporulated oocyst of *Eimeria auritanensis*. **3.6.** Photomicrograph of a sporulated oocyst of *E. auritanensis*. Both figures from Teixeira et al., 2007, with permission from the Editor-in-chief, *Revista Brasileira de Parasitologia Veterinária*.

Type host: *Didelphis aurita* (Wied-Neuwied, 1826), Big-eared Opossum.

Type locality: SOUTH AMERICA: Brazil: Mangaratiba, Rio de Janeiro and Sereopedica.

Other hosts: None to date.

Geographic distribution: SOUTH AMERICA: Brazil.

Description of sporulated oocyst: Oocyst shape: spheroidal to subspheroidal; number of walls: 2; wall characteristics: ~2.1 thick; outer membrane yellow and strongly ornamented with a prominently mammillated surface; inner layer is brown and smooth; L × W: 31.6 × 29.6 (ranges not given); L/W ratio: 1.1; M, OR: both absent, PG: present (?), as one or two granules according to Teixeira et al. (2007), but not visible in either their line drawing or in their photomicrograph. Distinctive features of oocyst: thick, mammillated oocyst wall.

Description of sporocyst and sporozoites: Sporocyst shape: ovoidal; L × W: 13.2 × 10.4 (ranges not given); L/W ratio: 1.7; SB: present, small and faint; SSB, PSB: both absent; SR: present; SR characteristics: composed of granules and spherules that fill the majority of the sporocyst obscuring the SZs; SZ, RB, and N not visible. Distinctive features of sporocyst: small, almost indistinct SB, and the SP has an SR that obscures the SZs.

Prevalence: Unknown.

Sporulation: Oocysts sporulated in 8–9 days in 2.5% potassium dichromate solution ($K_2Cr_2O_7$) (Teixeira et al., 2007).

Prepatent and patent periods: Unknown.

Site of infection: Unknown, oocysts were recovered from the feces.

Endogenous stages: Unknown.

Cross-transmission: None to date.

Pathology: Unknown.

Materials deposited: Oocysts in 10% formaldehyde–saline solution, phototypes, and line drawing are deposited in the Parasitology Collection, Department of Animal Parasitology, UFRRJ, Seropédica, Rio de Janeiro, Brazil, repository number P-012/2006.

Etymology: The specific epithet is derived from the specific epithet of the host.

Remarks: The oocysts described by Teixeira et al. (2007) were said to be different from all other eimerians previously described from the Didelphidae when they published their paper (see their Table 1). However, there are several discrepancies in their paper that make me question the accuracy of their description and, thus, the validity of this species. First, in their Table 1, they listed *this* species as *E. rugosa* (sic) rather than *E. auritanensis*. Second, they said that one or two PG were present within the oocyst, but these were not included in their line drawing, nor were they visible in their photomicrograph of a sporulated oocyst (their Figures 1, 2). Finally, they said the sporocysts "have a faint Stieda's body," but their photomicrograph showed a distinct SB, and likely an SSB, to be present. I am inclined to believe that the form observed by Teixeira et al. (2007) is actually *E. caluromydis* described by Lainson and Shaw (1989), because their measurements and photomicrographs are nearly identical (see above). However, it is described from a different host genus/species. Although we know that some eimerians (e.g., *E. marmosopos*), apparently, can be shared by species in several opossum genera (see below), it is probably best at this time not to synonymize *E. auritanensis* under *E. caluromydis*. Its actual identity will remain a curiosity until cross-transmission and/or molecular evidence can help sort out whether this is a distinct species or should become a junior synonym of *E. caluromydis*.

EIMERIA DIDELPHIDIS CARINI, 1936 EMEND. PELLÉRDY, 1974

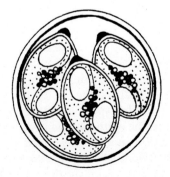

FIGURE 3.7 Line drawing of the sporulated oocyst of *Eimeria didelphis* modified from Carini, 1936, from Archivio Italiano di Scienze Medicina Tropical e di Parassitologia (Colon).

Synonym: *Eimeria didelphydis* Carini, 1936.

Type host: *Didelphis aurita* (Wied-Neuwied, 1826), Big-eared Opossum.

Type locality: SOUTH AMERICA: Brazil: São Paulo.

Other hosts: None to date.

Geographic distribution: SOUTH AMERICA: Brazil.

Description of sporulated oocyst: Oocyst shape: spheroidal; number of walls: 1 or 2; wall characteristics: smooth, colorless; L × W: 16 × 16; L/W ratio: 1.0; M, OR, PG: all absent. Distinctive features of oocyst: a small, spheroidal ball with a smooth, single-layered outer wall.

Description of sporocyst and sporozoites: Sporocyst shape: ovoidal, slightly pointed at one end; L × W: 10 × 6 (ranges not given); L/W ratio: 1.7; SB: present, as a small, knoblike structure at slightly pointed end; SSB, PSB: both absent; SR: present; SR characteristics: composed of small granules in a reasonably compact mass in the middle of the sporocyst (line drawing); SZ: banana-shaped, arranged head-to-tail and each SZ has one clear, spheroidal RB at its more rounded end; N: not visible. Distinctive features of sporocyst: small SB, SR granules in center of SP, and SZ with only one, round RB at its more rounded end.

Prevalence: Carini (1936) found it in 1/2 (50%) specimens of the type host.

Sporulation: Oocysts sporulated in 8 days, while in 1% chromic acid (Carini, 1936).

Prepatent and patent periods: Carini (1936) said the prepatent period is 15 days, but the methods he used makes this statement uncertain (see *Remarks*).

Site of infection: Unknown, oocysts were recovered from the feces.

Endogenous stages: Unknown.

Cross-transmission: Carini (1936) (apparently) successfully infected a second *D. aurita* with oocysts from the first one he examined (see *Remarks*).

Pathology: Unknown.

Materials deposited: None.

Remarks: The descriptive parameters noted above are taken from both Carini (1936) and Pellérdy (1974); the former said the oocyst wall was composed of a single layer, while the latter said it was bilayered. The first animal Carini (1936) examined died in the laboratory a few days after its arrival. He removed and fixed its intestine, and examined some of the fragments in different parts of the gut, but did not see any endogenous stages that resembled those of an *Eimeria* species. A few weeks later he received another opossum from the same locality, and he examined its feces daily, but did not find any oocysts. He then tried to infect that animal by making it swallow, on two consecutive days, feces from the first opossum that had been preserved in a chromic acid solution and had only a few "mature" oocysts. He examined the feces of this second opossum "almost daily," and 15 days after the first meal he saw a few oocysts for several days, but they were always rare. Given the reasonably cryptic description by Carini (1936), and the fact that no one has yet to report this eimerian in another opossum, the validity of this form seems questionable to me.

EIMERIA GAMBAI CARINI, 1938

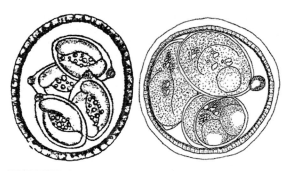

FIGURES 3.8, 3.9 Line drawings of the sporulated oocyst of *Eimeria gambai* Carini, 1938. **3.8.** Line drawing modified from Carini, 1938 (Figure 1(b)), *Archivos de Biologia (São Paulo)*. **3.9.** Line drawing from Teixeira et al., 2007 (Figure 3), with permission from the Editor-in-chief, *Revista Brasileira de Parasitologia Veterinária*.

Type host: *Didelphis aurita* (Wied-Neuwied, 1826), Big-eared Opossum.

Type locality: SOUTH AMERICA: Brazil: São Paulo.

Other hosts: None to date.

Geographic distribution: SOUTH AMERICA: Brazil.

Description of sporulated oocyst: Oocyst shape: ellipsoidal; number of walls: 2 (?); wall characteristics: light brown, radially striated, rough, ~2 thick, and outer layer of wall detaches easily (Pellérdy, 1974); L × W: 23–28 × 18–22; L/W ratio: 1.1 (Teixeira et al., 2007, see *Remarks*); M, OR: both absent, PG: may be absent (Carini, 1938) or one or more may often be present (Teixeira et al., 2007). Distinctive features of oocyst: thick striated wall, the outer layer of which detaches easily, and lacking M and OR.

Description of sporocyst and sporozoites: Sporocyst shape: ovoidal; L × W: 12 × 10; L/W ratio: 1.2; SB: present, small, knoblike (line drawing); SSB, PSB: both absent; SR: present; SR characteristics: composed of numerous granules of various sizes (line drawing) that are located between the SZ; SZ: banana-shaped, arranged head-to-tail and lacking RB; N: not visible. Distinctive features of sporocyst: small SB, SR granules nested between the SZ, and SZ without RB.

Prevalence: Unknown.

Sporulation: Oocysts sporulated in 6–7 days while in 1% chromic acid at room temperature (Carini, 1938).

Prepatent and patent periods: The prepatent period is 6–8 days according to Carini (1938), who experimentally infected opossums.

Site of infection: Small intestine.

Endogenous stages: Meronts in epithelial cells of the small intestinal villi were 16–18 × 14, some with 10–14 merozoites that were 8–10 long and others with 15–25 merozoites, 4–6 long. Merozoites were banana-shaped, with one end pointed and had a central N. Gamonts were in epithelial cells of the small intestinal villi, but were not measured (Carini, 1938).

Cross-transmission: None to date.

Pathology: Apparently none; Carini (1938) said that animals passing enormous numbers of oocysts in their feces had no signs of disease.

Materials deposited: None.

Remarks: This species resembles *E. haberfeldi*, but the fact that Carini (1937) could not infect *D. aurita* with *E. haberfeldi* while he (1938) readily infected *D. aurita* with *E. gambai*, suggested to him that the two eimerians were different species. Teixeira et al. (2007) redescribed the sporulated oocysts of this species from the same host species in southeastern Brazil (Mangaratiba, Rio de Janeiro, and Seropedica). Their ovoidal oocysts had two distinct walls that measured 2.1 thick, the outer was colorless to pale yellow and entirely pitted, while the inner was smooth and dark yellow; however, their line drawing showed a spheroidal oocyst with a smooth outer wall and a striated inner wall. Their oocysts were 26.5 × 24.8, with an L/W ratio 1.1, and the sporocysts were reported to be ovoidal or subspheroidal, 12.5 × 9.2, with a tiny SB and an SR composed of many granules and spherules. Unfortunately, their line drawing does not match their description, there are discrepancies between their written description and measurements given in their Table 1, and the only photomicrograph they presented of this eimerian is too dark to see any detail.

EIMERIA INDIANENSIS JOSEPH, 1974

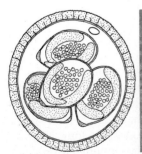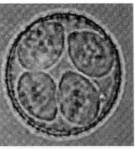

FIGURES 3.10, 3.11   **3.10.** Line drawing of the sporulated oocyst of *Eimeria indianensis*. **3.11.** Photomicrograph of a sporulated oocyst of *E. indianensis*. Both figures from Joseph, 1974, with permission from John Wiley & Sons, publisher of the *Journal of Eukaryotic Microbiology* (formerly, *Journal of Protozoology*).

Type host: *Didelphis virginiana* Kerr, 1792, Virginia Opossum.

Type locality: NORTH AMERICA: USA: Indiana.

Other hosts: None to date.

Geographic distribution: NORTH AMERICA: USA: Indiana.

Description of sporulated oocyst: Oocyst shape: spheroidal (63%) or slightly subspheroidal (37%); number of walls: 2; wall characteristics: outer layer ~1.5 thick, yellow, striated, with a rough and pitted outer surface; inner is ~0.3 thick and very difficult to separate from the outer layer; L × W: spheroidal oocysts were 16 (13–18) and subspheroidal oocysts were 18 × 16 (15–18 × 14–17); L/W ratio: 1.0–1.1; M, OR; both absent; PG: present in 85% of sporulated oocysts. Distinctive features of oocyst: thick striated wall, and lack of an M and OR, but with a PG usually present.

Description of sporocyst and sporozoites: Sporocyst shape: ovoidal; L × W: 9 × 6 (8–10 × 6–7); L/W ratio: 1.5; SB: present, small, knoblike (line drawing); SSB, PSB: both absent; SR: present; SR characteristics: composed of coarse granules occupying the center of the SP; excysted SZ: 13 (13–15) × 2, slightly curved and banana-shaped, with one end more blunt than the other and lacking visible RB and N. Distinctive features of sporocyst: small SB, SR granules centered within the SP, and SZ without visible RB and N.

Prevalence: Joseph (1974) found this form in 2/15 (13%) road-killed opossums in Indiana.

Sporulation: Oocysts sporulated in 10 days at room temperature (22–24 °C) while in 2.5% potassium dichromate ($K_2Cr_2O_7$) (Joseph, 1974).

Prepatent and patent periods: The prepatent period is 10 days and the patent period is 9–15 days according to Joseph (1974), who fed sporulated oocysts from two road-killed opossums to two live opossums maintained in his laboratory.

Site of infection: Unknown, oocysts were collected from fecal material.

Endogenous stages: Unknown.

Cross-transmission: Joseph (1974) tried a second time to infect the two opossums that he had previously infected with this species, but "two subsequent attempts to re-infect the same animals with large doses of sporulated oocysts were not successful, indicating the development of immunity." As a side note, Andrews (1927) tried to infect four opossums that he called "*Didelphis* sp." (likely *D. virginiana*) with sporulated oocysts of *Eimeria perforans* (Leuckart, 1879) Sluiter and Swellengrebel, 1912, a parasite of rabbits; their feces were checked for oocysts on 7, 8, 12, and 23 days PI, but no oocysts were found. All opossums were killed and their intestines were carefully examined for evidence of endogenous stages, but none were found.

Pathology: Experimentally infected opossums did not show any clinical signs.

Materials deposited: None.

Remarks: Joseph (1974) compared the sporulated oocyst *E. indianensis* to those of the three previously described (at that time) eimerians from opossums, *E. didelphidis*, *E. gambai*, and *E. haberfeldi*, and said they differed from *E. indianensis* as follows: those of *E. didelphidis* have a smooth oocyst wall, lack a PG, its SZ have RBs, and it has a longer prepatent period; oocysts of *E. gambai* are different in shape (ovoidal vs mostly spheroidal), have much larger oocysts and sporocysts, and lack a PG; *E. haberfeldi* oocysts also are different in shape (ovoidal vs mostly spheroidal), have much larger oocysts and sporocysts, and lack a PG.

EIMERIA MARMOSOPOS HECKSCHER, WICKESBERG, DUSZYNSKI, AND GARDNER, 1999

Type host: *Marmosops dorthea* Thomas, 1911, Mouse Opossum.

Remarks: Valerio-Campos et al. (2015) compared all known *Eimeria* species from three genera of marsupials that have overlapping ranges in Costa Rica, including *Didelphis*, *Marmosops*,

and *Philander*, and concluded that the mensural and qualitative characters of sporulated oocysts they recovered from *D. marsupialis* corresponded with those already described for *E. marmosopos* (Heckscher et al., 1999). Their comparative statistical analysis of their measurements to those of *E. marmosopos* showed no significant differences ($P = 0.0734$) between them. This led Valerio-Campos et al. (2015) to believe that *E. marmosopos*, previously described and reported only in *M. dorothea* from Bolivia, also infected *D. marsupialis* in Costa Rica. They also reiterated what Heckscher et al. (1999) had written, "…it is unclear to what extent *Eimeria* species from Bolivian marsupials are generalists or host specific," because so little is known about what coccidians are found in marsupials of the Americas, and the relationship(s) they have with their natural host species. Finally, Chinchilla et al. (2015) used oocysts of *E. marmosops* they had collected from *D. marsupialis* in Costa Rica to infect five, 2-month-old, laboratory-reared *D. marsupialis* to describe the endogenous stages of this eimerian (see details under *Marmosops*, below).

ISOSPORA ARCTOPITHECI (RODHAIN, 1933)

Synonym: *Isospora scorzai* Arcay-de-Peraza, 1967.

Type host: *Callithrix penicillata* (I. Geoffroy, 1812), (syn. *Hapale penicilatus*), Black Tufted-ear Marmoset.

Type locality: Unknown (see Remarks).

Other hosts: According to Hendricks (1974, 1977), other "natural" primate hosts include: *Alouatta pigra* Lawrence, 1933, Howler Monkey (syn. *Alouatta villosa*); *Aotus trivirgatus* (Humboldt, 1811), Night Monkey; *Ateles fuscips* Gray, 1866, Spider Monkey; *Cebus capucinus* (L., 1758), Capuchin; *Saguinus geoffroyi* (Pucheran, 1845), Marmoset; *Saimiri sciureus* (L., 1758), Squirrel Monkey. Hendricks (1977) also reported many nonprimate hosts could be infected and serve

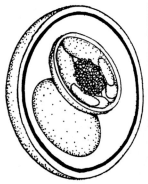 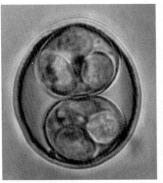 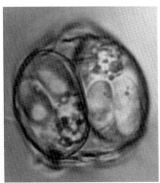

FIGURES 3.12–3.14   **3.12.** Line drawing of the sporulated oocyst of *Isospora arctopitheci*. **3.13.** Photomicrograph of a sporulated oocyst of *I. arctopitheci*. **3.14.** Photomicrograph of a sporulated oocyst of *I. arctopitheci* showing SZ and SR. All figures, original.

as definitive hosts: *Canis familiaris* L., 1758, Domestic Dog; *Nasua nasua* (L., 1766), Coatimundi; *Potos flavus* (Schreber, 1774), Kinkajou; *Eira barbara* (L., 1758), Tayra; *Felis catus* L., 1758, Domestic Cat; **Didelphis marsupialis L., 1758, Common Opossum**. Hendricks (1977) said that the laboratory mouse, *Mus musculus* L., 1758, and the chicken, *Gallus gallus* (L., 1758) can serve as transport hosts. Polema (1966) reported some isosporan oocysts "resembling *Isospora arctopitheci*" in *Galago senegalensis* É. Geoffroy, 1796, the African Bush Baby, which died the day after its arrival in the Amsterdam Zoo. Arcay-de-Peraza (1967) found oocysts of what is likely *I. arctopitheci* in the feces of *Cacajao calvus rubicundus* (I. Geoffrey, St. Helaire, and Deville, 1848), a Uakari, that was in captivity in the London Zoo. She said that she successfully infected *Cebus olivaceus* (syn. *nigrivittatus*) Schomburgk, 1848, Weeper Capuchin, from Venezuela with these oocysts.

Geographic distribution: EUROPE: Belgium (?); England (?); Holland (?); SOUTH AMERICA: Brazil; Colombia: Antioquia and Alto Magdalena Regions; Panamá: Provinces of Chiriqui, Panamá, Darien, and the Canal Zone, near Cardenas Village; Venezuela (?); AFRICA (?).

Description of sporulated oocyst: Oocyst shape: slightly subspheroidal; number of walls: 2, about 1 thick; wall characteristics: outer layer is colorless, smooth; inner is a light yellow-brown; L×W: 27.7×24.3 (23–33×20–27); L/W ratio: 1.1(1.05–1.3); M, OR, PG: all absent. Distinctive features of oocyst: subspheroidal shape, smooth outer wall that is easily deformed in handling, especially in concentrated sugar solution used for flotation, and M, OR, PG all absent.

Description of sporocyst and sporozoites: Sporocyst shape: ellipsoidal; L×W: 17.6×12.5 (13–20×10–16); L/W ratio: 1.4(1.2–1.6); SB, SSB, PSB: all absent; SR: present; SR characteristics: a compact mass of large globules; SZ: sausage or banana-shaped, with one end blunter than the other, and with a distinct RB. Distinctive features of sporocyst: voluminous SR, ~10.2×6.9, composed of spheroidal, coarse granules in middle of the SP.

Prevalence: In 1/1 of the type host; from 50 to 100% prevalence in other naturally infected hosts (Arccay-de-Peraza, 1967; Hendricks, 1974; Poelma, 1966).

Sporulation: Exogenous. Oocysts sporulated in 2 days at room temperature (? °C) in 1% chromic acid in Belgium; 4 days in 2.5% aqueous potassium dichromate ($K_2Cr_2O_7$) at 24 °C in Panamá.

Prepatent and patent periods: Prepatent period 5–9 days and the patent period is 3–55 days in experimentally infected primates (Hendricks, 1977).

Site of infection: Epithelial cells of the small intestinal villi, principally the jejunum; no parasites were found in any extra-intestinal tissue (Olcott et al., 1982).

Endogenous stages: Hendricks (1974) said he transmitted this species from *C. capucinus* to *S. geoffroyi* and Olcott et al. (1982) described the endogenous stages in *S. geoffroyi*. They found developmental stages 1–7 days PI and said that asexual development was principally by several cycles of endodyogeny that resulted in ~16 merozoites within one parasitophorous vacuole. Gamogony occurred 5–7 days PI. Oocysts were present only as early as the seventh day PI, when sloughing of the epithelium began to occur.

Cross-transmission: Rodhain (1933) was unable to infect six young white rats or a cynocephalus monkey (?) (possibly *Papio hamadryas cynocephalus*, Yellow Baboon) with oocysts from *Cal. penicillata*. Hendricks (1974), however, was able to transmit this species from *Cebus capucinus* to two male *Saguinus geoffroy*, a juvenile and an adult. He also reported that he successfully transmitted it, via oocysts, and achieved patent infections in six genera of New World primates, five genera of carnivores, and one opossum, *D. marsupialis*. Hendricks and Walton (1974) had evidence that lab mice and chicks could act as intermediate or transport hosts for *I. arctopitheci*; marmosets fed selected organs of white mice and 1-week-old chicks that had been given sporulated oocysts 21–40 days earlier, developed patent infections with *I. arctopitheci* on days 7–8 postfeeding, just as did those inoculated orally with oocysts.

Pathology: Olcott et al. (1982) had 4/13 (31%) of their marmosets die at three (1), five (1), and seven (2) days PI during their experimental infections to study endogenous development of this parasite.

Materials deposited: A photoneotype of a sporulated oocyst is in the United States National Parasite Collection as USNPC No. 87407.

Remarks: Rodhain (1933) first described oocysts of this isosporan from a marmoset held in captivity at the Prince Leopold Institute in Antwerp, Belgium; the natural origin of this host was unknown. The description used here is based on Rodhain (1933) and Hendricks (1974). Hendricks (1974) stated that the shape of the sporulated oocysts was subspheroidal to ellipsoidal and that the SR was "equatorial;" however, the photomicrographs he published show oocysts that are clearly ovoidal (slightly pointed at one end) and have sporocysts with an SR located at one end.

Evidence continues to accumulate (Barta et al., 2005) that *Isospora* species infecting mammals that have oocysts with thick walls and sporocysts without an SB should have their genus name emended to *Cystoisospora* Frenkel, 1977, which is placed in the Sarcocystidae. Whether or not such emendation should apply to this species is not clear, but it does illustrate how much basic work still needs to be done with this species.

GENUS MARMOSOPS MATSCHIE, 1916 (14 SPECIES)

EIMERIA COCHABAMBENSIS HECKSCHER, WICKESBERG, DUSZYNSKI, AND GARDNER, 1999

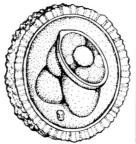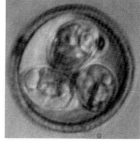

FIGURES 3.15, 3.16　**3.15.** Line drawing of the sporulated oocyst of *Eimeria cochabambensis*, from Heckscher et al., 1999, with kind permission from Elsevier, publisher of the *International Journal of Parasitology* and from the senior author. **3.16.** Photomicrograph of a sporulated oocyst of *E. cochabambensis*, original.

Type host: *Marmosops dorthea* Thomas, 1911, Mouse Opossum.

Type locality: SOUTH AMERICA: Bolivia: Cochabamba, 9.5 km by the road NE of Tablas Monte, Rio Jatun Mayu, 17° 2′ 29″ S, 65° 59′ 05″ W, elevation 1500 m.

Other hosts: *Monodelphis domestica* Wagner, 1842, Short-tailed Opossum; *Thylamys venustus* (Thomas, 1902), Mouse Opossum.

Geographic distribution: SOUTH AMERICA: Bolivia: Departments of Chuquisaca, Cochabamba, Santa Cruz, Tarija.

Description of sporulated oocyst: Oocyst subspheroidal; number of walls: 2; wall characteristics: ~2.0 (1.2–2.5) thick; outer is sculptured, yellow, appears slightly striated in cross-section, ~¾ of total thickness; inner is transparent; L × W (n = 150): 21.6 × 20.2 (17–27 × 17–24); L/W ratio: 1.1 (1.0–1.2); M, OR: both absent; PG: one, distinct. Distinctive features of oocyst: thick outer wall that is sculptured and appears striated in optical cross-section.

Description of sporocyst and sporozoites: Sporocyst shape: fusiform, slightly pointed at one end; L × W (n = 150): 11.0 × 7.2 (8–13 × 4–8); L/W ratio: 1.5 (1.2–2.0); SB: present as distinct nipplelike structure at pointed end of SP; SSB, PSB: both absent; SR: present; SR characteristics: appears as a slightly flattened globular mass between the SZ; SZ: sausage-shaped, located at each end of the SP, with the SR between them; each SZ has a large RB at each end. Distinctive features of sporocyst: arrangement of the SZs at the ends of the SP with the SR between them.

Prevalence: Found in 8/18 (44%) of the type host in Cochabamba and in 2/5 (40%) of the same host in the Santa Cruz district; also found in 7/19 (37%) *M. domestica* and in 9/28 (32%) *T. venustus* in the Chuquisaca district; in 3/18 (17%) *T. venustus* in the Santa Cruz district; and in 10/32 (31%) *T. venustus* at two localities in the Tarija district.

Sporulation: Unknown.

Prepatent and patent periods: Unknown, oocysts were collected from the feces.

Site of infection: Unknown.

Endogenous stages: Unknown.

Cross-transmission: None to date.

Pathology: Unknown.

Materials deposited: Photosyntype of sporulated oocysts in the United States National Parasite Collection as USNPC No. 88157. Symbiotype host, *M. dorothea*, in the University of New Mexico, Museum of Southwestern Biology, No. 87080 (NK 30323, female). Collected by M.L. Campbell, No. 2461, July 15, 1993.

Etymology: The nomen triviale is derived from the Departmento del Cochabamba, where the first infected host was collected and -*ensis* (L., belonging to).

Remarks: Prior to the work of Heckscher et al. (1999), only six *Eimeria* species were described from species in the Didelphidae and sporulated oocysts of *E. cochabambensis* could be easily distinguished from all of them. Teixeira et al. (2007) described sporulated oocysts with a similar morphology (*E. auritanensis*) in the black-eared opossum, *D. aurita*, from southeastern Brazil; however, their oocysts were distinctly larger (31.6 × 29.6 vs 21.6 × 20.2), among other differences.

Heckscher et al. (1999) noted that *E. cochabambensis* was unusual in that they found it to be present in three host species in different genera (*Marmosops*, *Monodelphis*, and *Thylamys*), and they were unable to distinguish between the oocysts from each host genus; *E. cochabambensis* also was the most common eimerian species encountered by them, being present in 28 hosts in 4 departments, and was collected in 3 of the 10 sampling years of their survey. Only molecular and/or cross-transmission studies can definitively determine if their oocysts represented one or more species from the different host genera.

EIMERIA MARMOSOPOS HECKSCHER, WICKESBERG, DUSZYNSKI, AND GARDNER, 1999

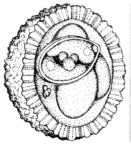 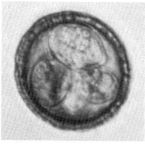

FIGURES 3.17, 3.18   **3.17.** Line drawing of the sporulated oocyst of *Eimeria marmosopos*, from Heckscher et al., 1999, with permission from Elsevier, publisher of the *International Journal of Parasitology* and from the senior author. **3.18.** Photomicrograph of a sporulated oocyst of *E. marmosopos*, original.

Type host: *Marmosops dorthea* Thomas, 1911, Mouse Opossum.

Type locality: SOUTH AMERICA: Bolivia: Santa Cruz, 15 km S of Santa Cruz, 17° 53' S, 67° 07' W, elevation 400 m.

Other hosts: *Didelphis marsupialis* L., 1758, Common Opossum.

Geographic distribution: CENTRAL AMERICA: Costa Rica; SOUTH AMERICA: Bolivia.

Description of sporulated oocyst: Oocyst subspheroidal; number of walls: 1; wall characteristics: ~2.2 (1.8–2.5), rough, and striated; L × W (n = 52): 22.2 × 19.9 (19–25 × 17–23); L/W ratio: 1.1 (1.0–1.2); M, OR: both absent; PG: one, highly refractive. Distinctive features of oocyst: thick, single-layered oocyst wall that is sculptured and appears striated in optical cross-section.

Description of sporocyst and sporozoites: Sporocyst shape: ovoidal, slightly pointed at one end; L × W (n = 52): 11.1 × 6.8 (8–13 × 5–8); L/W ratio: 1.7 (1.3–2.0); SB: present as distinct nipple-like structure at pointed end of SP; SSB: present, about same width as SB; PSB: absent; SR: present;

SR characteristics: consists of several large globules in center or to one side of SP; SZ: sausage-shaped, lying side-by-side along length of the SP; each SZ has one spheroidal RB at one end. Distinctive features of sporocyst: none.

Prevalence: Found in 2/9 (22%) of the type host in Santa Cruz district, Bolivia, and in 1/1 *D. marsupialis* in Costa Rica.

Sporulation: Exogenous, 6–7 days at 21 °C (Valerio-Campos et al., 2015).

Prepatent and patent periods: 7–8 days (Chinchilla et al., 2015).

Site of infection: Epithelial cells of villi throughout the small intestine (Chinchilla et al., 2015).

Endogenous stages: Chinchilla et al. (2015) described the endogenous stages from small intestine tissue of experimentally infected *D. marsupialis* that was prepared in two ways: fresh mucosal scrapings stained with Giemsa, and fixed, embedded, and sectioned intestinal tissues.

Trophozoites in mucosa scrapings, observed day 2 PI, were spheroidal to subspheroidal, 4.2 (3–5) wide, with a slightly vacuolated cytoplasm and a prominent eccentric N; spheroidal trophozoites in histological sections were 3.3 (2–4) wide, and had a vacuolated cytoplasm and an eccentric N.

Immature first-generation meronts (M_1) had many N (average ~11), each surrounded by cytoplasm, and were observed on day 2 PI in mucosal scrapings. Mature first-generation meronts (M_1) on day 3 PI were spheroidal to subspheroidal; those in mucosal scrapings (Figure 3.19) were 20.6 × 16.1 (17–25 × 17–24); L/W: 1.3 (1–3.5), and in histological sections were 12.5 × 10 (12–14 × 8–11); L/W: 1.3 (1–2). First-generation merozoites (m_1) were usually arranged parallel to each other within the M_1 and in the mucosal scrapings, the number of m_1 per M_1 was 12.2 (8–15). The m_1 (Figure 3.20) was tapered toward each end, sharply pointed at one end (anterior), and rounded in the other end (posterior). In fresh squash preparations, m_1 displayed movements described earlier by Ernst et al. (1977). The N of a stained m_1 was usually spheroidal and located in the middle of their posterior end; m_1s in mucosal scrapings were 14.1×2.2 ($13–15 \times 2–3$); L/W: 6.4 (4.5–7).

Immature and mature second-generation meronts (M_2) were observed both in mucosal scrapings and histological sections on days 3–6 PI. Immature stages were usually spheroidal, with a few N within their cytoplasm. Mature M_2s were spheroidal or subspheroidal and their merozoites (m_2) were arranged parallel to each other in each M_2. In mucosal scrapings (Figure 3.21) M_2s were 15.2×12.6 ($13–17 \times 9–17$); L/W: 1.2 (1–2), while in histological sections M_2s were 10.5×9.5 ($10–11 \times 8–11$); L/W: 1.1 (1.1–1.3). The M_2 in mucosal scrapings had 5.7 (4–9) m_2 and those in histological sections contained 6.5 (4–9) m_2. Stained m_2s in mucosal scrapings were basophilic, shorter than those seen in other meronts, curved, with a pointed anterior end and a rounded posterior end (Figure 3.22). Their N was located in a centric, or slightly eccentric, position and some vacuoles were present in the cytoplasm. In mucosal scrapings these m_2s were 10.1×2.1 ($7–13 \times 1.5–3$); L/W: 4.8 (3.5–7).

Both immature and mature third-generation meronts (M_3) were seen in mucosal scrapings and histological sections on day 6 PI. Immature M_3s were subspheroidal or ellipsoidal, with many rounded N scattered within the cytoplasm. Mature M_3s were subspheroidal to ovoidal, with many long and slender m_3s randomly arranged within the M_3 (Figure 3.23). In mucosal scrapings M_3s were 28×22.9 ($20–42 \times 11–31$); L/W: 1.2 (1–2), and in tissue sections they were 13.5×11 ($10–17 \times 8–16$); L/W: 1.2 (1–2). The number of m_3s observed in mucosal scrapings was 25 (22–30) and in histological sections was 14.7 (11–21). The m_3s were long, slender, and pointed at both ends. Their N was elongate-subspheroidal, and located in the posterior end. Some vacuoles were observed within their cytoplasm. In mucosal scrapings the m_3 were 16.1×2 ($14–18 \times 2–2.5$); L/W: 8 (5.8–8.5).

Gamonts are undifferentiated stages observed in mucosal scrapings and in tissue sections as early as 4 days PI. These early gamonts were highly variable in size and usually spheroidal. This stage has a homogeneous cytoplasm and it is distinguishable from some of the trophozoites seen by the presence of a prominent N. Gamonts in mucosal scrapings were 9.3 (7–12).

Macrogametes were recognized 6–7 days PI. Some young gametes in mucosal scrapings were basophilic and had a vacuolated cytoplasm and an eccentric N; others showed a dense cytoplasm. They were usually spheroidal, 16.5 (12–20). Intermediate macrogametes had eosinophilic wall-forming bodies (**WFB**), and as they matured, the WFBs increased in size and number and started their migration to the periphery of the wall. Mature macrogametes, usually spheroidal in mucosal scrapings (Figure 3.24), were 23.2 (20–43) and contained 33 (16–57) WFB. Mature macrogametes in histological sections were 16.8 (13–22). As in other eimerian species, WFB migrated to the periphery of the macrogamete to form the cyst wall; oocysts with fully formed walls were observed in mucosal scrapings and histological sections on day 7 PI.

Microgametocytes were studied in mucosal scrapings and histological sections on days 6–7 PI. Young microgametocytes had many N and were spheroidal to subspheroidal. Older microgametocytes were spheroidal and had the N characteristically located in their periphery (Figure 3.25). Immature microgametocytes in mucosal scrapings were 32×20.6 ($19–70 \times 12–40$) and in tissue sections they were 13.8×9.7 ($10–18 \times 6–15$). Immature microgametocytes in mucosal scrapings had 75.1 (41–144) N and in histological sections they had 19–71 (39.3) N. Mature microgametocytes were recognized by the presence of microgametes randomly arranged surrounding the residual body. The microgametocytes had a variable morphology (usually ellipsoidal) and in mucosal scrapings were 30.7×21 ($20–45 \times 14–35$) and in histological sections were 15.8×11.2 ($13–20 \times 9–14$). In mucosal scrapings, the number of microgametes in microgametocytes was 67.7 (44–104) and in histological sections it was 32.6 (23–44).

Microgametes in mucosal scrapings (Figure 3.26) were short and slender with both extremes slightly pointed and measured 4.6 × 1.1 (3–6 × 1–1.5). In tissue sections, the flagella of the microgametes were observed emerging from the microgametocyte, and these microgametes were 3 × 1.

Oocysts at different stages of development were observed in histological sections on day 7 PI (Figure 3.27). The oocysts were spheroidal or subspheroidal, and the more advanced stages presented the characteristic rough and striated outer wall. Unsporulated oocysts in mucosal scrapings were 22.6 × 20.9 (21–25 × 17–22) and in histological sections were 20.4 × 18.9 (20–24 × 16–22).

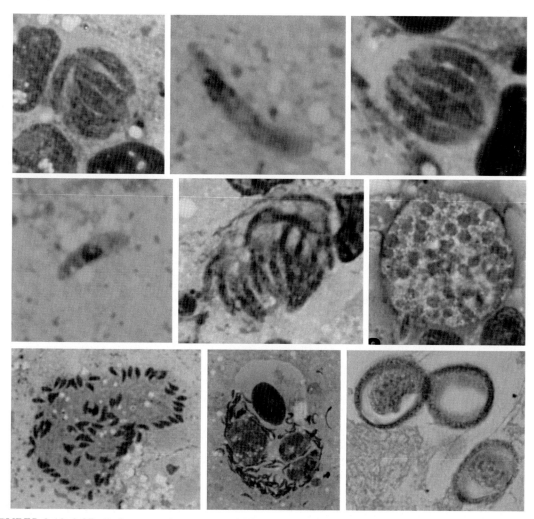

FIGURES 3.19–3.27 Endogenous tissue stages of *Eimeria marmosopos* in the intestinal epithelium of experimentally infected *Didelphis marsupialis*. Figures 3.19–3.26 are in stained mucosal tissue smears and Figure 3.27 is a paraffin-embedded tissue section. All figures are originals from Drs Misael Chinchilla and Idalia Valerio, Research Department, Universidad de Ciencias Médicas (UCIMED), San Jose, Costa Rica. **3.19.** Mature M_1 showing well-organized m_1. **3.20.** An m_1 released from its M_1. **3.21.** Matue M_2. **3.22.** An m_2 released from its M_2. **3.23.** A mature M_3 releasing its m_3; note how much longer they are than the m_1 and m_2 stages. **3.24.** Macrogametocyte with WFBs. **3.25.** Microgametocyte with the N of microgametes visible around the periphery. **3.26.** Free microgametes. **3.27.** Unsporulated oocysts with walls completely formed in tissue section.

Cross-transmission: None. Although *E. marmosopos* was initially discovered and described from *M. dorthea* in Bolivia (Heckscher et al., 1999), and later found in, and redescribed from, *D. marsupialis* in Costa Rica (Valerio-Campos et al., 2015), there have been no true experimental cross-transmission attempts in which sporulated oocysts recovered from one host species are administered to another host species or genus.

Pathology: Endogenous developmental stages produced severe intestinal lesions caused by cellular necrosis in two-month-old *D. marsupialis* opossums that were administered ~100,000 sporulated oocysts (Chinchilla et al., 2015).

Materials deposited: Photosyntype of sporulated oocysts in the United States National Parasite Collection as USNPC No. 88158. The symbiotype host, *M. dorthea*, is in the University of New Mexico, Museum of Southwestern Biology, No. 58512 (NK 15125, female). Collected by J. Salazar-Bravo, No. JSB-84, July 22, 1987.

Etymology: The nomen triviale is derived from the generic part of the scientific name of the host, in the genitive singular ending, meaning "of *Marmosops*."

Remarks: In addition to this species, Heckscher et al. (1999) found two other eimerians (*E. cochabambensis*, *E. micouri*) in Bolivian marsupials during their 10-year surveys and all species shared some similarities in size and wall thickness of their sporulated oocysts. To support their arguments for separate species status of all three, a multigroup discriminant analysis was performed on log-ten transformed variables (oocyst length and width, sporocyst length and width, and oocyst wall thickness) and centroids of all groups were found to be different, with 90.1% of the variation in the data being accounted for in the first canonical variate. A plot of discriminant scores indicated minimum polygons enclosing the spread of individuals for each of the three species they described. Their canonical analysis indicated that as the lengths of the oocysts and sporocysts decreased, their widths increased.

Chinchilla et al. (2015) worked out the details of the endogenous life cycle when they used

oocysts recovered from *D. marsupialis* in Costa Rica, and experimentally infected five, 2-month-old *D. marsupialis* and killed them at 24 h intervals beginning on day 2 PI.

GENUS *MICOUREUS* LESSON, 1842 (6 SPECIES)

EIMERIA MICOURI HECKSCHER, WICKESBERG, DUSZYNSKI, AND GARDNER, 1999

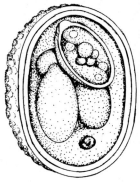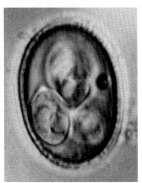

FIGURES 3.28, 3.29   **3.28.** Line drawing of the sporulated oocyst of *Eimeria micouri*, from Heckscher et al., 1999, with kind permission from Elsevier, publisher of the *International Journal of Parasitology* and from the senior author. **3.29.** Photomicrograph of a sporulated oocyst of *E. micouri*, original.

Type host: *Micoureus constantiae constantiae* Thomas, 1904, Mouse Opossum.

Type locality: SOUTH AMERICA: Bolivia: Cochabamba, 9.5 km by the road NE of Tablas Monte, Rio Jatun Mayu, 17° 02′ 29″ S, 65° 59′ 05″ W, elevation 1500 m.

Other hosts: *Micoureus constantiae budini* Thomas, 1919, Mouse Opossum.

Geographic distribution: SOUTH AMERICA: Bolivia: Departments of Cochabamba, Santa Cruz, and Tarija.

Description of sporulated oocyst: Oocyst ellipsoidal; number of walls: 2; wall characteristics: total thickness ~1.6 (1.2–2.0), both layers of equal thickness; outer is pitted, inner is transparent;

L×W (n=50): 24.6×18.2 (20–28×17–20); L/W ratio: 1.3 (1.2–1.5); M, OR: both absent; PG: one or two always present. Distinctive features of oocyst: thick, pitted outer oocyst wall and presence of a PG, but no OR.

Description of sporocyst and sporozoites: Sporocyst shape: fusiform, slightly pointed at one end; L×W (n=50): 11.5×6.7 (10–13×6–8); L/W ratio: 1.7 (1.5–1.8); SB: present as distinct nipplelike structure at pointed end of SP; SSB, PSB: both absent; SR: present; SR characteristics: several small globules usually along one side of SP wall; SZ: sausage-shaped, lying side-by-side along length of the SP; each SZ has one small spheroidal RB at its more pointed end and a larger RB at its more rounded end. Distinctive features of sporocyst: SZ with two distinct RBs of different sizes.

Prevalence: Found in 4/6 (67%) of the type host in Cochabamba district; in 1/1 *M. c. budini* in the Santa Cruz district; and in 1/1 *M. c. budini* in the Tarija district.

Sporulation: Unknown.

Prepatent and patent periods: Unknown, oocysts were collected from the feces.

Site of infection: Unknown.

Endogenous stages: Unknown.

Cross-transmission: None to date.

Pathology: Unknown.

Materials deposited: Photosyntype of sporulated oocysts in the United States National Parasite Collection as USNPC No. 88159. Symbiotype host, *M. c. constantiae*, in the Collection Boliviana de Fauna, La Paz, Bolivia, No. 3569 (NK 30341, male). Collected by J.P. Téllez, No. 25, July 16, 1993.

Etymology: The nomen triviale is derived from the generic part of the scientific name of the host, in the genitive singular ending, meaning "of *Micoureus*."

Remarks: This is the only eimerian found in any of the six species in this host genus to date. Arguments for how its sporulated oocysts differs from those of *E. cochabambensis* and *E. marmosopos*, also found in Bolivian marsupials (Didelphimorphia), are given in Heckscher et al. (1999). Oocysts of this species also somewhat resemble those of *E. haberfeldi* described (above) from *Caluromys philander*

by Carini (1937) because of the ellipsoidal shape, absence of an OR, and presence of an SB. However, the oocysts differ from those of *E. haberfeldi* by being smaller (25×18 vs 30×20), by having a two-layered wall (vs one), and by having PGs, which *E. haberfeldi* lacks.

EIMERIA COCHABAMBENSIS HECKSCHER, WICKESBERG, DUSZYNSKI, AND GARDNER, 1999

Type host: *Marmosops dorthea* Thomas, 1911, Mouse Opossum.

Remarks: Heckscher et al. (1999) reported on a 10-year survey (1984–1993) of 330 marsupials from seven districts of Bolivia. They reported this eimerian in 7/21 (33%) *M. domestica* (Wagner, 1842) from the Chuquisaca district, but found no coccidian oocysts in five *M. domestica* from two localities in the Department of Santa Cruz.

EIMERIA PHILANDERI LAINSON AND SHAW, 1989

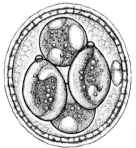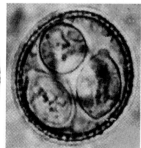

FIGURES 3.30, 3.31 **3.30.** Line drawing of the sporulated oocyst of *Eimeria philanderi*. **3.31.** Photomicrograph of a sporulated oocyst of *E. philanderi*. Both figures slightly modified from Lainson and Shaw, 1989, from the *Bulletin du Museum National d'Histoire Naturalle (Paris)* and with permission from the senior author.

Type host: *Philander opossum opossum* (L., 1758), Gray Four-eyed Opossum.

Type locality: SOUTH AMERICA: Brazil: Pará State, Island of Tocantins, 4° 49′ S, 49° 49′ W, now submerged beneath the waters of the Tucurui Reservoir.

Other hosts: None to date.

Geographic distribution: SOUTH AMERICA: Brazil.

Description of sporulated oocyst: Oocyst spheroidal to subspheroidal; number of walls: 2; wall characteristics: total thickness ~1.9, both layers are striated and of equal thickness (line drawing); outer is mammillated, colorless; inner is yellow-brown; L×W (n=50): 23.5×22.4 (21–27.5×19–25); L/W ratio: 1.0+; M, OR: both absent; PG: distinct, ~4×2. Distinctive features of oocyst: thick, two-layered mammillated outer oocyst wall.

Description of sporocyst and sporozoites: Sporocyst shape: ovoidal to ellipsoidal; L×W (n=50): 11.4×8.1 (10–12.5×7.5–9); L/W ratio: 1.4; SB: present as a prominent, nipplelike structure at pointed end of SP; SSB, PSB: both absent; SR: present; SR characteristics: composed of granules and spherules, usually concentrated between the SZ; SZ: sausage-shaped, recurved, each without visible RB. Distinctive features of SP: SZ without RBs and longer than the length of the sporocyst, which causes them to become recurved (line drawing).

Prevalence: Found in 7/13 (54%) of the type host; two of the infected opossums also were passing isosporan-type oocysts that Lainson and Shaw (1989) thought might be *I. boughtoni*, but which we now know was a *Sarcocystis* species, possibly *S. falcatula* or *S. lindsayi* (see Chapter 7), both of which have been found in *Didelphis* species in Brazil and Argentina.

Sporulation: Lainson and Shaw (1989) said sporulation took 5 days at ~24°C.

Prepatent and patent periods: Unknown, oocysts were collected from the feces.

Site of infection: Unknown.

Endogenous stages: Unknown.

Cross-transmission: None to date.

Pathology: Unknown.

Materials deposited: Phototypes are deposited with the Department of Parasitology, the Instituto Evandro Chagas, Belém, Pará, Brazil, and with the Muséum National d'Histoire Naturelle (Laboratoire des Vers), Paris, P 6555.

Remarks: Lainson and Shaw (1989) compared the mensural characteristics of the sporulated oocysts of this species to those of *E. didelphidis* Carini, 1936 (from *D. auritus*), to *E. gambai* Carini, 1938 (from *D. auritus*), and to those of *E. haberfeldi* Carini, 1937 (from *Cal. philander*), and they are all very different. Lainson and Shaw (1989) also compared sporulated oocysts of this species to those of *E. indianensis* Joseph, 1974, from the North American opossum, *D. virginiana*. The shape and sculptured outer wall of the two species are quite similar, but the oocysts of *E. indianensis* are much smaller than those of *E. philanderi*, averaging only 16.3 (spheroidal forms) or 17.6×16.4 (subspheroidal forms) vs 23.5×22.4 (21–27.5×19–25) for *E. philanderi*; their sporocysts are also comparatively different in size.

GENUS *THYLAMYS* GRAY, 1843 (10 SPECIES)

EIMERIA COCHABAMBENSIS HECKSCHER, WICKESBERG, DUSZYNSKI, AND GARDNER, 1999

Type host: *Marmosops dorthea* Thomas, 1911, Mouse Opossum.

Remarks: Heckscher et al. (1999) reported on a 10-year survey (1984–1993) of 330 marsupials from seven districts of Bolivia. They reported this eimerian in 9/28 (32%) *T. venustus* (Thomas, 1902) from the Chuquisaca district, 3/20 (15%) from the Santa Cruz district, and in 10/39 (26%) from the Tarija district.

There are no other eimerians described from this genus as far as I know.

DISCUSSION AND SUMMARY

The following **subfamilies** (-inae), genera, and species (number) in this order of New World marsupials either have no Apicomplexa: Eimeriidae parasites described from them, or they have never been examined/surveyed for them: **Subfamily** Caluromyinae: *Caluromysiops* (1), *G,lironia* (1); **Subfamily** Didelphinae: *Chironectes* (1), *Gracilinanus* (9), *Hyladelphys* (1), *Lestodelphys* (1), *Lutreolina* (1, but see Chapter 10, *Species Inquirendae*), *Marmosa* (9), *Metachirus* (1), and *Tlacuatzin* (1). In addition, in the Caluromyinae, only one of three *Caluromys* species has been examined. In the Didelphinae, only 3 of 6 *Didelphis* species, only 1 of 6 *Micoureus* species, only 1 of 14 *Monodelphis* species, only 1 of 4 *Philander* species, and only 1 of 10 *Thylomys* species have been examined for coccidia. Put another way, only 7 of the 17 (41%) genera and only 9 of the 87 (10%) species in the New World's Didelphimorphia opossums have ever been examined for intestinal coccidians. From this very modest sample, 10 *Eimeria* and 1 *Isospora* species have been identified, of which a few may not be valid. In addition, more than a dozen other apicomplexan species, found in either the intestinal tract or muscles have been found in Didelphimorphia species; these include *Besnoitia*, *Cryptosporidium*, *Isospora*, and *Sarcocystis*-like forms, but these must be relegated to *Species Inquirendae* for reasons given elsewhere (see Chapter 10, Tables 11.1 and 11.2). Of the nine opossum species that have been examined, only very small sample numbers from limited geographic areas have been surveyed to date, and these factors certainly contribute to the fact that more than one valid coccidium was found in only four opossum species: *C. philander* (2), *D. aurita* (3), *D. marsupialis* (2), and *M. dorothea* (2). Clearly, there is still a *great deal* of work to

accomplish before we can begin to have even a clue about the biodiversity of intestinal coccidians in New World opossums.

The data presented above reveal precious little about the biology of these intestinal coccidians from New World opossums. The amount of time it takes for oocysts to sporulate once they leave the confines of their host's intestinal tract is reasonably well known for 6 of the 11 (54.5%) known species: *E. haberfeldi*, *E. auritanensis*, *E. didelphidis*, *E. gambai*, *E. philanderi*, and *I. arctopitheci*. We know the prepatent and/or patent periods only for 3 of the 11 (27%). We know the site of infection for only 3 of the 11 (27%). We know only a few details of one or more endogenous stages in *E. haberfeldi*; however, on the bright side, and most importantly, we know the complete life cycle of endogenous development in *E. marmosopos*. This is a landmark study because it is the only complete life cycle known for any marsupial intestinal coccidian. Only two species, *E. haberfeldi* and *I. arctopitheci*, have been cross-transmitted to other host species, and we know only that *E. marmosopos* can be pathogenic in one opossum species, *D. marsupialis*. The only category in which we have done a reasonable job is that 7 of these 11 (64%) coccidia species have been archived into accredited museums as phototypes: *E. auritanensis*, *E. caluromydis*, *E. cochabambensis*, *E. marmosopos*, *E. micouri*, *E. philanderi*, and *I. arctopitheci* and the **symbiotype** host (see Frey et al., 1992) has been archived for 4 of the 11 (36%) species: *E. caluromydis*, *E. cochabambensis*, *E. marmosopos*, and *E. micouri*.

A tremendous amount of work remains to be started and completed; wide geographic surveys sampling many localities in each didelphid species known geographic range should be undertaken, and the sooner the better, before they are gone forever. I hope that this synopsis of what is, but mostly what is not, known will stimulate such efforts among North, Central, and South American parasitologists and mammalogists.

4

Order Diprotodontia—Eimeriidae

ORDER DIPROTODONTIA
OWEN, 1866

INTRODUCTION

The Diprotodontia includes a wide variety of uniquely Australian and familiar marsupials including kangaroos, wallabies, possums, wombats, and koalas, along with many less-recognized groups/names (e.g., antechinids, dasyurids, quolls, and more). Almost all **extant** Diprotodontia are **herbivores**, with a few **insectivores** and **omnivores** in the group, but the latter two are thought to have arisen as relatively recent adaptations from the mainstream herbivorous lifestyle. Wilson and Reeder (2005) list the Diprotodontia as having 11 families, with 39 genera and 143 species. It is one of four Australian orders of marsupials (along with Dasyuromorphia, Notoryctemorphia, Peramelemorphia).

Szalay (1982) proposed that the seven marsupial orders be divided into two cohorts, Ameridelphia for the three orders in the Americas, and Australidelphia for the four Australian orders, based on the distinction between the continuous lower ankle joint pattern (**CLAJP**) and the separate lower ankle joint pattern (**SLAJP**). The Australidelphia (along with the American order Microbiotheria) are characterized by CLAJP, which is thought to be a derived condition versus SLAJP, the primitive condition that characterizes the Ameridelphia. Meredith et al. (2008) emphasized that molecular data sets, including mitochondrial and nuclear genome sequences, are diverse and extensive, confirming the Australidelphia as a unique evolutionary lineage. However, resolving relationships *within* the Australidelphia has been difficult and sometimes contentious (e.g., Kirsch et al., 1997; Nilsson et al., 2003, 2004 versus Amrine-Madsen et al., 2003; Phillips et al., 2006), with much of the debate involving the relationship of the Microbiotheria relative to the other Australidelphia.

Diprotodontia is the largest and most diverse order of Australidelphian marsupials, and historically, relationships between subdivisions (e.g., suborders, families, subfamilies, tribes) within it have been difficult to resolve. Members of the order are united by distinctive shared traits (**synapomorphies**), the most obvious of which is having two front teeth (**diprotodonty**), a pair of large incisors on the lower jaw, but no canines. Other unifying traits include having only a superficial thymus, and as many as 22 morphological traits unique to this group (**apomorphies**) (Horovitz and Sánchez-Villagra, 2003; Meredith et al., 2008). These characters provide overwhelming morphological evidence to support this clade, and recent molecular evidence now available (Amrine-Madsen et al., 2003; Meredith et al., 2008, 2009) lends very strong support for it.

Wilson and Reeder (2005) recognized three suborders within the Diprotodontia: Macropodiformes (kangaroos, wallabies, and kin), Phalangeriformes (possums) and Vombatiformes (wombats and koalas). Meredith et al. (2008), using a nuclear five-gene data set, strongly supported the monophyly of the Vombatiformes (Vombatus + Phascolarctos), consistent with several previous supporting studies that range from their hook-shaped spermatozoa (Harding, 1987), to serological data (Kirsch, 1977), mitochondrial DNA (Munemasa et al., 2006), DNA hybridization (Springer et al., 1997a,b), and morphological similarities (Horovitz and Sánchez-Villagra, 2003). Meredith et al. (2008) also found strong molecular support of monophyly for Macropodiformes (+Phalangeriformes), which was consistent with previous morphological evidence and mitochondrial genome sequences.

Below, I list the Diprotodontia genera, and the species in those genera, that have apicomplexan Eimeriidae species described from them. The host taxonomic order I followed for the suborders, families, and genera is that of Wilson and Reeder (2005).

SPECIES DESCRIPTIONS

SUBORDER VOMBATIFORMES BURNETT, 1830 (2 FAMILIES, 3 GENERA, 4 SPECIES)

FAMILY VOMBATIDAE BURNETT, 1830 (2 GENERA, 3 SPECIES)

GENUS LASIORHINUS GRAY, 1863 (2 SPECIES)

EIMERIA URSINI SUPPERER, 1957

Synonym: *Eimeria* (*Eimeria*) *ursini* Supperer, 1957.

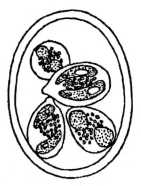

FIGURE 4.1   Line drawing of the sporulated oocyst of *Eimeria ursini* from Supperer, 1957, with kind permission of Springer Science + Business Media, publishers of *Zeitschrift für Parasitenkunde*.

Type host: *Lasiorhinus latifrons* (Owen, 1845), Southern Hairy-nosed Wombat (Supperer, 1957, said the type host was *Vombatus ursinus* (Shaw, 1800), the common wombat, but Barker et al. 1979, said that he had misidentified the host; see *Remarks* under *E. wombati*, below.

Type locality: AUSTRALIA: South Australia.

Other hosts: None to date.

Geographic distribution: AUSTRALIA: South Australia; EUROPE: Austria.

Description of sporulated oocyst: Oocyst shape: ellipsoidal (Supperer, 1957) or subspheroidal to ellipsoidal (Barker et al., 1979); number of walls: 1; wall characteristics: ~1 thick, colorless (Supperer, 1957), or clear, and purple-pink (Barker et al., 1979); L×W ($n=45$): 22–27×17–22 (Supperer, 1957) or 23.9×19.6 (20–29×17–21) (Barker et al., 1979); L/W ratio: 1.2; M, OR, PG: all absent (Supperer, 1957) or M: absent; OR: present, small; PG: present, small (Barker et al., 1979). Distinctive features of oocyst: thin, clear, single-layered wall, without M, but small OR and small PG may be present.

Description of sporocyst and sporozoites: Sporocyst shape: ovoidal; tapering slightly toward SB; L×W: 12×7 (Supperer, 1957) or 10.0×7 (8–11×7) (Barker et al., 1979); L/W ratio: 1.4–1.7; SB: present, small, knob-like (line drawing) or described as protuberant (Barker et al., 1979); SSB, PSB: both absent; SR: present; SR characteristics: composed of a more-or-less compact, irregular mass of granules scattered around equator; SZ: sausage-shaped, with one clear RB at more rounded end. Distinctive features of sporocyst: none, a typical eimerian SP, with an SB and an SR.

Prevalence: Barker et al. (1979) examined feces from *L. latifrons* from five localities: one wombat had been held in a sanctuary near Melbourne; two were removed from the wild in South Australia and used in a study at the University of Adelaide; three wombats were from the Adelaide Zoo; and two pools of fecal samples were examined, one pool from wombats at the Cleland Wildlife Park, Adelaide, and a second pool from widely separated warrens in a natural habitat near Blanchetown, South Australia. The feces from each individual *L. latifrons* and all samples from the selected pools, except one, contained oocysts of *E. ursini*.

Sporulation: Oocysts sporulated in 4–5 days at 25 °C (Supperer, 1957).

Prepatent and patent periods: Unknown.

Site of infection: Unknown, oocysts found in the fecal material, although Doube (1981) listed the small intestine as the site of infection.

Endogenous stages: Unknown.

Cross-transmission: None to date.

Pathology: Unknown.

Materials deposited: None.

Remarks: There was considerable variation in the shape of oocysts seen by Barker et al. (1979) ranging from subspheroidal to ellipsoidal. They attributed this as a function of oocyst length, which varied continuously within the geographic ranges sampled. On the basis of the measurements of 15 sporulated oocysts from each of three different animals (see above), they felt that most features, except sporocyst length, conformed closely with the description of *E. ursini* by Supperer (1957).

EIMERIA WOMBATI (GILRUTH AND BULL, 1912) BARKER, MUNDAY, AND PRESIDENTE, 1979

Synonyms: *Ileocystis wombati* Gilruth and Bull, 1912; *Gastrocystis wombati* (Gilruth and Bull, 1912) Chatton, 1912; *Globidium wombati* (Gilruth

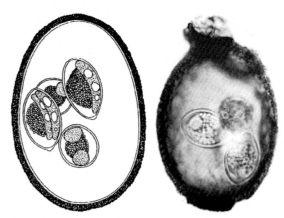

FIGURES 4.2, 4.3 **4.2.** Line drawing of a sporulated oocyst of *Eimeria wombati* from Supperer, 1957 (his Figure 2, as *E. tasmaniae*), with kind permission of Springer Science+Business Media, publishers of *Zeitschrift für Parasitenkunde*. **4.3.** Photomicrograph of a sporulated oocyst of *E. wombati* from Barker et al., 1979, with permission from the senior author and from the Editor of the *Journal of Parasitology*.

and Bull, 1912) Wenyon, 1926; *Eimeria tasmaniae* Supperer, 1957; *Eimeria* (*Globidium*) *tasmaniae* Supperer, 1957.

Type host: *Lasiorhinus latifrons* (Owen, 1845), Southern Hairy-nosed Wombat.

Type locality: AUSTRALIA: South Australia: Melbourne Zoo.

Other hosts: None to date.

Geographic distribution: AUSTRALIA: South Australia; EUROPE: Austria: Vienna Zoo.

Description of sporulated oocyst: Oocyst shape: broadly ovoidal; number of walls: 2; wall characteristics: outer layer ~5–7 thick, yellow to dark brown, brittle, coarsely granular; inner is thin, colorless (Supperer, 1957), while Barker et al. (1979) said the outer wall was irregular, thick, brown, rough, radially striated, and broke away readily from the inner wall, which was 1.5 thick; L×W: 73–94 × 48–63 (Supperer, 1957) or (*n* = 6) 75.1 × 57.4 (73–77 × 56–59) (Barker et al., 1979, who said their oocysts corresponded with those of Supperer's (1957) *E. tasmaniae*); oocysts without their outer wall were 63.0 × 49.4 (62–64 × 49–50) (Barker et al., 1979); L/W ratio: 1.3; M, OR, PG: all absent. Distinctive features of oocyst: very large size and extremely thick, striated outer wall.

Description of sporocyst and sporozoites: Sporocyst shape: ovoidal, broader at one end than the other, tapering toward both, but more sharply toward SB; L×W: 25.2×16.8 (24–27×16–18); L/W ratio: 1.5; SB: present, prominent, nipple-like (photomicrograph); SSB, PSB: both absent; SR: present; SR characteristics: composed of many granules in a compact, irregular mass, usually at the equator of the SP; SZ: banana-shaped, with one large RB at its wider end. Distinctive features of sporocyst: ovoidal shape, one end broader than the other, with a prominent SB and the four SP only occupy about half the space inside the oocyst.

Prevalence: Barker et al. (1979) found this species only four times: three times in a pool of fecal samples obtained from the *L. latifrons* held at the Cleland Wildlife Park, Adelaide, South Australia, and once in another pool of fecal samples obtained from widely separated warrens in a natural habitat near Blanchetown, South Australia. They were only able to study and measure six sporulated oocysts.

Sporulation: Oocysts sporulated in 7 days at 25°C (Supperer, 1957).

Prepatent and patent periods: Unknown.

Site of infection: Small intestine, mainly in the lamina propria of the duodenum, jejunum, and ileum.

Endogenous stages: Gilruth and Bull (1912) reported only on some endogenous "forms," but not oocysts, of what are likely stages of this species (see *Remarks*). According to them, these "cysts" were 93–113 in diameter, with a thin wall, and contained many small nuclei. Barker et al. (1979) identified mature microgametocytes that were 208×177 in their tissue sections. Macrogametocytes contained many round, regular amorphous, eosinophilic wall-forming granules; the largest macrogametocyte seen was 65×39.

Cross-transmission: None to date.

Pathology: According to Gilruth and Bull (1912), the villi were greatly distorted by spheroidal or ellipsoidal cysts of *E. wombati* that generally attached to their surface, but also crowded and distended the glands of Lieberkühn.

Materials deposited: None.

Remarks: Gilruth and Bull (1912) reported only on endogenous stages of a parasite they called *Ileocystis wombati*. Barker et al. (1979) looked at Gilruth and Bull's (1912) illustrations and concluded that it was a microgametocyte of a coccidium in the lamina propria of the small intestine, very similar to their own. They also produced a photomicrograph of a tissue section with a developing oocyst (their Figure 4) that is of a size consistent with that of *E. tasmaniae*, described by Supperer (1957), from a male and female *V. ursinus*. Professor Ian Barker wrote to Rudolf Supperer, and in a private correspondence, learned that the female died in 1957, and was not studied further, but when the male died in 1963, it was examined by a new curator, who noted in his records that the male was possibly *L. latifrons*. This evidence allowed Barker et al. (1979) to suggest that the type host for *E. tasmaniae* (and *E. ursini*) was really the **allopatric** *L. latifrons*. On the basis of this evidence, Barker et al. (1979) considered it probable that *Il. wombati* of Gilruth and Bull (1912) is the microgametogonous stage of *E. tasmaniae* of Supperer (1957). According to the *International Code of Zoological Nomenclature*, the specific epithet *wombati* used by Gilruth and Bull (1912) has priority, *E. tasmaniae* becomes a junior synonym, and their new combination, as I have cited above, becomes *Eimeria wombati* (Gilruth and Bull, 1912) Barker, Munday, and Presidente, 1979.

GENUS VOMBATUS É. GEOFFROY, 1803 (MONOTYPIC)

EIMERIA ARUNDELI BARKER, MUNDAY, AND PRESIDENTE, 1979

Type host: *Vombatus ursinus* (Shaw, 1800), Common Wombat.

Type locality: AUSTRALIA: Tasmania.

Other hosts: None to date.

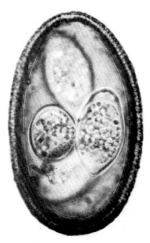

FIGURE 4.4   Photomicrograph of the sporulated oocyst of *Eimeria arundeli* from Barker et al., 1979, with permission from the senior author and from the Editor of the *Journal of Parasitology*.

Geographic distribution: AUSTRALIA: Tasmania; Victoria.

Description of sporulated oocyst: Oocyst shape: slightly ovoidal to sometimes ellipsoidal; number of walls: 2; wall characteristics: outer layer granular, dark brown, but occasionally opaque, 4–7 thick, inner is clear, ~1.5 thick; L×W: 63.7×43.4 (60–67×41–48); L/W ratio: 1.5; M: present, ~3 wide; OR: present, small; PG: absent. Distinctive features of oocyst: large size, a thick two-layered wall, with an M and small OR.

Description of sporocyst and sporozoites: Sporocyst shape: ovoidal; tapering toward SB and slightly pointed at the opposite end; L×W: 25.8×14.1 (22–29×13–15); L/W ratio: 1.8; SB: present, protuberant; SSB, PSB: both absent; SR: present; SR characteristics: large, composed of numerous granules that obscure SZ. Distinctive features of sporocyst: large protuberant SB, end opposite SB is often pointed, large granular SR that obscures SZ.

Prevalence: Found in the feces of 4/18 (22%) and in the tissues of 3/5 (60%) of the type host (Barker et al., 1979); Hum et al. (1991) found *E. arundeli* oocysts in the feces, and observed both micro- and macrogametocytes in the intestinal mucosa of 2/2 (100%) female, captive, juvenile *V. ursinus*.

Sporulation: Unknown.

Prepatent and patent periods: Unknown.

Site of infection: Lamina propria of the intestinal mucosa below the villi of the entire small intestine.

Endogenous stages: Interestingly, meronts have not yet been found in this species (Barker et al., 1979; Hum et al., 1991), even though they have been searched for throughout the gastrointesinal tract, liver, biliary epithelium, and lungs. Barker et al. (1979) found large numbers of gamonts and developing oocysts distending the lamina propria of the villi of the lower small intestine. Microgamonts within **hypertrophic** host cells were up to 150 wide and had many complex infoldings, along which microgametes developed. Hum et al. (1991) said that microgametocytes formed cysts up to 190 wide, similar to those described by Barker et al. (1979). Mature microgamonts contained many microgametes and irregular dense inclusions. Macrogametes were also in hypertrophic cells of the lamina propria and contained large, deeply eosinophilic wall-forming bodies (Hum et al., 1991). Developing oocysts were up to 56×32 in size. There were many mononuclear inflammatory cells among the gamonts.

Cross-transmission: None to date.

Pathology: Barker et al. (1979) noted that the villi over extensive areas of the small intestine were white and hypertrophied, projecting above uninfected mucosa, and that there were many mononuclear inflammatory cells among the gamonts. Presidente (1982) said that diarrhea was not present in young animals he examined when infected with *E. arundeli* and passing oocysts; thus, *E. arundeli* was generally considered to be nonpathogenic. However, Hum et al. (1991) described severe coccidiosis in two captive, juvenile wombats, both females. One had diarrhea, while the second had mucoid soft feces, but both lost weight over several weeks before their deaths. They found masses of gametocytes in hypertrophic cells in the lamina propria with distended villi, causing grossly visible, raised and pale thickened regions over extensive areas of the mucosa of the small intestine. Neutrophils infiltrated the infected mucosa, resulting in inflammatory exudate being discharged into the intestinal lumen. The crypts of Lieberkühn were distended by necrotic debris and the epithelium on the villi was extremely attenuated (Hum et al., 1991), while oocysts consistent with *E. arundeli* were present in tissue sections, and in the diarrheic feces of both animals. Hum et al. (1991) also said that the lamina propria of affected villi was noticeably edematous, had dilated lymphatics, and became infiltrated with mononuclear cells, eosinophils, and large numbers of neutrophils. In some of the sections, they found proteinaceous exudate containing neutrophils, epithelial cells, and necrotic debris in the lumen of the small intestine. No pathogenic bacteria were found on aerobic culture of lung and portions of both small and large intestine, and selective culture for *Salmonella* and *Yersinia* species were negative, leading Hum et al. (1991) to conclude that coccidiosis was the cause of death of the two wombats. They also found it noteworthy that the two wombats were shedding large numbers of oocysts in their feces, because according to Barker et al. (1979), the number of oocysts in the feces is relatively small, while gametocytes are more commonly encountered in tissue than oocysts in the feces. Clearly, *E. arundeli* may be pathogenic to wombats under certain circumstances, even in their natural environments.

Materials deposited: Tissue sections of infected intestine from a female wombat are deposited in the National Registry of Zoo Animal Pathology (Taronga Park Zoological Gardens, P.O. Box 20, Mosman, New South Wales 2066, Australia), accession number C-0086.

Remarks: Barker et al. (1979) felt that the qualitative and quantitative characteristics of the oocysts they studied were sufficiently distinctive to warrant its consideration as a species. Presidente (1982) occasionally found oocysts of *E. arundeli* in the feces of wild-caught *V. ursinus*, especially in younger animals.

SUBORDER PHALANGERIFORMES SZALAY, 1982 (6 FAMILIES, 20 GENERA, 63 SPECIES)

FAMILY PHALANGERIDAE THOMAS, 1888 (6 GENERA, 27 SPECIES)

SUBFAMILY PHALANGERINAE THOMAS, 1888

TRIBE TRICHOSURINI FLYNN, 1911

GENUS *TRICHOSURUS* LESSON, 1828 (5 SPECIES)

EIMERIA TRICHOSURI O'CALLAGHAN AND O'DONOGHUE, 2001

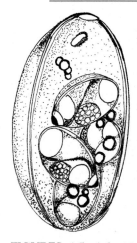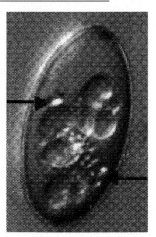

FIGURES 4.5, 4.6 **4.5.** Line drawing of a sporulated oocyst of *Eimeria trichosuri*. **4.6.** Photomicrograph of a sporulated oocyst of *E. trichosuri*. Both figures from O'Callaghan and O'Donoghue, 2001, with permission of both authors and from the Editor of the *Transaction of the Royal Society of South Australia*.

Type host: *Trichosurus vulpecula* (Kerr, 1792), Common Brushtail Possum.

Type locality: AUSTRALIA: Queensland: Townsville (19° 16′ S, 146° 49′ E).

Other hosts: *Trichosurus caninus* (Ogilby, 1836), Short-eared Possum; *Trichosurus cunninghami* Lindenmayer, Dubach, and Viggers, 2002, Mountain Brushtail Possum (see *Remarks*).

Geographic distribution: AUSTRALIA: Queensland, South Australia, Tasmania, Victoria; NEW ZEALAND.

Description of sporulated oocyst: Oocyst shape: ellipsoidal to cylindroidal; number of walls: 2; wall characteristics: outer layer smooth, occasionally stippled at pole near M, 1.6–2.0 thick; inner layer clear, colorless, 1.0 thick; L×W (*n*=120): 41.4×22.7 (34–49×18–28); L/W ratio: 1.8 (1.3–2.6); M: present, 3.3–4.0 wide; OR: present, consists of globules, up to 3.0 wide, occurring either as a loose aggregate or scattered throughout oocyst; PG: 1–2 present or occasionally disintegrated. Distinctive features of oocyst: large size with distinct M, OR, and PG and highly variable L/W ratio.

Description of sporocyst and sporozoites: Sporocyst shape: ellipsoidal to pyriform; L×W (*n*=110): 15.6×9.9 (13–18×8–12); L/W ratio: 1.6 (1.1–2.0); SB: present at pointed end of sporocyst, cap- or knoblike; SSB: present, slightly wider than SB (line drawing); PSB: absent; SR: present; SR characteristics: an accumulation of small globules, 5.0–5.8 wide, at equator of SP and these appear to be membrane bound (line drawing); SZ: lie head-to-tail filling SP, each with one large RB, 5.0 wide, and a second smaller RB, 2.5 wide. Distinctive features of sporocyst: a relatively large ovoid, with SB, SSB, and membrane-bound SR (as seen in line drawing).

Prevalence: Eimeria trichosuri was found in 50/212 (24%) fecal samples collected from the type host from five localities between 1994 and 2001; these included 11/51 (21.5%) collected in Tasmania, 9/40 (22.5%) collected in Victoria, 6/40 (15%) collected in South Australia, 16/64 (25%) collected in Queensland, and 8/17 (47%) collected in New Zealand. Power et al. (2009) also found it in 2/15 (13%) *T. cunninghami* in Victoria.

Sporulation: Could not be determined because oocysts were stored in 2% (w/v) potassium dichromate ($K_2Cr_2O_7$) solution at room temperature for 12 weeks.

Prepatent and patent periods: Unknown.

Site of infection: Unknown.

Endogenous stages: Unknown.

Cross-transmission: None to date.

Pathology: There was no evidence seen by O'Callaghan and O'Donoghue (2001) to suggest that this species is pathogenic.

Materials deposited: Holotype from feces of *T. vulpecula*, Townsville, Queensland; paratype from feces of *T. vulpecula* Launceston, Tasmania, is in the United States National Parasite Collection, USNPC No. 91524. Nucleotide sequences were submitted to GenBank under Accession Nos. FJ829320–FJ829323.

Remarks: This is the only eimerian described from this host genus. When compared to other eimerians described from the Diprotodontia in Australia, these oocysts most closely resemble those of *E. gaimardi* from *Bettongia gaimardi*, the Tasmanian bettong. Oocysts of *E. trichosuri* differ, however, by being larger (41.4×22.7 vs 34.6×24.3), and by possessing an M, which the latter lacks. Also, the oocyst wall of *E. gaimardi* is thinner than that of *E. trichosuri*. Presidente et al. (1982) reported on the effects of habitat, host sex, and age on helminth and ectoparasites of 57 congeners of *T. caninus*, trapped in rural and urban areas of Melbourne. Although they were interested in arthropod and helminth parasites, they did examine the feces of seven *T. caninus* for oocysts and found three that were passing oocysts; after they sporulated, the oocysts were L×W (*n*=42): 39.1×19.7; L/W ratio: 2.0; M: present, 3.8 wide; and sporocysts were L×W (*n*=7): 15.4×10.0; L/W ratio: 1.5. The dimensions of the oocysts they reported (1982) correspond well with those of *E. trichosuri*.

Power et al. (2009) examined 15 *T. cunninghami* caught at Boho South in northeast Victoria, Australia (36° 48′ S, 145° 45′ E) and found oocysts of this species in two animals that measured, L×W: 40.3×20.8 (31.5–46×18–24); L/W ratio: 1.9 (1.5–2.5); M: present, 3.0–4.4 wide; and sporocysts were L×W: 13.9×9.6 (10–19×7–12); L/W ratio: 1.4 (1.0–1.8). Qualitative characters of the sporulated oocysts and their sporocysts, such as number of walls and presence/absence of M, OR, PG, SB, SSB, SR, and RB, all confirmed that they were dealing with *E. trichosuri*. Most importantly, Power et al. (2009) provided *the first gene sequence* of a marsupial coccidium. They amplified genomic DNA to generate a clear 18S rDNA sequence of about 1600 bp and used these data to assess its phylogenetic position relative to *Eimeria* sequences in GenBank from birds, reptiles, and placental mammals. Their analysis placed *E. trichosuri* clones in a clade that diverged before the major clade comprising species from placental mammals. They suggested that the position of *E. trichosuri* is consistent with host phylogeny where marsupials represent an ancient evolutionary lineage that predates the placental mammal line.

SUPERFAMILY PETAUROIDEA BONAPARTE, 1838

FAMILY PETAURIDAE BONAPARTE, 1838 (3 GENERA, 11 SPECIES)

GENUS *PETAURUS* SHAW, 1791 (6 SPECIES)

There are no eimeriid coccidia described from this genus, as far as I know. However, recent molecular works by Merino et al. (2010) and Zhu et al. (2009) to identify an intraerythrocytic parasite that, based on morphology alone, would be classified as a *Hematozoan* species, appear to have partial SSU- and LSU rDNA sequences that align with members of the Sarcocystidae; this unusual apicomplexan is likely in an, as yet, unnamed genus with an, as yet, unknown life cycle. There is some very interesting work to be done here.

SUBORDER MACROPODIFORMES AMEGHINO, 1889 (3 FAMILIES, 16 GENERA, 76 SPECIES)

FAMILY HYPSIPRYMNODONTIDAE COLLETT, 1877 (1 GENUS, 1 SPECIES)

GENUS *HYPSIPRYMNODON* RAMSAY, 1876 (MONOTYPIC)

EIMERIA HYPSIPRYMNODONTIS BARKER, O'CALLAGHAN, AND BEVERIDGE, 1988a

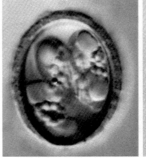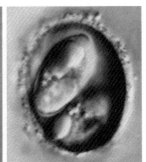

FIGURES 4.7, 4.8 **4.7.** Photomicrograph of a sporulated oocyst of *Eimeria hypsiprymnodontis*, original (from M. O'Callaghan); **4.8.** Photomicrograph of a second sporulated oocyst of *E. hypsiprymnodontis* from Barker et al., 1988a (their Figure 2), with permission from all authors and with kind permission from Elsevier, publishers of the *International Journal for Parasitology*.

Type host: *Hypsiprymnodon moschatus* Ramsey, 1876, Musky Rat-kangaroo.

Type locality: AUSTRALIA: Queensland: Atherton Tableland.

Other hosts: None to date.

Geographic distribution: AUSTRALIA: Queensland.

Description of sporulated oocyst: Oocyst shape: bluntly ellipsoidal; number of walls: 2; wall characteristics: outer layer tan with an irregular, rough surface, 2.4–3.2 thick, occasionally thinner at one pole, but no clear M; inner layer ~0.4; L×W ($n=15$): 28.6×22.7 (26–32×21–24); L/W ratio: 1.3; M, OR: both absent; PG: present, 1.2 wide. Distinctive features of oocyst: bluntly ellipsoidal shape and possessing a distinct PG.

Description of sporocyst and sporozoites: Sporocyst shape: ellipsoidal, slightly pointed at one end; L×W ($n=15$): 17.0×8.3 (16–18×8–9); L/W ratio: 2.0; SB: present at pointed end of sporocyst and is sometimes asymmetrical; SSB: present, 2.4

high × 3.2 wide; PSB: absent; SR: present; SR characteristics: ~1.6 wide, composed of a cluster of 10–20 granules loosely aggregated at the equator of the SP; SZ: described as large, filling the sporocyst, "recurved," with finely granular cytoplasm, each with one large RB, 7.2 × 4.8. Distinctive features of sporocyst: large L/W ratio (2.0), long SZ that fill the space within the sporocyst, and each SZ with a large RB at its more rounded end.

Prevalence: This species was found in 3/5 (60%) specimens of the type host.

Sporulation: Could not be determined because of the transit time from the field until they reached the lab.

Prepatent and patent periods: Unknown.

Site of infection: Unknown.

Endogenous stages: Unknown.

Cross-transmission: None to date.

Pathology: Not described.

Materials deposited: None.

Remarks: Barker et al. (1988a) said that oocysts of this species were rare in the feces of *H. moschatus*. They decided to name this a new species (in spite of the fact that they found and could measure only 15 oocysts) based on the combination of dimensions of oocysts and sporocysts, with the suite of morphologic characters described. The large oocyst size and thick wall composed of two layers distinguish this form from other eimerians known to parasitize *H. moschatus*. Although *Hypsiprymnodon* is a monotypic genus, it has demonstrated a rich cohort of relatively homogenous *Eimeria* species when all their qualitative and quantitative features are considered. A group demonstrating such homogeneity suggested to Barker et al. (1988a) that these various species may be a result of radiation within this host, of one or two lineages of *Eimeria* isolated by the unique characteristics of this host.

EIMERIA KAIRIENSIS BARKER, O'CALLAGHAN, AND BEVERIDGE, 1988a

Type host: *Hypsiprymnodon moschatus* Ramsey, 1876, Musky Rat-kangaroo.

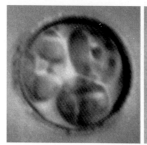 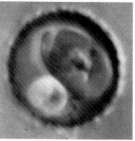

FIGURES 4.9, 4.10 Photomicrographs of two sporulated oocyst of *Eimeria kairiensis*, both originals from M. O'Callaghan. **4.9.** Shows the SB on one sporocyst; **4.10.** Shows RB in the SZ.

Type locality: AUSTRALIA: Queensland: Atherton Tableland.

Other hosts: None to date.

Geographic distribution: AUSTRALIA: Queensland.

Description of sporulated oocyst: Oocyst shape: spheroidal to subspheroidal; number of walls: 2; wall characteristics: outer layer with a finely mammillated surface, ~0.6 thick; inner layer is clear; L × W (*n* = 44): 13.4 × 12.9 (11–15 × 10–15); L/W ratio: 1.0; M, OR: both absent; PG: present. Distinctive features of oocyst: very small size.

Description of sporocyst and sporozoites: Sporocyst shape: ellipsoidal; L × W (*n* = 44): 8.2 × 5.2 (6–10 × 4–6); L/W ratio: 1.6; SB: present, knoblike; SSB, PSB: both absent; SR: present; SR characteristics: a few granules, each ~0.8 wide, scattered at equator of SP; SZ: "elongate (?)" and fill the sporocyst, each with one RB, 3.2 × 1.6. Distinctive features of sporocyst: small size with a knoblike SB, but lacking an SSB.

Prevalence: This species was found in 5/5 (100%) specimens of the type host.

Sporulation: Could not be determined because of the transit time from the field until they reached the lab.

Prepatent and patent periods: Unknown.

Site of infection: Unknown.

Endogenous stages: Unknown.

Cross-transmission: None to date.

Pathology: Not described.

Materials deposited: None.

Etymology: This species was named by Barker et al. (1988a) for the town Kairi, on the Atherton Tableland, which has an architecturally unique pub.

Remarks: Oocysts of this species were common in all five hosts examined. Barker et al. (1988a) distinguished this form from the others they found in *H. moschatus* based on oocyst and sporocyst dimensions, and the suite of qualitative and quantitative characters they observed. Although *Hypsiprymnodon* is a monotypic genus, it has demonstrated a rich cohort of relatively homogenous *Eimeria* species when all their qualitative and quantitative features are considered. A group demonstrating such homogeneity suggested to Barker et al. (1988a) that these various species may be a result of radiation within this host, of one or two lineages of *Eimeria* isolated by the unique characteristics of this host.

EIMERIA SPEAREI BARKER, O'CALLAGHAN, AND BEVERIDGE, 1988a

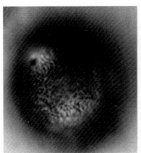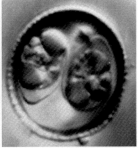

FIGURES 4.11, 4.12 Photomicrographs of two sporulated oocysts of *Eimeria spearei*, both originals, from M. O'Callaghan. **4.11.** Shows sculptured outer oocyst wall; **4.12.** Shows two sporocysts with SB and SSB.

Type host: *Hypsiprymnodon moschatus* Ramsey, 1876, Musky Rat-kangaroo.

Type locality: AUSTRALIA: Queensland: Atherton Tableland.

Other hosts: None to date.

Geographic distribution: AUSTRALIA: Queensland.

Description of sporulated oocyst: Oocyst shape: spheroidal to subspheroidal; number of walls: 2; wall characteristics: outer layer, ~0.8 thick, with a finely pebbled surface; inner layer is ~0.4 thick; L×W (*n*=47): 16.9×16.3 (15–20×14–18); L/W ratio: 1.0; M, OR: both absent; PG: present. Distinctive features of oocyst: pebbled surface of outer wall.

Description of sporocyst and sporozoites: Sporocyst shape: ellipsoidal; L×W (*n*=47): 10.4×6.4 (8–12×5–7); L/W ratio: 1.6; SB: present, small and knoblike; SSB: present, as a small lenticular body; PSB: absent; SR: present; SR characteristics: an aggregate of large granules/globules, ~4.8 wide, at equator of the SP; SZ: with finely granular cytoplasm, and they fill the SP; each SZ has two RB, the larger 4.8×2.4, the smaller is 2.4 wide. Distinctive features of SP: small SB and SZ each with two RB.

Prevalence: This species was found in 5/5 (100%) specimens of the type host.

Sporulation: Could not be determined because of the transit time from the field until they reached the lab.

Prepatent and patent periods: Unknown.

Site of infection: Unknown.

Endogenous stages: Unknown.

Cross-transmission: None to date.

Pathology: Not described.

Materials deposited: None.

Etymology: This species was named in recognition of Dr Richard Speare, Postgraduate School of Tropical Veterinary Science, James Cook University, Townsville, Queensland.

Remarks: *Eimeria spearei* was found commonly in all five *H. moschatus* examined by Barker et al. (1988a). They felt that it was distinct from the other four eimerians they described from *H. moschatus* based on both oocyst and sporocyst size, and the suite of qualitative and quantitative characters seen. Although *Hypsiprymnodon* is a monotypic genus, it has demonstrated a rich cohort of relatively homogenous *Eimeria* species when all their qualitative and quantitative features are considered. A group demonstrating such homogeneity suggested to Barker et al. (1988a) that these various species may be a result of radiation within this host, of one or two lineages of *Eimeria* isolated by the unique characteristics of this host.

EIMERIA SPRATTI BARKER, O'CALLAGHAN, AND BEVERIDGE, 1988a

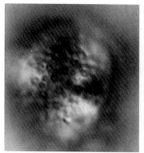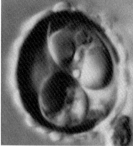

FIGURES 4.13, 4.14 Photomicrographs of two sporulated oocyst of *Eimeria spratti*; **4.13.** Shows the sculptured outer surface of the oocyst wall, original, from M. O'Callaghan. **4.14.** Photomicrograph of a sporulated oocyst of *E. spratti* from Barker et al., 1988a (their Figure 5), with permission of all authors and kind permission from Elsevier, publisher of the *International Journal for Parasitology*.

Type host: *Hypsiprymnodon moschatus* Ramsey, 1876, Musky Rat-kangaroo.

Type locality: AUSTRALIA: Queensland: Atherton Tableland.

Other hosts: None to date.

Geographic distribution: AUSTRALIA: Queensland.

Description of sporulated oocyst: Oocyst shape: subspheroidal; number of walls: 2; wall characteristics: outer layer, ~1.6 thick, composed of flattened granules up to 3.2 wide and ~1.6 thick, giving the surface a cobblestone-like appearance; inner layer is clear, ~0.4 thick; L × W ($n = 30$): 21.3 × 19.4 (18–24 × 16–23); L/W ratio: 1.1; M, OR: both absent; PG: present, 2.4 wide. Distinctive features of oocyst: unique cobblestone-like appearance of the outer wall.

Description of sporocyst and sporozoites: Sporocyst shape: ellipsoidal to elongated ovoidal; L × W ($n = 30$): 13.1 × 7.6 (11–15 × 6–9); L/W ratio: 1.7; SB: present, but inconspicuous at more pointed end of sporocyst; SSB: described as clear; PSB: absent; SR: present; SR characteristics: a mass of granules, 1.6 wide, dispersed about the equator of the SP; SZ: completely fill sporocyst, each with a large, clear RB, 6.4 × 3.2 in size. Distinctive features of sporocyst: size, L/W ratio, and inconspicuous nature of the SB and SSB.

Prevalence: This species was found in 5/5 (100%) specimens of the type host.

Sporulation: Could not be determined because of the transit time from the field until they reached the lab.

Prepatent and patent periods: Unknown.

Site of infection: Unknown.

Endogenous stages: Unknown.

Cross-transmission: None to date.

Pathology: Not described.

Materials deposited: None.

Etymology: This species was named in recognition of Dr D.M. Spratt, C.S.I.R.O. Division of Ecology and Wildlife Research, Canberra.

Remarks: Barker et al. (1988a) distinguished the oocysts of this form from others present in the five *H. moschatus* they examined based on the size of oocyst and sporocyst measurements and the suite of structural characteristics they observed, particularly the unique structure of the oocyst outer wall. Although *Hypsiprymnodon* is a monotypic genus, it has demonstrated a rich cohort of relatively homogenous *Eimeria* species when all their qualitative and quantitative features are considered.

EIMERIA TINAROOENSIS BARKER, O'CALLAGHAN, AND BEVERIDGE, 1988a

Type host: *Hypsiprymnodon moschatus* Ramsey, 1876, Musky Rat-kangaroo.

Type locality: AUSTRALIA: Queensland: Atherton Tableland.

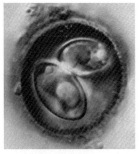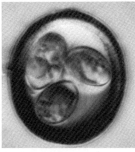

FIGURES 4.15, 4.16 Photomicrographs of two sporulated oocysts of *Eimeria tinarooensis*, both originals from M. O'Callaghan.

Other hosts: None to date.

Geographic distribution: AUSTRALIA: Queensland.

Description of sporulated oocyst: Oocyst shape: subspheroidal to bluntly ellipsoidal; number of walls: 2; wall characteristics: outer layer is tan, with radial striations and a finely mammillated outer surface, 2.0–2.4 thick, but thinning to 1.6 at the poles; L×W ($n=22$): 26.0×23.8 (24–28×22–26); L/W ratio: 1.1; M, OR: both absent; PG: present, 1.6 wide. Distinctive features of oocyst: sculptured outer oocyst wall with radial striations.

Description of sporocyst and sporozoites: Sporocyst shape: ellipsoidal, slightly pointed at one end; L×W ($n=22$): 12.3×7.9 (11–14×7–8); L/W ratio: 1.6; SB: present as small, clear knob; SSB: present, about same size as SB; PSB: absent; SR: present; SR characteristics: a loose aggregate of granules, ~1.6 wide, scattered about the equator of the SP; SZ: they completely fill the sporocyst and were described as "recurved," with finely granular cytoplasm; each contains a clear RB, 4.8×3.2 in size. Distinctive features of sporocyst: presence of SB, SSB, and SR, and SZ each have a large RB.

Prevalence: This species was found in 4/5 (80%) specimens of the type host.

Sporulation: Could not be determined because of the transit time from the field until they reached the lab.

Prepatent and patent periods: Unknown.
Site of infection: Unknown.
Endogenous stages: Unknown.
Cross-transmission: None to date.

Pathology: Not described.
Materials deposited: None.
Etymology: This species name was derived from the type locality, Tinaroo, on the Atherton Tableland of Queensland.

Remarks: Barker et al. (1988a) distinguished this form from the oocysts of *E. hypsiprymnodontis* by its more irregular shape, more regular outer surface of the oocyst wall, and by its smaller sporocysts. Although *Hypsiprymnodon* is a monotypic genus, it has demonstrated a rich cohort of relatively homogenous *Eimeria* species when all their qualitative and quantitative features are considered.

FAMILY POTOROIDAE GRAY, 1821 (4 GENERA, 10 SPECIES)

GENUS *AEPYPRYMNUS* GARROD, 1875 (MONOTYPIC)

EIMERIA AEPYPRYMNI BARKER, O'CALLAGHAN, AND BEVERIDGE, 1988a

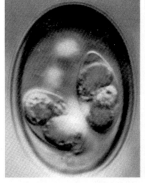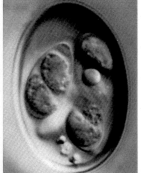

FIGURES 4.17, 4.18 Photomicrographs of two sporulated oocysts of *Eimeria aepyprymni*, both originals from M. O'Callaghan.

Type host: *Aepyprymnus rufescens* (Gray, 1837), Rufous Rat-kangaroo.

Type locality: AUSTRALIA: South Australia: Adelaide, Adelaide Zoo.

Other hosts: None to date.

Geographic distribution: AUSTRALIA: South Australia.

Description of sporulated oocyst: Oocyst shape: ellipsoidal; number of walls: 2; wall characteristics: outer layer colorless, smooth, ~1.5 thick; inner is clear, ~0.5 thick; L × W (*n* = 35): 36.7 × 21.9 (32–43 × 18–25); L/W ratio: 1.7; M, PG: both absent; OR: present as a few scattered granules (not mentioned in the original description). Distinctive features of oocyst: it is a large ellipsoid, with an OR of scattered granules, but no PG.

Description of sporocyst and sporozoites: Sporocyst shape: ellipsoidal to ovoidal, slightly pointed at one end; L × W (*n* = 35): 15.8 × 9.5 (14–18 × 8–11); L/W ratio: 1.7; SB: present as a small cap on the more pointed end of SP; SSB: present, lenticulate; PSB: absent; SR: present; SR characteristics: a compact, finely granular mass, ~5.6 wide, at the equator of SP; SZ: shape not mentioned, but with finely granular cytoplasm, and they do not fill the space within SP; each SZ with one RB, 5.6 wide. Distinctive features of SP: distinct ovoidal shape, with a small caplike SB covering the lenticulate SSB.

Prevalence: Oocysts of this species were found in a single *A. rufescens* in the Adelaide Zoo, while four other *A. rufescens* from north Queensland had no oocysts in their feces.

Sporulation: Unknown.

Prepatent and patent periods: Unknown.

Site of infection: Unknown.

Endogenous stages: Unknown.

Cross-transmission: None to date.

Pathology: Not described.

Materials deposited: None.

Remarks: Barker et al. (1988a) based their naming this a new species on "oocyst and sporocyst dimensions and the suite of morphologic characters described," and because no eimerian had been previously described from this host genus. They felt that there were no defined similarities among the four eimerian oocysts found parasitizing the three genera (*Aepyprymnus*, *Bettongia*, and *Potorous*) in the Potoroidae they examined.

GENUS BETTONGIA GRAY, 1837 (4 SPECIES)

EIMERIA GAIMARDI BARKER, O'CALLAGHAN, AND BEVERIDGE, 1988a

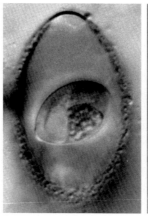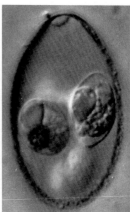

FIGURES 4.19, 4.20 Photomicrographs of two sporulated oocysts of *Eimeria giamardi*, both originals from M. O'Callaghan.

Type host: *Bettongia gaimardi* (Desmarest, 1822), Eastern Bettong.

Type locality: AUSTRALIA: Tasmania: Launceston.

Other hosts: None to date.

Geographic distribution: AUSTRALIA: Tasmania.

Description of sporulated oocyst: Oocyst shape: ovoidal to pyriform; number of walls: 2; wall characteristics: outer is colorless, mammillated, ~1.2 thick, and thins at apex of oocyst, but no clear M was seen; inner layer clear, ~0.4 thick; L × W (*n* = 15): 34.6 × 24.3 (32–39 × 21–26); L/W ratio: 1.4; M, OR, PG: all absent. Distinctive features of oocyst: large pyriform size and lacking M, OR, and PG.

Description of sporocyst and sporozoites: Sporocyst shape: ellipsoidal to slightly ovoidal, slightly pointed at one end; L × W (*n* = 15): 15.0 × 9.6 (14–16 × 9–10); L/W ratio: 1.6; SB: present as a small caplike structure; SSB: present, lenticulate; PSB: absent; SR: present; SR characteristics: a loose aggregate of granules at equator of SP; SZ:

have finely granular cytoplasm, and they do not fill the SP; each SZ has two RB, the smaller is 2.4 wide and the larger is 6.4 wide. Distinctive features of SP: a large ovoid structure with both SB and SSB and the SZ have two RB each.

Prevalence: Barker et al. (1988a) found oocysts of this form in 5/13 (38%) *B. gaimardi*.

Sporulation: Unknown.

Prepatent and patent periods: Unknown.

Site of infection: Unknown.

Endogenous stages: Unknown.

Cross-transmission: None to date.

Pathology: Not described.

Materials deposited: None.

Remarks: Barker et al. (1988a) based their naming this a new species on "oocyst and sporocyst dimensions in combination with the suite of morphologic characters described," and because no eimerian previously had been described from this host genus. They felt that there were no defined similarities among the oocysts of the four eimerians found parasitizing the three genera (*Aepyprymnus*, *Bettongia*, and *Potorous*) in the Potoroidae they examined.

GENUS *POTOROUS* DESMAREST, 1804 (4 SPECIES)

EIMERIA MUNDAYI BARKER, O'CALLAGHAN, AND BEVERIDGE, 1988a

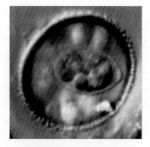

FIGURE 4.21   Photomicrograph of a sporulated oocyst of *Eimeria mundayi* showing one sporocyst and its distinct SB; original from M. O'Callaghan.

Type host: *Potorous tridactylus* (Kerr, 1792), Long-nosed Potoroo.

Type locality: AUSTRALIA: Tasmania: near Launceston.

Other hosts: None to date.

Geographic distribution: AUSTRALIA: Tasmania.

Description of sporulated oocyst: Oocyst shape: spheroidal to subspheroidal; number of walls: 2; wall characteristics: outer is tan, ~1 thick, with a mammillated surface; inner is clear, ~0.4 thick; L×W (*n*=40): 16.9×16.2 (14–21×14–19); L/W ratio: 1.0; M, OR: both absent; PG: present. Distinctive features of oocyst: a relatively small subspheroidal shape, with a mammillated surface.

Description of sporocyst and sporozoites: Sporocyst shape: ellipsoidal to ovoidal; L×W (*n*=40): 9.7×6.2 (8–12×5–8); L/W ratio: 1.6; SB: present; SSB: present; PSB: absent; SR: present; SR characteristics: a few scattered granules, 0.8–1.6 wide, at equator of the SP; SZ: described as "curved (?)" and not filling sporocyst; each with one RB, ~2.4–4.0 wide. Distinctive features of SP: None.

Prevalence: Barker et al. (1988a) did not state how many of the three *P. tridactylus* they examined passed oocysts of this eimerian.

Sporulation: Could not be determined because of the transit time from the field until they reached the lab.

Prepatent and patent periods: Unknown.

Site of infection: Unknown.

Endogenous stages: Unknown.

Cross-transmission: None to date.

Pathology: Not described.

Materials deposited: None.

Etymology: This species was named in recognition of Dr Barry L. Munday, former Director of the Mt. Pleasant Laboratories, Tasmanian Department of Agriculture, Launceston, Tasmania.

Remarks: Barker et al. (1988a) named this form as new based "on oocyst and sporocyst dimensions, and the suite of morphologic characteristics described;" they mentioned that this species has a wide range in size of both oocysts and sporocysts, and a positive correlation between length of oocyst and sporocyst. They felt that there were no defined similarities among the sporulated oocysts of the four eimerians found parasitizing the three genera (*Aepyprymnus*, *Bettongia*, and *Potorous*) in the Potoroidae they examined.

EIMERIA POTOROI BARKER, O'CALLAGHAN, AND BEVERIDGE, 1988a

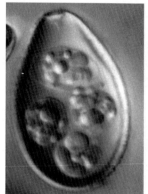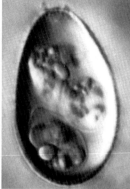

FIGURES 4.22, 4.23   Photomicrographs of two sporulated oocysts of *Eimeria potoroi*, both clearly show the M at the pointed end of the oocyst; both originals from M. O'Callaghan.

Type host: *Potorous tridactylus* (Kerr, 1792), Long-nosed Potoroo.

Type locality: AUSTRALIA: Tasmania: near Launceston.

Other hosts: None to date.

Geographic distribution: AUSTRALIA: Tasmania.

Description of sporulated oocyst: Oocyst shape: pointed-ovoidal to pyriform; number of walls: 2; wall characteristics: outer layer tan, ~1.0 wide, radially striated with a mammillated surface; inner is clear, ~0.4 thick; L×W (*n*=20): 26.2×18.5 (24–30×17–22); L/W ratio: 1.4; M: present, 4 wide; OR: present as an aggregate of two to six granules, ~1.6 wide; PG: absent. Distinctive features of oocyst: pyriform shape and having a distinct M and OR.

Description of sporocyst and sporozoites: Sporocyst shape: ellipsoidal; L×W (*n*=20): 11.9×7.6 (11–14×6–9); L/W ratio: 1.6; SB: present as a protuberant bump; SSB: present, lenticulate; PSB: absent; SR: present; SR characteristics: loose aggregate of granules, up to 2.0 wide, scattered about equator of SP; SZ: described as "curved (?)," not filling sporocyst, each with one RB, 3.2 wide. Distinctive features of SP: large SB that appears as a protuberant bump, with a lenticulate SSB beneath it.

Prevalence: Barker et al. (1988a) did not state how many of the three *P. tridactylus* they examined were passing oocysts of this eimerian.

Sporulation: Could not be determined because of the transit time from the field until they reached the lab.

Prepatent and patent periods: Unknown.

Site of infection: Unknown.

Endogenous stages: Unknown.

Cross-transmission: None to date.

Pathology: Not described.

Materials deposited: None.

Remarks: Barker et al. (1988a) distinguished the oocysts of this form from the other eight eimerians named in their (1988a) paper, "based on oocyst and sporocyst dimensions, and the suite of morphologic characteristics described." They felt that there were no defined similarities among the four eimerian oocysts found parasitizing the three genera (*Aepyprymnus*, *Bettongia*, and *Potorous*) in the Potoroidae they examined.

FAMILY MACROPODIDAE GRAY, 1821 (11 GENERA, 65 SPECIES)

SUBFAMILY MACROPODINAE GRAY, 1821

GENUS DENDROLAGUS MÜLLER, 1840 (12 SPECIES)

EIMERIA DENDROLAGI BARKER, O'CALLAGHAN, AND BEVERIDGE, 1988b

Type host: *Dendrolagus lumholtzi* Collett, 1884, Lumholtz's Tree-kangaroo.

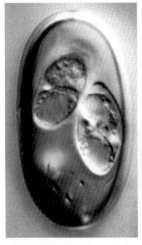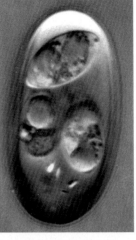

FIGURES 4.24, 4.25 Photomicrographs of two sporulated oocyst of *Eimeria dendrolagi*, both originals from M. O'Callaghan.

Type locality: AUSTRALIA: Queensland: Townsville, Pallarenda (captive animal, originally from Herberton Range).

Other hosts: None to date.

Geographic distribution: AUSTRALIA: Queensland.

Description of sporulated oocyst: Oocyst shape: bluntly ellipsoidal to cylindroidal; number of walls: 2; wall characteristics: outer layer smooth, colorless, ~1.6 thick, thinning at apex of oocyst; inner layer ~0.4 thick; L×W: 33.5×17.9 (30–37×16–21); L/W ratio: 1.9; M: 1.6–2.4 wide, evident in some oocysts (original description), but not in all oocysts (Figures 4.24 and 4.25); OR: absent; PG: present, highly refractile. Distinctive features of oocyst: large ellipsoidal to cylindroidal shape, with a refractile PG, but an indistinct M.

Description of sporocyst and sporozoites: Sporocyst shape: ellipsoidal; L×W: 14.2×8.7 (13–16×7–11); L/W ratio: 1.6; SB: present; SSB: present; PSB: absent; SR: present; SR characteristics: a cluster of granules, 1.6–2.4 wide; SZ: have finely granular cytoplasm and each has one RB, 4.0–6.4 wide. Distinctive features of SP: presence

of SB, SSB, SR, and SZ that fill the SP, and each SZ has a large RB.

Prevalence: Barker et al. (1988b) said they found this form in 1/2 (50%) *D. lumholtzi* examined from the type locality.

Sporulation: Could not be determined because specimens in 2.5% (w/v) potassium dichromate ($K_2Cr_2O_7$) solution spent varying periods in transit before reaching the lab.

Prepatent and patent periods: Unknown.

Site of infection: Unknown.

Endogenous stages: Unknown.

Cross-transmission: None to date.

Pathology: Not described.

Materials deposited: None.

Remarks: Barker et al. (1988b) distinguished the oocysts of this form "based on oocyst and sporocyst dimensions, combined with the suite of morphologic characteristics described." In particular, this species has much larger oocysts and sporocysts than those of *E. lumholtzi*, also reported from Lumholtz's Tree-kangaroo. These are the only two eimerians yet described from this host species and they are different enough from each other, and from other eimerians found in other genera of the Macropodinae, that their reasoning was justified. Barker et al. (1988b,c) hypothesized that as eimerians coevolved with their Australian marsupial hosts, they would be relatively conservative in their morphology, and that such evidence (if it existed) could provide clues to phylogenetic relationships among Macropodoidea. Their earlier work (1988c) suggested there may be value in this hypothesis for rock wallabies (*Petrogale* spp.), but the evidence garnered from their limited examination of coccidia from the Potoroidae failed to show morphologic similarities that, if present, might suggest relatedness of groups of hosts at the generic level. Overall, these studies were unable to demonstrate any obvious patterns of oocyst morphology that could suggest phylogenetic relationships among genera of Macropodidae they examined.

EIMERIA LUMHOLTZI BARKER, O'CALLAGHAN, AND BEVERIDGE, 1988b

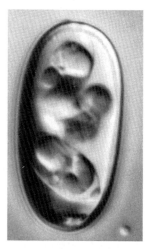

FIGURE 4.26 Photomicrograph of a sporulated oocyst of *Eimeria lumholtzi* from Barker et al., 1988b (their Figure 15), with permission from all authors and with kind permission from Elsevier, publisher of the *International Journal for Parasitology*.

Type host: *Dendrolagus lumholtzi* Collett, 1884, Lumholtz's Tree-kangaroo.

Type locality: AUSTRALIA: Queensland: Townsville, Pallarenda (captive animal, originally from Herberton Range).

Other hosts: None to date.

Geographic distribution: AUSTRALIA: Queensland.

Description of sporulated oocyst: Oocyst shape: irregularly ellipsoidal, often flattened on one side; number of walls: 2; wall characteristics: outer layer smooth, colorless, ~0.8 thick; inner layer, ~0.4 thick; L×W: 21.6×11.1 (18–26×10–13); L/W ratio: 2.0; M, OR: both absent; PG: present. Distinctive features of oocyst: distinct ellipsoidal shape with PG near one end of oocyst along inner wall.

Description of sporocyst and sporozoites: Sporocyst shape: ellipsoidal, but slightly pointed at one end; L×W: 9.1×5.4 (7–13×4–6); L/W ratio:

1.7; SB: present, knoblike, at pointed end of sporocyst; SSB, PSB: both absent; SR: present; SR characteristics: a few small granules scattered at equator of SP; SZ: recurved, seem to fill most of space in SP, and each SZ has one RB, ~3.2 wide. Distinctive features of sporocyst: relatively small size, presence of SB and SR, and SZ that fill most of the space in their SP, each with one RB.

Prevalence: Barker et al. (1988b) found this form in 2/2 (100%) *D. lumholtzi* examined from the type locality.

Sporulation: Could not be determined because specimens in 2.5% (w/v) potassium dichromate ($K_2Cr_2O_7$) solution spent varying periods in transit before reaching the lab.

Prepatent and patent periods: Unknown.

Site of infection: Unknown.

Endogenous stages: Unknown.

Cross-transmission: None to date.

Pathology: Not described.

Materials deposited: None.

Remarks: Barker et al. (1988b) distinguished the oocysts of this form from *D. lumholtzi*, "based on dimensions of oocysts and sporocysts, combined with morphologic features described." Specifically, this species has much smaller oocysts and sporocysts than those of *E. dendrolagi*. These are the only two eimerians described from Lumholtz's Tree-kangaroo, and they are different enough from each other, and from eimerians from other genera in the subfamily, that the reasoning to consider them to represent separate species is justified. Barker et al. (1988b,c) hypothesized that as eimerians coevolved with their Australian marsupial hosts, they would be relatively conservative in their morphology and that such evidence (if it existed) could provide clues to phylogenetic relationships among Macropodoidea. Their earlier work (1988c) suggested there may be value in this hypothesis for rock wallabies (*Petrogale* spp.), but the evidence garnered from their limited examination of coccidia from the Potoroidae failed to show morphologic similarities that might suggest relative relatedness of groups of hosts at the generic level. Thus, there seem to be no obvious patterns of oocyst morphology suggesting phylogenetic relationships among the genera of Macropodidae they examined.

GENUS *LAGORCHESTES* GOULD, 1841 (4 SPECIES)

EIMERIA LAGORCHESTIS BARKER, O'CALLAGHAN, AND BEVERIDGE, 1988b

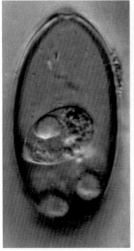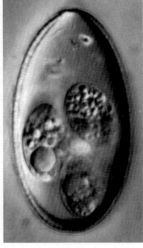

FIGURES 4.27, 4.28 Photomicrographs of two sporulated oocysts of *Eimeria lagorchestis*, both originals from M. O'Callaghan.

Type host: *Lagorchestes conspicillatus* Gould, 1842, Spectacled Hare-wallaby.

Type locality: AUSTRALIA: Queensland: Townsville, Pallarenda (hosts had been relocated from Inkerman).

Other hosts: None to date.

Geographic distribution: AUSTRALIA: Queensland.

Description of sporulated oocyst: Oocyst shape: ellipsoidal to elongate-ovoidal; number of walls: 2; wall characteristics: outer layer is mammillated and striated in optical section, colorless with a brown tinge, ~2.4 thick; inner layer is clear, ~0.4 thick; L×W: 48.2×27.4 (42–54×25–30); L/W ratio: 1.8; M: present, ~3.2 wide at pointed end; OR: absent; PG: present as several scattered granules, each ~1.0 wide. Distinctive features of oocyst: large size with distinct M.

Description of sporocyst and sporozoites: Sporocyst shape: ellipsoidal, slightly pointed at one end; L×W: 18.5×11.4 (17–20×10–12); L/W ratio: 1.6; SB: small and inconspicuous, present at slightly pointed end of SP; SSB: prominent, much wider than SB; PSB: absent; SR: present; SR characteristics: composed of a loose aggregate of granules, 2.4–3.6 wide, scattered throughout sporocyst, largely obscuring SZ; SZ: completely fill the SP, and each has a large RB, 6.0 wide. Distinctive features of sporocyst: large size and SZ with a very large RB.

Prevalence: Barker et al. (1988b) found this form in the only specimen of *L. conspicillatus* they were able to examine.

Sporulation: Could not be determined because specimens in 2.5% (w/v) potassium dichromate ($K_2Cr_2O_7$) solution spent varying periods in transit before reaching the lab.

Prepatent and patent periods: Unknown.

Site of infection: Unknown.

Endogenous stages: Unknown.

Cross-transmission: None to date.

Pathology: Not described.

Materials deposited: None.

Remarks: Barker et al. (1988b) distinguished the oocysts of this form "based on oocyst and sporocyst dimensions, combined with morphologic features described." To date, this is the only eimerian from *L. conspicillatus*, and its sporulated oocysts are different enough from eimerians from other genera in the family, that their reasoning to name it as a distinct species was justified. Barker et al. (1988b,c) hypothesized that as eimerians coevolved with their Australian marsupial hosts, they would be relatively conservative in their morphology and that such evidence (if it existed) could provide clues to phylogenetic relationships among Macropodoidea. Their earlier work (1988c) suggested there may be value in this hypothesis for rock wallabies (*Petrogale* spp.) but, as noted previously (above), there seem to be no patterns of oocyst morphology that suggest phylogenetic relationships among the genera of Macropodidae they examined.

GENUS *MACROPUS* SHAW, 1790 (14 SPECIES)

EIMERIA DESMARESTI BARKER, O'CALLAGHAN, AND BEVERIDGE, 1989

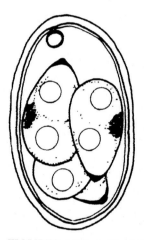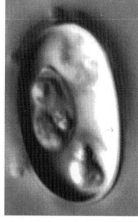

FIGURES 4.29, 4.30 **4.29.** Line drawing of the sporulated oocyst of *Eimeria desmaresti*. **4.30.** Photomicrograph of a sporulated oocyst of *E. desmaresti*. Both figures from Barker et al., 1989, with permission from all authors and with kind permission from Elsevier, publisher of the *International Journal for Parasitology*.

Type host: *Macropus rufogriseus* (Desmarest, 1817), Red-necked Wallaby (syn. *Macropus bennetti* Waterhouse, 1838).

Type locality: AUSTRALIA: Tasmania: Connerville.

Other hosts: None to date.

Geographic distribution: AUSTRALIA: Tasmania.

Description of sporulated oocyst: Oocyst shape: irregular, blunt ellipsoidal, sometimes flattened on one side; number of walls: 2; wall characteristics: outer layer smooth, clear, colorless, 0.8 thick; inner layer is thin, colorless, ~0.4 thick; L × W (*n* = 22): 16.8 × 10.3 (15–18 × 10–11); L/W ratio: 1.6; M, OR: both absent; PG: present. Distinctive features of oocyst: relatively small, blunt-ellipsoidal shape, and lacking both M and OR, but having a distinct PG.

Description of sporocyst and sporozoites: Sporocyst shape: ellipsoidal, slightly pointed at one end; L × W (*n* = 22): 7.5 × 4.5 (7–10 × 4–5); L/W ratio: 1.7; SB: present at pointed end; SSB, PSB: both absent; SR: a few granules scattered at equator of SP; SZ: fill all the space within the SP and each has a small RB, ~1.6 wide. Distinctive features of SP: very small size.

Prevalence: Barker et al. (1989) found this species in 3/18 (17%) *M. rufogriseus* from three locations in Tasmania.

Sporulation: Unknown.

Prepatent and patent periods: Unknown.

Site of infection: Unknown. Oocysts recovered only from the feces.

Endogenous stages: Unknown.

Cross-transmission: None to date.

Pathology: Not described.

Materials deposited: None.

Etymology: This species was named in honor of Anselme Gaetan Desmarest, French zoologist and veterinarian, who described several species of wallabies and kangaroos, including the type host of *E. desmaresti*.

Remarks: The sporulated oocysts of this species are differentiated from those of *E. macropodis* and *E. marsupialium* based on their smaller size, shape, and more prominent SB. They are differentiated from those of *E. gungahlinensis* on the basis of their shape and smooth oocyst surface, and from those of *E. parma* on the basis of small oocyst and sporocyst dimensions.

EIMERIA FLINDERSI BARKER, O'CALLAGHAN, AND BEVERIDGE, 1989

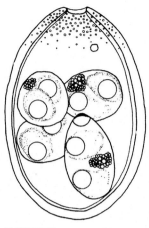
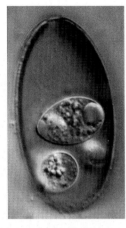

FIGURES 4.31, 4.32   **4.31.** Line drawing of the sporulated oocyst of *Eimeria flindersi* from Barker et al., 1989, with permission from all authors and with kind permission from Elsevier, publisher of the *International Journal for Parasitology*. **4.32.** Photomicrograph of a sporulated oocyst of *E. flindersi*, original from M. O'Callaghan.

Type host: *Macropus eugenii* (Desmarest, 1817), Tammar Wallaby.

Type locality: AUSTRALIA: South Australia: Kangaroo Island.

Other hosts: *Macropus antilopinus* (Gould, 1842), Antilopine Kangaroo; *Macropus rufogriseus* (Desmarest, 1817), Red-necked Wallaby (syn. *Macropus bennetti* Waterhouse, 1838).

Geographic distribution: AUSTRALIA: Queensland; South Australia; Tasmania.

Description of sporulated oocyst: Oocyst shape: ovoidal to nearly ellipsoidal; number of walls: 2; wall characteristics: outer layer finely mammillated at more pointed end surrounding M, otherwise smooth, clear, dark tan, 1.4 thick; inner layer is thin, colorless, ~0.4 thick; L×W (n=20): 44.2×29.2 (42–49×27–32); L/W ratio: 1.5; M: present, up to 5.6 wide, at more pointed end of oocyst; OR: absent; PG: present, usually in anterior part of the oocyst near M. Distinctive

features of oocyst: large size with distinct M and a PG present in its anterior part near M, but lacking an OR.

Description of sporocyst and sporozoites: Sporocyst shape: ellipsoidal to slightly ovoidal, typically distributed in basal part of oocyst; L×W: 18.1×10.6 (17–19×10–12); L/W ratio: 1.7; SB: present at more pointed end of SP; SSB: prominent, lenticular; PSB: absent; SR: a granular aggregate, up to 8 wide, at equator of SP; SZ: with finely granular cytoplasm, they nearly fill SP and each has an RB, ~4 wide. Distinctive features of SP: all four SP are usually distributed in the basal, more rounded, portion of the oocyst, opposite the M.

Prevalence: Barker et al. (1989) found this species in 7/20 (35%) *M. eugenii* from the type locality, in 1/5 (20%) *M. antilopinus* from Queensland, and in 4/18 (22%) *M. rufogriseus* from Tasmania.

Sporulation: Unknown.

Prepatent and patent periods: Unknown.

Site of infection: Unknown, oocysts recovered only from the feces.

Endogenous stages: Unknown.

Cross-transmission: None to date.

Pathology: Not described.

Materials deposited: None.

Etymology: This species was named for Matthew Flinders, who charted the waters of much of the Australian coast, including Kangaroo Island and Tasmania.

Remarks: Barker et al. (1989) distinguished the sporulated oocysts of this species from those of the two other *Eimeria* species with the most similar structural features; the larger oocyst and sporocyst sizes and their tan hue distinguish them from those of *E. toganmainensis*, and although oocysts of *E. lagorchestes* overlap the upper end of oocyst size range, they differ in having a thicker, diffusely mammillated wall. They also noted that sporulated oocysts recovered from *M. antilopinus* (one animal) lacked the mammillated pattern and tan color of the oocyst wall and were intermediate in oocyst and sporocyst dimensions between those oocysts recovered from *M. eugenii*, those from *M. rufogriseus*, and those of *E. toganmainensis*. They argued that since the sporocysts are relatively wider than those in *E. toganmainensis*, the oocysts they studied from *M. antilopinus* should be included, "with reservation," as *E. flindersi*.

The oocyst and sporocyst dimensions given above are those measured from the type host, *M. eugenii*. Barker et al. (1989) also measured oocysts from the two other *Macropus* species in which they found it. The oocysts and sporocysts, respectively, in *M. antilopinus* (n=18), were 41.2×24.3 (38–47×21–28), L/W ratio: 1.7, and 15.0×11.1 (14–16×10–12), L/W ratio: 1.35, while those measured from *M. rufogriseus* (n=21) were 46.8×26.0 (42–49×25.5–27.5), L/W ratio: 1.8, and 17.6×11.1 (14–22×10–13), L/W ratio: 1.6.

EIMERIA GUNGAHLINENSIS MYKYTOWYCZ, 1964

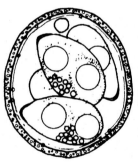 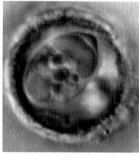

FIGURES 4.33, 4.34 **4.33.** Line drawing of the sporulated oocyst of *Eimeria gungahlinensis* from Barker et al., 1989, with permission from all authors and with kind permissiion from Elsevier, publisher of the *International Journal for Parasitology*. **4.34.** Photomicrograph of a sporulated oocysts of *E. gungahlinensis*, original from M. O'Callaghan.

Type host: *Macropus fuliginosus* (Desmarest, 1817), Western Grey Kangaroo.

Type locality: AUSTRALIA: New South Wales: Yathong Nature Reserve, near Mount Hope.

Other hosts: *Macropus giganteus* Shaw, 1790, Eastern Grey Kangaroo.

Geographic distribution: AUSTRALIA: New South Wales; South Australia; Victoria.

Description of sporulated oocyst: Oocyst shape: spheroidal to subspheroidal; number of walls: 2; wall characteristics: outer layer slightly mammillated, clear, colorless, ~0.8, thick; inner layer is clear, colorless, ~0.4 thick; L×W (n=50): 16.5×14.6 (13–20.5×12–18); L/W ratio: 1.1 (Mykytowycz, 1964); or, L×W (n=70): 18.1×16.6 (13–21×12–20); L/W ratio: 1.1 (Barker et al., 1989); M, OR: both absent; PG: present, ~1.6 wide. Distinctive features of oocyst: small nearly spheroidal shape lacking M and OR, but with a distinct PG.

Description of sporocyst and sporozoites: Sporocyst shape: ovoidal–ellipsoidal, slightly pointed and thickened at one end; L×W (n=50): 8.8×5.9 (7–11×4–7.5); L/W ratio: 1.5 (Mykytowycz, 1964); or, L×W (n=70): 9.1×6.3 (7–11×5–8); L/W ratio: 1.4 (Barker et al., 1989); SB: present, distinct; SSB, PSB: both absent; SR: a granular aggregate up to 4.8 wide; SZ: fill the SP and each has an RB, ~1.6×2.4 wide. Distinctive features of sporocyst: SP occupy almost the entire space within the oocyst, their elongate ovoidal shape, and the presence of a distinct SB.

Prevalence: Mykytowycz (1964) found this species in 69/102 (68%) *M. fuliginosus* (syn. *M. canguru*) near Mt Hope, in New South Wales. Barker et al. (1989) found this species in 3/133 (2%) *M. giganteus* from the type locality, from "Pine Plains," via Patchewollock, Victoria, and near Kersbrook, Kangaroo Island, South Australia, and in 37/180 (20.5%) *M. giganteus* from Yan Yean, Victoria.

Sporulation: Unknown.

Prepatent and patent periods: Unknown.

Site of infection: Unknown, oocysts recovered only from the feces.

Endogenous stages: Unknown.

Cross-transmission: None to date.

Pathology: Not described.

Materials deposited: None.

Remarks: Barker et al. (1989) distinguished the sporulated oocysts of this species from other eimerians in *Macropus* by its small size and its spheroidal to subspheroidal shape. The oocysts of *E. marsupialium* overlap in size, but the sporocyst size is smaller in *E. gungahlinensis.*

The oocyst and sporocyst dimensions given above are those measured from the type host, *M. fuliginosus.* Barker et al. (1989) measured oocysts from *M. giganteus* in which they also found it. The oocysts and sporocysts, respectively, in *M. giganteus* (n=50) were 18.8×16.1 (17–22×14–19), L/W ratio: 1.2, and 8.4×7.0 (7–10.5×6–8), L/W ratio: 1.2.

EIMERIA HESTERMANI MYKYTOWYCZ, 1964

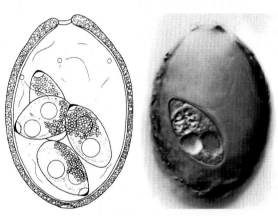

FIGURES 4.35, 4.36   **4.35.** Line drawing of the sporulated oocyst of *Eimeria hestermani* from Barker et al., 1989, with permission from all authors and with kind permission from Elsevier, publisher of the *International Journal for Parasitology.* **4.36.** Photomicrograph of a sporulated oocyst of *E. hestermani,* original from M. O'Callaghan.

Synonym: Globidium mucosum of Zwart and Strik, 1964 (see Pellérdy, 1974 and Barker et al., 1989).

Type host: Macropus giganteus Shaw, 1790 (syn. *Macropus canguru* aka Mykytowycz, 1964), Eastern Grey Kangaroo. However, as Barker et al. (1989) pointed out, Mykytowycz (1964) sampled a population of grey kangaroos that was comprised both *M. giganteus* (Eastern) and *M. fuliginosus* (Western), as later distinguished by Kirsch and Poole (1972), but which Mykytowycz (1964)

identified as *M. canguru*; thus, with no way to determine the true type host, Barker et al. (1989) simply "nominated" the former species.

Type locality: AUSTRALIA: New South Wales: Mount Hope, Yathong Nature Reserve.

Other hosts: Macropus dorsalis (Gray, 1817), Black-striped Wallaby; *Macropus eugenii* (Desmarest, 1817), Tammar Wallaby; *Macropus fuliginosus* (Desmarest, 1817), Western Grey Kangaroo; *Macropus rufogriseus* (Desmarest, 1817), Red-necked Wallaby (syn. *Macropus bennetti* Waterhouse, 1838).

Geographic distribution: AUSTRALIA: New South Wales; Queensland.

Description of sporulated oocyst: Oocyst shape: ellipsoidal; number of walls: 2; wall characteristics: outer layer grayish brown, granulated, 2.1–3.2 thick, slightly thicker around the M; inner layer is relatively thin, colorless, ~0.8 thick, and can be readily separated from the outer; L×W (n=50): 66.1×46.6 (63–69×45–49), L/W ratio: 1.4 (Mykytowycz, 1964) or (n=26) 64.7×45.3 (62–69×42–48), L/W ratio: 1.4 (Barker et al., 1989); M: present, 4–6 wide, at more pointed end of oocyst; OR: absent; PG: variable; was not mentioned in the original description by Mykytowycz (1964), but was reported as "variably present" by Barker et al. (1989). Distinctive features of oocyst: very large size with distinct M.

Description of sporocyst and sporozoites: Sporocyst shape: distinctly ovoidal, slightly pointed at one end; L×W: 24.5×14 (22–27×13–15), L/W ratio: 1.75 (Mykytowycz, 1964) or L×W (n=26): 24.9×13.4 (23–27×12–15), L/W ratio: 1.9 (Barker et al., 1989); SB: present; it was not mentioned by Mykytowycz (1964), but well described and pictured by Barker et al. (1989); SSB: prominent, lenticular; PSB: absent; SR: a tight aggregate of granules, up to 8 wide, or loose aggregate of granules scattered about equator of SP; SZ: fill most of the space within the SP, and each SZ has finely granular cytoplasm and contains a large RB, 9.2×5.6–6.8. Distinctive features of SP: they are relatively small compared to the size of the oocyst, and combined, fill ≤50% of the space within the oocyst.

Prevalence: Mykytowycz (1964) reported this species in 4/102 (4%) *M. giganteus* (= *M. canguru*) in Mount Hope, Yathong Nature Reserve, New South Wales, but did not find it in 456 *M. rufus* from the same state. Barker et al. (1989) examined fecal samples from 514 kangaroos and wallabies from New South Wales, South Australia, Victoria, Tasmania, and Queensland, and found this species in 11/133 (8%) *M. giganteus* from New South Wales and Victoria, in 31/180 (17%) *M. fuliginosus* from South Australia and Victoria, in 8/18 (44%) *M. rufogriesus* from Tasmania, in 7/20 (35%) *M. eugenii* from South Australia, and in 3/14 (21%) *M. dorsalis* from Queensland.

Sporulation: Unknown.

Prepatent and patent periods: Unknown.

Site of infection: Unknown, oocysts recovered only from the feces.

Endogenous stages: Unknown.

Cross-transmission: None to date.

Pathology: Not described.

Materials deposited: None.

Remarks: Prior to the work of Mykytowycz (1964), all knowledge on the four eimerians previously known from kangaroos was gleaned from animals in captivity (Wenyon and Scott, 1925; Prasad, 1960; Yakimoff and Matschoulsky, 1936). Mykytowycz collected fecal samples from 516 red (*M. rufus*) and 157 grey (*M. giganteus*) kangaroos taken from four localities in New South Wales and one in Queensland, from which he described and named seven species of *Eimeria*, including *E. hestermani*. His description of this form (as with the others) was somewhat incomplete, but he did include a photomicrograph of four sporulated oocysts (his Figure 7) from which some structural information not included in his written description (e.g., SB, SSB) could be found. This species was more fully described, along with a line drawing and four photomicrographs (their Figures 1, 16–19), by Barker et al. (1989).

Barker et al. (1989) also measured oocysts from the four other *Macropus* species in which they found *E. hestermani*. The oocysts and sporocysts, respectively, in *M. fuliginosus* (*n*=85) were 71.1 × 50.3 (63–77 × 43–56), L/W ratio: 1.4, and 24.6 × 14.2 (19–29 × 13–16), L/W ratio: 1.7; those measured from *M. rufogriseus* (*n*=23)

were 64.9 × 40.5 (61–72 × 38–45), L/W ratio: 1.6, and 25.2 × 13.1 (22–31 × 12–15), L/W ratio: 1.9; those measured from *M. dorsalis* (*n*=20) were 63.5 × 44.2 (60–67 × 42–46), L/W ratio: 1.4, and 25.9 × 13.3 (25–28 × 12–14), L/W ratio: 1.9; and those measured from *M. eugenii* (*n*=20) were 59.8 × 39.2 (57–62 × 36–41), L/W ratio: 1.5, and 24.6 × 13.3 (22–27 × 12–14), L/W ratio: 1.8.

EIMERIA MACROPODIS WENYON AND SCOTT, 1925

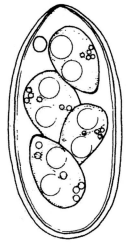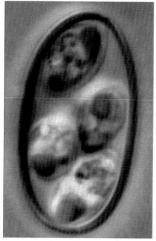

FIGURES 4.37, 4.38 **4.37.** Line drawing of the sporulated oocyst of *Eimeria macropodis* from Barker et al., 1989, with permission from all authors and with kind permission from Elsevier, publisher of the *International Journal for Parasitology*. **4.38.** Photomicrograph of a sporulated oocyst of *E. macropodis*, original from M. O'Callaghan.

Synonyms: *Eimeria fausti* Yakimoff and Matschoulsky, 1936; *Eimeria cunnamullensis* Mykytowycz, 1964; *Eimeria purchasei* Mykytowycz, 1964.

Type host: *Macropus rufogriseus* (Desmarest, 1817), Red-necked Wallaby (syn. *Macropus bennetti* Waterhouse, 1838).

Type locality: EUROPE: United Kingdom: London, Zoological Gardens. Obviously, however, the wallaby originated in Australia, but it is not possible to pinpoint the state or exact locality.

Other hosts: *Macropus dorsalis* (Gray, 1817), Black-striped Wallaby; *Macropus eugenii* (Desmarest, 1817), Tammar Wallaby; *Macropus fuliginosus* (Desmarest, 1817), Western Grey Kangaroo; *Macropus giganteus* Shaw, 1790, Eastern Grey Kangaroo; *Macropus irma* (Jourdan, 1837), Western Brush Wallaby; *Macropus parma* Waterhouse, 1846, Parma Wallaby; *Macropus parryi* Bennett, 1835, Pretty-faced Wallaby; *Macropus rufus* (Desmarest, 1822), Red Kangaroo.

Geographic distribution: AUSTRALIA: New South Wales; South Australia; Queensland; Tasmania; Victoria; Western Australia.

Description of sporulated oocyst: Oocyst shape: highly variable in shape ranging from ovoidal, to ellipsoidal, to cylindroidal, and often slightly asymmetric or flattened on one side (Triffitt, 1926; Prasad, 1960; Barker et al., 1989); number of walls: 2 (Barker et al., 1989) or 3 (Triffitt, 1926; Prasad, 1960); wall characteristics: outer layer smooth, clear, colorless, ~0.8 thick, and thinning at more pointed end, often with slight concave indentation of inner wall; inner is clear, colorless, ~0.4 thick; middle layer with transverse striations (Prasad, 1960); L×W of larger oocysts: 30×15 or 32×16; L/W ratio: 2.0, and smaller oocysts: 22–23×10–11, with overall range 22–34×10–17 (Triffitt, 1926) or L×W (n=30): 25.5×13.1 (23–28×12–17); L/W ratio: 1.9; M: present, ~3 wide, or as a "slight concave inward distortion of inner wall, but no clear cut M" (Barker et al., 1989); OR: absent; PG: present. Distinctive features of oocyst: the wide variation in shape and size of oocysts having the specific characters described within a particular host individual (see *Remarks*, below).

Description of sporocyst and sporozoites: Sporocyst shape: ovoidal to slightly ellipsoidal, pointed at one end; L×W: 7–11×6–8 (Triffitt, 1926) or L×W (n=30): 8.8×6.3 (8–10×5–7); L/W ratio: 1.4 (Barker et al., 1989); SB: present; SSB, PSB: both absent; SR: finely granular material scattered near the equator of SP; SZ: club-shaped, slightly curved, ~5–6×2–3, and they fill most of the space within the SP; each SZ contains a distinct RB, ~1.6–3.2 wide, at their broader end and an N about mid-body. Distinctive features of sporocyst: typical SP with an SB, SR, and club-shaped SZ.

Prevalence: Wenyon and Scott (1925) found this species in a single *M. rufogriseus* that died in the Zoological Gardens of London. Prasad (1960) reported *E. macropodis* in one *M. rufogriseus* (syn. *M. bennetti*) from the London Zoological Gardens. Barker et al. (1989) examined fecal samples from 514 kangaroos and wallabies from New South Wales, Queensland, South Australia, Tasmania, and Victoria, and found this species in 9/18 (50%) *M. rufogriesus* from Tasmania and New South Wales. In addition, Barker et al. (1989) also found it in 2/97 (2%) *M. rufus* from New South Wales; in 62/133 (47%) *M. giganteus* from New South Wales, Victoria, and South Australia; in 48/180 (27%) *M. fuliginosus* from New South Wales, Victoria, and South Australia; in 20/20 (100%) *M. eugenii* from South Australia; in 6/11 (55%) *M. parryi* from Queensland and South Australia; in 11/14 (79%) *M. dorsalis* from Queensland; in 5/8 (62.5%) *M. parma* from New South Wales and South Australia; and in 4/4 (100%) *M. irma* from Western Australia.

Sporulation: Triffitt (1926) said, "Forty-eight hours after the faeces were passed the sporocysts were fully developed," but she did not mention how the oocysts were preserved during that time. Prasad (1960) also said that sporulation was completed in 48 h.

Prepatent and patent periods: Unknown.

Site of infection: Epithelial cells of the small intestine.

Endogenous stages: Triffitt (1926) examined fixed, embedded, stained tissue sections and found a small area with an intense infection in which she measured some of the endogenous developmental stages. Small trophozoites (young meronts), ~2.5 wide, increased in size to an ovoidal form of 10×8.5, with homogenous cytoplasm and an N that was either central or eccentrically placed. Nuclear division and merozoite formation commenced before the completion of growth. Merozoites varied in number from 8 to 32, each ~8×2–2.5, with granular cytoplasm and an N in the thicker end of their club-shaped body.

Immature microgametocytes were distinguishable from early meronts by the greater number and more deeply staining character of their N. Mature microgametocytes were ~32×22; each microgamete measured 3.5×0.75. In mature macrogametocytes, their granules became more definite and arranged themselves at regular intervals in the most superficial layer of the cytoplasm, ultimately coalescing to form the oocyst wall.

Cross-transmission: None to date.

Pathology: Triffitt (1926) examined the intestinal tissue sections supplied to her by Dr Scott (of Wenyon and Scott, 1925) from which she described the following pathological effects of this eimerian. The surface epithelium she examined was heavily parasitized such that virtually every host epithelial cell harbored multiple endogenous stages, and where the mature meronts and gametocytes occurred in groups, these cells were "completely obliterated." Portions of the intestinal tissue showed an acute inflammatory response accompanied by edema and a heavy infiltration of cells, most of which were polymorphonuclear leukocytes; where the epithelium had become denuded, numerous petechial hemorrhages were seen. This denudation of the mucous layer was accompanied by the formation of a "pseudo-membrane" and a marked thickening of the tissues immediately below it.

Materials deposited: Nucleotide sequences identified were submitted to GenBank under the accession numbers JQ392574–JQ392580.

Remarks: In March, 1925, at a laboratory meeting of the Royal Society of Tropical Medicine and Hygiene, Wenyon and Scott exhibited tissue sections of the small intestine of a Bennett's wallaby, *M. bennetti* (now a junior synonym of *M. rufogriseus*), that had died in the Zoological Gardens in London (thus, technically, London, UK, is the type locality). In those sections, they discovered and described meronts and gametocytes of a coccidium they named *E. macropodis*. Marjorie Triffitt, a field officer at the Institute of Agricultural Parasitology, London, received the material from Dr Scott and studied the endogenous stages of *E. macropodis*, measuring some of them, and the oocysts they produced (Triffitt, 1926). The shape of oocysts of *E. macropodis* seem to possess the most extreme variation in the dimensions of oocysts studied and measured from any other species of *Macropus*. Prasad (1960) also found this species in one *M. rufogriseus* in the Zoological Gardens, London. Barker et al. (1989) documented the shape(s) and ranges of oocyst dimensions from five *Macropus* species including, *M. rufogriseus* (type host), *M. dorsalis*, *M. irma*, *M. parma*, and *M. parryi*. On the basis of their broad range of measurements, they were unable to confidently discriminate more than a single species within any of these hosts. This led them to conclude, "that the strong homology among the oocysts present in the various hosts of the genus *Macropus*, despite differences in mean oocyst length and other parameters, justifies lumping them as a single species, in the absence of experimental information on host specificity." Clearly, molecular characterization of the oocysts from these various *Macropus* species will help verify their conclusion, or not.

Barker et al. (1989) used their observations and measurements to distinguish *E. macropodis* from many other eimerians described from *Macropus* as follows: *E. macropodis* has shorter, narrower oocysts than *E. wilcanniensis*, *E. mykytowyczi*, and the other larger species in *Macropus*, and in their view, no M; it has shorter SP than does *E. parryi*; it has a more elongate, irregular shape than oocysts of *E. marsupialium*; it has a generally larger, less regular shape than oocysts of *E. yathongensis*, which are consistently ovoidal; it has larger oocysts and SP than those of *E. parma*; it has a larger, more elongate shape compared to *E. gungahlinensis*; and it has larger oocysts than those of *E. desmaresti*. They acknowledged that the smaller-type oocysts of *E. macropodis* share similarities with oocysts of *E. petrogale* (in *Petrogale*), *E. bicolor* (in *Wallabia*), and *E. lumholtzi* (in *Dendrolagus*), but considered them separate species on the basis of host generic differences. The larger-type oocysts of *E. macropodis* share similarities with oocysts of *E. obendorfi* (in *Thylogale*), but differ by the size and shape of their

SP and the possession of an SB, and are similar to those of *E. ringaroomaensis* (in *Thylogale*), but differ by having smaller SP that lack an SSB.

In addition to the measurements given above for oocysts from *M. rufogriseus*, Barker et al. (1989) also measured oocysts of *E. macropodis* from eight other *Macropus* species in which they found it. The oocysts and sporocysts, respectively, in *M. fuliginosus* (*n* = 30) were 24.6 × 13.4 (18–28 × 11–16), L/W ratio: 1.8, and 9.2 × 6.3 (8–10 × 6–7), L/W ratio: 1.5; those measured from *M. rufus* (*n* = 40) were 25.2 × 13.5 (21–28 × 12–15), L/W ratio: 1.9, and 9.2 × 6.0 (8–11 × 5–7), L/W ratio: 1.5; those measured from *M. eugenii* (*n* = 20) were 24.3 × 13.6 (19–29 × 12–15), L/W ratio: 1.8, and 9.3 × 6.5 (8–10 × 6–7), L/W ratio: 1.4; those measured from *M. giganteus* (*n* = 50) were 26.0 × 13.0 (22–30 × 11–14), L/W ratio: 2.0, and 9.5 × 6.2 (8–11 × 6–7), L/W ratio: 1.5; those in *M. irma* (*n* = 25) were 27.6 × 13.3 (24–31 × 12–14), L/W ratio: 2.1, and 9.8 × 7.5 (9–11 × 6–9), L/W ratio: 1.3; those in *M. parryi* (*n* = 33) were 25.5 × 12.8 (21–28 × 11–14), L/W ratio: 2.0, and 8.3 × 6.3 (7–10 × 5–8), L/W ratio: 1.3; those in *M. dorsalis* (*n* = 42) were 24.5 × 14.2 (18–29 × 10–16), L/W ratio: 1.7, and 9.1 × 6.3 (7–11 × 5–7), L/W ratio: 1.4; and those in *M. parma* (*n* = 30) were 21.1 × 11.9 (17–25 × 10–14), L/W ratio: 1.8, and 8.0 × 5.6 (6–10 × 5–6), L/W ratio: 1.4.

In addition to these size distributions of oocysts and sporocysts of *E. macropodis* between host species, Barker et al. (1989) found wide variation in shape of the oocysts having the characters described (above), within a particular host species and individual, along with the broader range in oocyst size among host species. Nonetheless, they were unable to confidently differentiate more than a single species. This led them to conclude that the strong homology among the oocysts present in the various *Macropus* species, despite differences in mean oocyst lengths and other parameters, justified their lumping them as variations in a single species in the absence of evidence (e.g., cross-transmission experiments at that time) to refute their idea.

Hill et al. (2012) sought to improve the taxonomic resolution of *E. macropodis* by contributing both morphological and molecular data on oocysts shed by the Tammar wallaby, *M. eugenii*, collected from a captive population at the Macquarie University Fauna Park. The oocysts and sporocysts they measured occurred in both small and large forms even within this single host, *M. eugenii*, and their L×W (*n* = 43) were: 24.4 × 13.7 (19–30 × 11–17), L/W ratio: 1.8, and 8.9 × 6.3 (6–11 × 4–7), L/W ratio: 1.4; their measurements are nearly identical to those recorded from *M. eugenii* by Barker et al. (1989). Their paper, however, is extremely important and timely because of their phylogenetic analysis of multiple gene markers (18S SSU and cytochrome *c* oxidase subunit I (COI)). Initially, their phylogenetic analysis of 18S SSU alleles separated *E. macropodis* into two lineages, causing them to suspect the presence of multiple species. However, incorporating their analysis of the COI gene showed the two lineages shared 99.9% similarity and originated from the same species. Their work highlights that molecular analysis of a single gene may not be adequate to uncover the full genetic diversity within one *Eimeria* species. Thus, their analysis of multiple genes and statistical analysis of oocyst morphological traits seemed to confirm the occurrence of a single polymorphic species.

Putting together the evidence at their disposal, they noted that *E. macropodis* has been found in all six states of Australia, from both free-ranging and captive populations, as well as in a zoo in the Ukraine (Yakimoff and Matschoulsky, 1936). Given the ubiquity of *E. macropodis* across multiple *Macropus* species, and such large geographic scales, it certainly highlights how important it is to be able to make accurate identifications of this and the other eimerians that infect *Macropus*. This challenge is complicated by the polymorphic nature of *E. macropodis* that may lead to misclassification and underestimation of its true host ranges. Molecular parasitologists need to become involved in the solution of this dilemma.

On the basis of their acceptance of a wide range of dimensions, shapes, and other characters (e.g., tiny SB, "weak" M), Barker et al. (1989, p. 256) concluded that *E. fausti*, described by Yakimoff and Matschoulsky (1936), and *E. cunnamullensis* and *E. purchasei*, described by Mykytowycz

(1964), were junior synonyms of *E. macropodis.* This means that *E. macropodis* is the most prevalent eimerian, and has the broadest host range, of any coccidium among *Macropus* species. The only *Macropus* species in which it has not yet been found inhabits xeric habitats and had a low overall prevalence of other coccidial infections.

EIMERIA MARSUPIALIUM YAKIMOFF AND MATSCHOULSKY, 1936

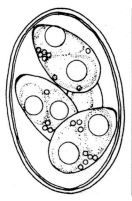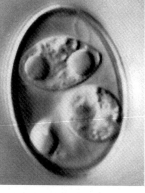

FIGURES 4.39, 4.40 **4.39.** Line drawing of the sporulated oocyst of *Eimeria marsupialium.* **4.40.** Photomicrograph of a sporulated oocyst of *E. marsupialium.* Both figures from Barker et al., 1989, with permission from all authors and with kind permission from Elsevier, publisher of the *International Journal for Parasitology.*

Type host: *Macropus giganteus* Shaw, 1790, Eastern Grey Kangaroo.

Type locality: ASIA: Ukraine (former USSR): Kharkov, Kharkov Zoo.

Other hosts: *Macropus fuliginosus* (Desmarest, 1817), Western Grey Kangaroo.

Geographic distribution: ASIA: Ukraine (former USSR); AUSTRALIA: New South Wales; South Australia; Victoria.

Description of sporulated oocyst: Oocyst shape: ellipsoidal to subspheroidal to ovoidal; number of walls: 2; wall characteristics: outer is smooth, clear, colorless, ~1.0 thick; inner is clear, ~0.4 thick; L × W ($n = 77$): 22 × 18 (20–26 × 16–20); L/W

ratio: 1.2 (Yakimoff and Matschoulsky, 1936), or L × W ($n = 44$): 22.5 × 16.3 (19–26 × 14–18); L/W ratio: 1.4 (Barker et al., 1989, from *M. giganteus* in Australia); M, OR, PG: all absent. Distinctive features of oocyst: mostly subspheroidal shape and lacking M, OR, and PG.

Description of sporocyst and sporozoites: Sporocyst shape: ellipsoidal–ovoidal; L × W ($n = 77$): 8–12 × 6–8; L/W ratio: unknown (Yakimoff and Matschoulsky, 1936), or L × W ($n = 44$): 10.8 × 6.9 (10–12 × 6–8); L/W ratio: 1.6 (Barker et al., 1989 from *M. giganteus* in Australia); SB: present; SSB, PSB: both absent; SR: present as an irregular granular aggregate scattered throughout SP; SZ: fill the space within the SP and each has an RB, 2.4–3.2 wide. Distinctive features of SP: ovoidal shape with an SR of only a few dispersed granules, and a small, but distinct SB.

Prevalence: Yakimoff and Matschoulsky (1936) found this species in 2/2 *M. giganteus* in a Zoo in the Ukraine (former USSR). Barker et al. (1989) found it in 23/133 (17%) *M. giganteus* from five locations in New South Wales, South Australia, and Victoria, and in 37/180 (20.5%) *M. fuliginosus* from six locations in New South Wales, South Australia, and Victoria.

Sporulation: Unknown.

Prepatent and patent periods: Unknown.

Site of infection: Unknown. Oocysts recovered only from the feces.

Endogenous stages: Unknown.

Cross-transmission: None to date.

Pathology: Not described.

Materials deposited: None.

Remarks: Yakimoff and Matschoulsky (1936) only had to compare the oocysts they discovered and described to those of *E. macropodis* from which it is quite different, when they named this a new species (1936). Barker et al. (1989) also separated the oocysts they redescribed as *E. macropodis* on the basis of shorter oocysts, higher L/W ratios, greater SP length, relative symmetry of the oocyst, and lack of any suggestion of an M. They also separated this species from *E. parryi*, *E. parma*, and *E. gungahlinensis* for structural reasons that are clear from their presentations made elsewhere in this chapter.

The oocyst and sporocyst dimensions given above are those measured from the type host, *M. giganteus*, in Australia, by Barker et al. (1989). Barker et al. (1989) also measured oocysts from *M. fuliginosus*. The oocysts and sporocysts, respectively, in *M. fuliginosus* ($n = 35$) were 22.3×16.6 (19–25 × 15–18), L/W ratio: 1.3, and 11.0×6.8 (10–12 × 6–7), L/W ratio: 1.6.

EIMERIA MYKYTOWYCZI BARKER, O'CALLAGHAN, AND BEVERIDGE, 1989

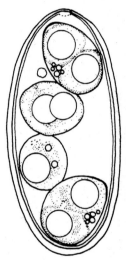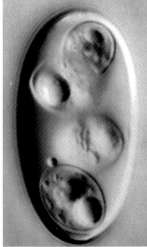

FIGURES 4.41, 4.42 **4.41.** Line drawing of the sporulated oocyst of *Eimeria mykytowyczi* from Barker et al., 1989, with permission from all authors and with kind permission from Elsevier, publisher of the *International Journal for Parasitology*. **4.42.** Photomicrograph of a sporulated oocyst of *E. mykytowyczi*, original from M. O'Callaghan.

Type host: *Macropus agilis* (Gould, 1842), Agile Wallaby.

Type locality: AUSTRALIA: Northern Territory: "Tipperary."

Other hosts: *Macropus antilopinus* (Gould, 1842), Antilopine Kangaroo; *Macropus parryi* Bennett, 1835, Pretty-faced Wallaby.

Geographic distribution: AUSTRALIA: Northern Territory; Queensland; South Australia.

Description of sporulated oocyst: Oocyst shape: irregular, elongate-ellipsoidal/ovoidal, often flattened on one or both sides; number of walls: 2; wall characteristics: outer layer is smooth, clear, colorless, 0.8–1.0 thick, and thins at slightly pointed end; inner layer is thin, colorless, ~0.4 thick, and protrudes at more pointed end; L × W ($n = 21$): 31.3×17.5 (30–34 × 17–18); L/W ratio: 1.8; M: present/absent, described as "equivocal;" OR: absent; PG: variably present. Distinctive features of oocyst: irregularly ellipsoid shape that flattens on one or both sides.

Description of sporocyst and sporozoites: Sporocyst shape: ellipsoidal, slightly pointed and thickened at one end; L × W ($n = 21$): 10.5×7.8 (10–12 × 7–9); L/W ratio: 1.3; SB: likely present at thickened, more pointed end; SSB, PSB: both absent; SR: a loose aggregate of granules usually scattered at equator of SP; SZ: nearly fill SP and each has an RB, ~3.2×4.0 wide. Distinctive features of sporocyst: the four SP are distributed such that they occupy the entire space in the oocyst and they have a small, thickened end that is likely an SB.

Prevalence: Barker et al. (1989) found this species in 1/2 (50%) *M. agilis* from the type locality, in 1/5 (20%) *M. antilopinus* from Queensland, and in 2/11 (18%) *M. parryi* from South Australia.

Sporulation: Unknown.

Prepatent and patent periods: Unknown.

Site of infection: Unknown, oocysts recovered only from the feces.

Endogenous stages: Unknown.

Cross-transmission: None to date.

Pathology: Not described.

Materials deposited: None.

Etymology: This species epithet was used to honor Dr Roman Mykytowycz, formerly of the C.S.I.R.O. Division of Wildlife Research, who first studied coccidia in kangaroos.

Remarks: Barker et al. (1989) separated the sporulated oocysts of this species from those of *E. wilcanniensis* on the basis of a consistently irregular oocyst shape, and a combination of smaller oocyst and sporocyst dimensions, as well as presumed host specificity. They separated it from other coccidia of *Macropus* species with overlapping oocyst size ranges on the basis of its tiny (? if present) SB and lacking an SSB. They also noted that *E. obendorfi* is smaller and lacks an M, and *E. godmani* is similar, but has a much thinner, tan, oocyst wall.

The oocyst and sporocyst dimensions given above are those measured from the type host, *M. agilis*. Barker et al. (1989) also measured oocysts from the two other *Macropus* species in which they found them. The oocysts and sporocysts, respectively, in *M. parryi* (n = 29) were 32.7 × 18.6 (28–36.5 × 16–20), L/W ratio: 2.0, and 11.3 × 8.2 (10–12 × 7–9), L/W ratio: 1.4; and those measured from *M. antilopinus* (n = 20) were 28.6 × 15.9 (26–34 × 15–16), L/W ratio: 1.8, and 10.5 × 7.7 (10–11 × 7–8), L/W ratio 1.4.

EIMERIA PARMA BARKER, O'CALLAGHAN, AND BEVERIDGE, 1989

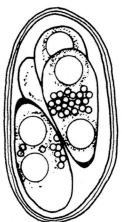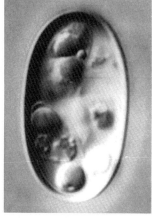

FIGURES 4.43, 4.44   **4.43.** Line drawing of the sporulated oocyst of *Eimeria parma*. **4.44.** Photomicrograph of a sporulated oocyst of *E. parma*. Both figures from Barker et al., 1989, with permission from all authors and with kind permission from Elsevier, publisher of the *International Journal for Parasitology*.

Type host: *Macropus parma* Waterhouse, 1846, Parma Wallaby.

Type locality: AUSTRALIA: South Australia: Adelaide, Adelaide Zoo.

Other hosts: None to date.

Geographic distribution: AUSTRALIA: South Australia.

Description of sporulated oocyst: Oocyst shape: blunt ellipsoidal, sometimes slightly pointed at one end, or flattened on one side; number of walls: 2; wall characteristics: outer layer smooth, clear, colorless, 0.8 thick; inner layer is thin, colorless, ~0.4 thick; L × W (n = 12): 20.7 × 11.6 (20–22 × 11–12); L/W ratio: 1.8; M, OR, PG: all absent. Distinctive features of oocyst: small ellipsoidal shape with blunt ends and lacking M, OR, and PG.

Description of sporocyst and sporozoites: Sporocyst shape: ellipsoidal, slightly pointed at one end; L × W (n = 12): 11.7 × 5.1 (11–12 × 5–6); L/W ratio: 2.3; SB: present at pointed end, but inconspicuous; SSB, PSB: both absent; SR: an aggregate of small granules at equator of SP; SZ: do not fill all the space in the SP and each has a small RB, ~2.4 wide. Distinctive features of SP: elongate ellipsoidal shape, which gives it an L/W ratio >2.2.

Prevalence: Barker et al. (1989) found this species in 1/8 (12.5%) *M. parma* from the Adelaide Zoo in South Australia.

Sporulation: Unknown.

Prepatent and patent periods: Unknown.

Site of infection: Unknown, oocysts recovered only from the feces.

Endogenous stages: Unknown.

Cross-transmission: None to date.

Pathology: Not described.

Materials deposited: None.

Remarks: This species resembles *E. parryi* in that their sporocysts both have an L/W ratio >2.1, but its oocysts are significantly shorter. The sporulated oocysts of *E. parma* also are similar to those of *E. volckertzooni*, but the generic and geographic/ecologic separation of the hosts was considered by Barker et al. (1989) to justify separate species status.

EIMERIA PARRYI BARKER, O'CALLAGHAN, AND BEVERIDGE, 1989

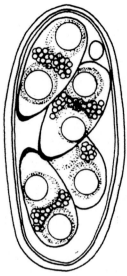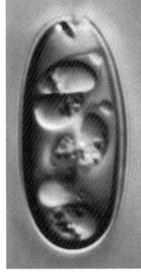

FIGURES 4.45, 4.46 **4.45.** Line drawing of the sporulated oocyst of *Eimeria parryi* from Barker et al., 1989, with permission from all authors and with kind permission from Elsevier, publisher of the *International Journal for Parasitology*. **4.46.** Photomicrograph of a sporulated oocyst of *E. parryi*, original from M. O'Callaghan.

Type host: *Macropus parryi* Bennett, 1835, Pretty-faced Wallaby.

Type locality: AUSTRALIA: South Australia, Adelaide, Adelaide Zoo.

Other hosts: None to date.

Geographic distribution: AUSTRALIA: South Australia; Queensland: 78 km north of Rockhampton.

Description of sporulated oocyst: Oocyst shape: elongate-ellipsoidal; number of walls: 2; wall characteristics: outer layer smooth, clear, colorless, 1.0 thick; inner is thin, colorless; L×W (*n*=21): 28.7×13.1 (26–30×12–14); L/W ratio: 2.2; M, OR: both absent; PG: present. Distinctive features of oocyst: elongated-ellipsoidal shape with an L/W ratio >2.0, lack of M and OR, and presence of PG.

Description of sporocyst and sporozoites: Sporocyst shape: elongate-ovoidal, pointed at one end; L×W (*n*=21): 12.3×6.0 (11–14×6); L/W ratio: 2.0; SB: inconspicuous as an indistinct thickening at the more pointed end; SSB, PSB: both absent; SR: present as a few scattered granules, up to 1.6 wide; SZ: nearly fill SP and each has an RB, ~3.2×2.4 wide. Distinctive features of sporocyst: an indistinct SB and SZs that occupy the entire space in the SP.

Prevalence: Barker et al. (1989) found this species in 3/11 (27%) *M. parryi* (their Table 1). It can only be presumed that two of the three infected wallabies were collected in Queensland and the third in South Australia from the Adelaide Zoo, because their "type locality" designation is ambiguous: "Localities: captive, Adelaide Zoo, Adelaide*, S.A.; 78 km north of Rockhampton, Qld." The asterisk (*) indicates the host from which oocysts were measured, according to their Materials and Methods. Thus, 1/1 *M. parryi* in the Adelaide Zoo and 2/10 (20%) *M. parryi* in Queensland were found to be infected. Since oocysts were only measured from the captive wallaby in the Adelaide Zoo, this is designated the type host locality.

Sporulation: Unknown.

Prepatent and patent periods: Unknown.

Site of infection: Unknown, oocysts recovered only from the feces.

Endogenous stages: Unknown.

Cross-transmission: None to date.

Pathology: Not described.

Materials deposited: None.

Etymology: This species epithet was chosen to mimic the host's species epithet.

Remarks: Barker et al. (1989) separated the sporulated oocysts of this species from those of most other eimerians in *Macropus* species on the basis of both its oocysts and sporocysts having an L/W ratio of 2.0 or greater. They separated it from *E. parma* by its larger oocysts, and from *E. sharmani* by its narrower oocysts and shorter sporocysts. There was another inconsistency in their (Barker et al., 1989) paper regarding this species in that their written description stated the SP tapered "slightly to inconspicuous Stieda body," while their Table 12 listed the SB as absent.

EIMERIA PRIONOTEMNI BARKER, O'CALLAGHAN, AND BEVERIDGE, 1989

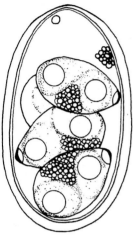
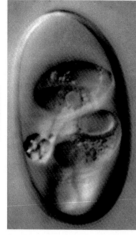

FIGURES 4.47, 4.48 **4.47.** Line drawing of the sporulated oocyst of *Eimeria prionotemni*. **4.48.** Photomicrograph of a sporulated oocyst of *E. prionotemni*. Both figures from Barker et al., 1989, with permission from all authors and with kind permission from Elsevier, publisher of the *International Journal for Parasitology*.

Type host: *Macropus eugenii* (Desmarest, 1817), Tammar Wallaby.

Type locality: AUSTRALIA: South Australia: Adelaide, Flinders University.

Other hosts: *Macropus agilis* (Gould, 1842), Agile Wallaby; *Macropus dorsalis* (Gray, 1817), Black-striped Wallaby; *Macropus parryi* Bennett, 1835, Pretty-faced Wallaby; *Macropus rufogriseus* (Desmarest, 1817), Red-necked Wallaby (syn. *Macropus bennetti* Waterhouse, 1838).

Geographic distribution: AUSTRALIA: Queensland; South Australia; Tasmania.

Description of sporulated oocyst: Oocyst shape: bluntly ellipsoidal to slightly ovoidal; number of walls: 2; wall characteristics: outer layer smooth,

clear, light tan, 1.2–1.6 thick, thinning at one pole of oocyst; inner layer is thin, colorless, ~0.4–0.8 thick; L×W (*n*=20): 37.1×22.0 (32–41×20–23); L/W ratio: 1.7; M: absent; OR: present, comprising a cluster of 3–8 granules; PG: apparently present as one small granule. Distinctive features of oocyst: ellipsoid shape that thins at one end, but without a distinct M, and the presence of a discrete OR of several granules in one mass along with one tiny PG.

Description of sporocyst and sporozoites: Sporocyst shape: ellipsoidal to slightly ovoidal; L×W (*n*=20): 15.7×10.1 (14–16×10–11); L/W ratio: 1.6; SB: present at more pointed end of SP; SSB: present, lenticular; PSB: absent; SR: a finely granular clump, up to 5.6 wide, at equator of SP; SZ: with finely granular cytoplasm, nearly filling SP and each has an RB, ~5.6×4.0 wide. Distinctive features of sporocyst: SP distributed such that they typically occupy the lower 75% of the space in the oocyst and each one has both a small SB and SSB.

Prevalence: Barker et al. (1989) found this species in 5/20 (25%) *M. eugenii* from the type locality, in 1/18 (5.5%) *M. rufogriseus* from Tasmania, in 4/11 (36%) *M. parryi* from South Australia and Queensland, in 1/2 (50%) *M. agilis* from South Australia, and in 1/14 (7%) *M. dorsalis* in Queensland.

Sporulation: Unknown.

Prepatent and patent periods: Unknown.

Site of infection: Unknown, oocysts recovered only from the feces.

Endogenous stages: Unknown.

Cross-transmission: None to date.

Pathology: Not described.

Materials deposited: None.

Etymology: This species epithet is based on the host distribution, which includes most of the "brush wallaby" species formerly included in the putative subgenus *Prionotemnus* (Bartholomai, 1975), as per Barker et al. (1989).

Remarks: Barker et al. (1989) separated the sporulated oocysts of this species from those of *E. toganmainensis* by the disposition of sporocysts within the oocyst, in lacking an M, and by usually possessing an OR. They separated them from those of *E. wilcanniensis* and *E. mykytowyczi* in lacking an M, but possessing an SB and SSB. They also pointed out that sporulated oocysts of *E. thylogale* have thicker, irregular oocyst walls. Both *E. aepyprymni* and *E. inornata* are similar, but are considered distinct on the basis of phylogenetic separation of their hosts from the genus *Macropus*.

The oocyst and sporocyst dimensions given above are those measured from the type host, *M. eugenii*. Barker et al. (1989) also measured oocysts from the four other *Macropus* species in which they found them. The oocysts and sporocysts, respectively, in *M. parryi* (*n*=45) were 35.2×21.2 (30–41×20–24), L/W ratio: 1.7, and 14.3×8.6 (13–16.5×7–10), L/W ratio: 1.7; those measured from *M. rufogriseus* (*n*=20) were 33.7×21.4 (32–36×20–22), L/W ratio: 1.6, and 13.4×8.6 (12–14×8–9), L/W ratio: 1.6; those in *M. agilis* (*n*=31) were 35.1×21.3 (31–39×18–23), L/W ratio: 1.6, and 14.4×8.3 (12–16.5×8–9), L/W ratio: 1.7; and those measured from *M. dorsalis* (*n*=2) were 32.4×22.6 (32–33×22–23), L/W ratio: 1.4, and 14.4×8.4 (14–15×8–9), L/W ratio: 1.7.

EIMERIA TOGANMAIENSIS MYKYTOWYCZ, 1964

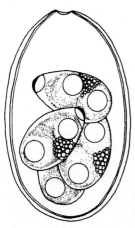
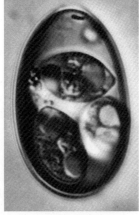

FIGURES 4.49, 4.50 **4.49.** Line drawing of the sporulated oocyst of *Eimeria toganmaiensis* from Barker et al., 1989, with permission from all authors and with kind permission from Elsevier, publisher of the *International Journal for Parasitology*. **4.50.** Photomicrograph of a sporulated oocyst of *E. toganmaiensis*, original from M. O'Callaghan.

Type host: *Macropus rufus* (Desmarest, 1822), Red Kangaroo.

Type locality: AUSTRALIA: New South Wales: Mount Hope, Yathong Nature Reserve.

Other hosts: *Macropus eugenii* (Desmarest, 1817), Tammar Wallaby; *Macropus fuliginosus* (Desmarest, 1817), Western Grey Kangaroo; *Macropus giganteus* Shaw, 1790, Eastern Grey Kangaroo; *Macropus rufogriseus* (Desmarest, 1817), Red-necked Wallaby (syn. *Macropus bennetti* Waterhouse, 1838).

Geographic distribution: AUSTRALIA: New South Wales; Queensland; South Australia; Tasmania; Victoria.

Description of sporulated oocyst: Oocyst shape: elongate-ovoidal with walls being parallel in the center and curvature of poles nearly equal (Mykytowycz, 1964) or bluntly ellipsoidal to ovoidal, slightly flattened on one side (Barker et al., 1989); number of walls: 2; wall characteristics: outer layer smooth, clear, slight purple–pink cast, 1.2 thick, and it thins at more pointed end forming an M; inner is clear, colorless, ~0.4 thick; L×W (*n*=50): 38.7×24.9 (34–44×23–27); L/W ratio: 1.6 (Mykytowycz, 1964) or (*n*=65) 41.0×26.2 (35–45×22–30); L/W ratio: 1.7 (Barker et al., 1989); M: present, 3.4–4.8, but not strongly delineated and is almost indistinguishable in some oocysts (Mykytowycz, 1964) or 3.2–4.0 wide, at more pointed end of oocyst (Barker et al., 1989); OR: absent; PG: present, Mykytowycz (1964) noticed a few disbursed granules in the anterior half of the some oocysts and Barker et al. (1989) said a PG was variably present. Distinctive features of oocyst: relatively large size, smooth outer wall, distinct M, and PG of a few dispersed granules.

Description of sporocyst and sporozoites: Sporocyst shape: ellipsoidal, slightly pointed at one end; L×W (*n*=50): 15.8×9.7 (13–18×8–11); L/W ratio: 1.6 (Mykytowycz, 1964) or L×W (*n*=65): 15.5×9.8 (14–17×9–11.5); L/W ratio: 1.6 (Barker et al., 1989); SB: present (not mentioned by Mykytowycz, 1964), but well described and pictured by Barker et al. (1989); SSB: prominent, lenticular; PSB: absent; SR: a granular aggregate, up to 6.4 wide, near the equator of SP; SZ: fill most of the space within the SP, they have finely granular cytoplasm, and each contains a large RB, ~5.6 wide. Distinctive features of sporocyst: the four SP usually are located in the lower half of the oocyst, opposite the M.

Prevalence: Mykytowycz (1964) found this species in 143/509 (28%) *M. rufus* in New South Wales and Queensland. He did not find it in 149 *M. giganteus* (syn. *M. conguru*) from the same states. Barker et al. (1989) examined fecal samples from 514 kangaroos and wallabies from New South Wales, Queensland, South Australia, Victoria, and Tasmania, and found this species in 7/97 (7%) *M. rufus* from New South Wales and South Australia, in 2/89 (2%) *M. giganteus* from New South Wales and South Australia, in 14/135 (10%) *M. fuliginosus* from South Australia, in 13/18 (72%) *M. rufogriseus* from Tasmania, and in 6/20 (30%) *M. eugenii* from South Australia.

Sporulation: Unknown.

Prepatent and patent periods: Unknown.

Site of infection: Unknown, oocysts recovered only from the feces.

Endogenous stages: Unknown.

Cross-transmission: None to date.

Pathology: Not described.

Materials deposited: None.

Remarks: Prior to the work of Mykytowycz (1964), all knowledge on the four eimerians previously known from kangaroos was gleaned from animals in captivity (Wenyon and Scott, 1925; Prasad, 1960; Yakimoff and Matschoulsky, 1936). Mykytowycz (1964) collected fecal samples from 516 red (*M. rufus*) and 157 grey (*M. giganteus*) kangaroos taken from four localities in New South Wales and one in Queensland from which he described seven new species of *Eimeria*, including *E. toganmainensis*. His description of all seven was grossly incomplete, but he did include two photomicrographs of sporulated oocysts (top oocysts in his Figures 1 and 2) from which some structural information not included in his written description (e.g., SB, SSB) could be found. The species was more fully described, along with a line drawing and four photomicrographs by Barker et al. (1989, Figures 2, 23–26).

Barker et al. (1989) also measured oocysts from the four other *Macropus* species in which they found *E. toganmainensis*. The oocysts and sporocysts, respectively, in *M. fuliginosus* (*n*=35)

were 37.2×21.4 (34–40×19–24), L/W ratio: 1.7, and 16.1×9.0 (14–18×8–10), L/W ratio: 1.8; those measured from *M. rufogriseus* (*n*=24) were 36.4 (sic)×21.2 (33–36×19–24), L/W ratio: 1.7, and 14.2×8.5 (12–16×8–10), L/W ratio: 1.7; those measured from *M. eugenii* (*n*=20) were 35.5×21.3 (33–36×19–22), L/W ratio: 1.7, and 14.1×8.7 (13–16×8–10), L/W ratio: 1.6; and those measured from *M. giganteus* (*n*=20) were 35.2×19.9 (32–38×18–22), L/W ratio: 1.8, and 14.6×9.0 (14–16×8–10), L/W ratio: 1.6.

Sporulated oocysts of this species differ from those of *E. flindersi* by having smaller oocysts and sporocysts. They differ from those of *E. prionotemni* by having an M, the location of the four SP within the oocyst, and by lacking an OR. Oocysts of *E. toganmaiensis* are larger than those of *E. wilcanniensis* and *E. mykytowyczi*, and further differ from them by having sporocysts with both SB and SSB. Finally, these oocysts differ from those of *E. lagorchestes* by having smaller oocysts with a thinner wall.

EIMERIA WILCANNIENSIS MYKYTOWYCZ, 1964

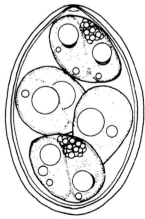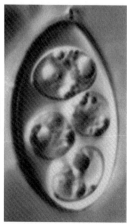

FIGURES 4.51, 4.52 **4.51.** Line drawing of the sporulated oocyst of *Eimeria wilcanniensis* from Barker et al., 1989, with permission from all authors and with kind permission from Elsevier, publisher of the *International Journal for Parasitology*. **4.52.** Photomicrograph of a sporulated oocyst of *E. wilcanniensis*, original from M. O'Callaghan.

Type host: *Macropus rufus* (Desmarest, 1822), Red Kangaroo.

Type locality: AUSTRALIA: New South Wales: Mount Hope, Yathong Nature Reserve.

Other hosts: *Macropus fuliginosus* (Desmarest, 1817), Western Grey Kangaroo; *Macropus giganteus* Shaw, 1790, Eastern Grey Kangaroo; *Macropus robustus* Gould, 1841, Wallaroo; *Macropus rufogriseus* (Desmarest, 1817), Red-necked Wallaby (syn. *Macropus bennetti* Waterhouse, 1838).

Geographic distribution: AUSTRALIA: New South Wales; South Australia.

Description of sporulated oocyst: Oocyst shape: almost ellipsoidal or ovoidal, slightly pointed at end with M; number of walls: 2; wall characteristics: outer layer smooth, clear, colorless, 0.8–1.0 thick, it begins to thin at more pointed end of oocyst forming the M; inner is clear, ~0.4 thick, and often protrudes at more pointed end of oocyst; L × W (*n* = 100): 31.8 × 20.3 (28–38 × 18–24); L/W ratio: 1.6 (Mykytowycz, 1964) or (*n* = 25) 32.2 × 20.3 (30–34 × 18–22); L/W ratio: 1.6 (Barker et al., 1989); M: present, 2.7–5.5, but not strongly delineated (Mykytowycz, 1964) and sometimes it is "equivocal" at more pointed end of oocyst (Barker et al., 1989); OR, PG: both absent. Distinctive features of oocyst: moderate sized oocyst with a smooth outer wall, an indistinct M, and lacking both OR and PG.

Description of sporocyst and sporozoites: Sporocyst shape: ellipsoidal to ovoidal, slightly pointed at one end; L × W (*n* = 100): 11.9 × 9.3 (9.5–14 × 8–11); L/W ratio: 1.3 (Mykytowycz, 1964) or L × W (*n* = 25): 13.1 × 9.8 (12–14 × 9–11); L/W ratio: 1.3 (Barker et al., 1989); SB: probably present as a small bump at more pointed end; it was not mentioned by Mykytowycz (1964), and Barker et al. (1989) said there was no "clear-cut" SB; SSB, PSB: both absent; SR: an aggregate of small granules, usually scattered near the equator and filling about half of the SP; SZ: fill most of the space within the SP and each has a large RB, ~3.2–4.0 wide. Distinctive features of sporocyst: a tiny, generally indistinct SB, and SZ pack the space within the SP.

Prevalence: Mykytowycz (1964) found this species in 381/523 (73%) *M. rufus* in New South Wales and Queensland. He did not find it in 149 *M. giganteus* (syn. *M. conguru*) from the same states. Barker et al. (1989) examined fecal samples from 514 kangaroos and wallabies from New South Wales, Queensland, South Australia, Victoria, and Tasmania, and found this species in 12/97 (12%) *M. rufus* from New South Wales and South Australia; in 2/89 (2%) *M. giganteus* from New South Wales; in 3/22 (14%) *M. robustus* from South Australia; and in 7/135 (5%) *M. fuliginosus* from South Australia.

Sporulation: Unknown.

Prepatent and patent periods: Unknown.

Site of infection: Unknown, oocysts recovered only from the feces.

Endogenous stages: Unknown.

Cross-transmission: None to date.

Pathology: Not described.

Materials deposited: None.

Remarks: Prior to the work of Mykytowycz (1964), all knowledge on the four eimerians previously known from kangaroos was gleaned from animals in captivity (Wenyon and Scott, 1925; Prasad, 1960; Yakimoff and Matschoulsky, 1936). Mykytowycz (1964) collected fecal samples from 523 red (*M. rufus*) and 157 grey (*M. giganteus*) kangaroos taken from four localities in New South Wales and one in Queensland from which he described seven *Eimeria* species, including *E. wilcanniensis*. His description was incomplete, but he did include two photomicrographs showing three sporulated oocysts (bottom two oocysts in his Figure 1, and bottom oocyst in his Figure 2) from which some structural information not included in his written description could be found. The species was more fully described, along with a line drawing and two photomicrographs by Barker et al. (1989, Figures 7, 29, 30, respectively).

Barker et al. (1989) also measured *E. wilcanniensis* oocysts from the three other *Macropus* species in which they found it. The oocysts and sporocysts, respectively, in *M. fuliginosus*

($n=40$) were 34.8×20.4 (31–38×19–22), L/W ratio: 1.7, and 14.3×9.3 (13–15×9–10), L/W ratio: 1.5; those measured from *M. giganteus* ($n=20$) were 35.4×21.0 (31–38×19–23), L/W ratio: 1.7, and 12.9×9.7 (11–14×9–10), L/W ratio: 1.3; and those measured from *M. robustus* ($n=20$) were 32.8×21.4 (31–36×21–22), L/W ratio: 1.5, and 11.4×9.0 (10–12×8–10), L/W ratio: 1.3.

Barker et al. (1989) separated the oocysts of *E. wilcanniensis* from other oocysts with overlapping size ranges on the basis of the indistinct SB on the sporocysts and the lack of an SSB. They differentiated it from *E. mykytowyczi* on the basis of oocyst shape and sporocyst size. Oocysts with similar form were also described by Mykytowycz (1964) and named *E. kogoni*, which is considered here, and by Barker et al. (1989), to be a *species inquirenda* (Chapter 10).

EIMERIA YATHONGENSIS BARKER, O'CALLAGHAN, AND BEVERIDGE, 1989

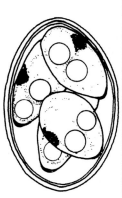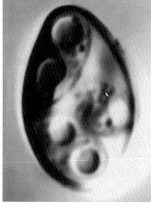

FIGURES 4.53, 4.54.　**4.53.** Line drawing of the sporulated oocyst of *Eimeria yathongensis*. **4.54.** Photomicrograph of a sporulated oocyst of *E. yathongensis*. Both figures from Barker et al., 1989, with permission from all authors and with kind permission from Elsevier, publisher of the *International Journal for Parasitology*.

Type host: *Macropus fuliginosus* (Desmarest, 1817), Western Grey Kangaroo.

Type locality: AUSTRALIA: New South Wales: Yathong Nature Reserve, near Mount Hope.

Other hosts: *Macropus giganteus* Shaw, 1790, Eastern Grey Kangaroo.

Geographic distribution: AUSTRALIA: New South Wales; South Australia.

Description of sporulated oocyst: Oocyst shape: ovoidal; number of walls: 2; wall characteristics: outer layer is smooth, clear, colorless, 0.6 thick; inner layer is thin, colorless, ~0.3 thick; L×W ($n=30$): 21.2×13.8 (19–23×13–15); L/W ratio: 1.5; M, OR, PG: all absent. Distinctive features of oocyst: small ovoidal shape and lacking M, OR, and PG.

Description of sporocyst and sporozoites: Sporocyst shape: ellipsoidal, slightly pointed at one end; L×W ($n=30$): 10.7×5.9 (10–12×5.5–7); L/W ratio: 1.8; SB: present at pointed end, but inconspicuous; SSB, PSB: both absent; SR: a loose aggregate of small granules scattered throughout SP; SZ: nearly fill SP and each has an RB, ~3.2 wide. Distinctive features of sporocyst: small size and a small, thickened end that is likely an SB.

Prevalence: Barker et al. (1989) found this species in 2/89 (2%) *M. giganteus* from the type locality, in 35/135 (26%) *M. fuliginosus* also from the type locality and from Kangaroo Island, South Australia.

Sporulation: Unknown.

Prepatent and patent periods: Unknown.

Site of infection: Unknown, oocysts recovered only from the feces.

Endogenous stages: Unknown.

Cross-transmission: None to date.

Pathology: Not described.

Materials deposited: None.

Etymology: This species epithet is based on the locality where it was present in both species of grey kangaroos.

Remarks: Barker et al. (1989) differentiated the sporulated oocysts of *E. yathongensis* on the combination of oocyst size and shape, and greater sporocyst length from *E. macropodis* in grey kangaroos. It had a thinner, less refractile oocyst wall and a lower L/W ratio than the oocysts of *E. marsupialium*, and larger oocyst and sporocyst size, different shape, and smooth surface, when compared to oocysts of *E. gungahlinensis*. Both oocysts and sporocysts differ in shape from those of *E. parma*. The authors found that this species was always present in relatively small numbers, in animals infected with one or the other, or both, of *E. macropodis* or *E. marsupialium*, never alone, and that it was much more prevalent in *M. fuliginosus* than in *M. giganteus* at Mount Hope.

The oocyst and sporocyst dimensions given above are those measured from the type host, *M. fuliginosus*. Barker et al. (1989) measured oocysts from *M. giganteus*, in which they also found them. The oocysts and sporocysts, respectively, in *M. giganteus* ($n=20$), were 21.4 × 14.1 (20–23 × 13–15), L/W ratio: 1.5, and 10.6 × 5.9 (10–11 × 5–7), L/W ratio: 1.8.

GENUS *PETROGALE* GRAY, 1837 (16 SPECIES)

EIMERIA BOONDEROOENSIS BARKER, O'CALLAGHAN, BEVERIDGE, AND CLOSE, 1988c

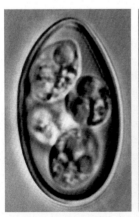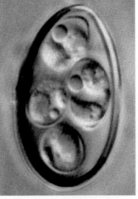

FIGURES 4.55, 4.56 Two photomicrographs of sporulated oocysts of *Eimeria boonderooensis*, both originals from M. O'Callaghan.

Type host: *Petrogale assimilis* Ramsay, 1877, Allied Rock-wallaby.

Type locality: AUSTRALIA: Queensland: Hughenden, "Boonderoo," Springlawn Creek Gorge.

Other hosts: *Petrogale inornata* Gould, 1842, Unadorned Rock-wallaby.

Geographic distribution: AUSTRALIA: Queensland.

Description of sporulated oocyst: Oocyst shape: elongate-ovoidal; number of walls: 2; wall characteristics: outer layer is smooth, clear, colorless, 1.0 thick; inner layer is thin, colorless, ~0.4 thick; L × W ($n=20$): 26.6 × 16.2 (24–28 × 15–18); L/W ratio: 1.6; M, OR: both absent; PG: present, up to 1.6 wide, usually located at more pointed end of oocyst. Distinctive features of oocyst: lacking M and OR (apparently, but not stated in original description), and with a PG usually located near the narrow end.

Description of sporocyst and sporozoites: Sporocyst shape: ellipsoidal, slightly tapering to one end; L × W ($n=20$): 10.8 × 6.8 (10–12 × 6–8); L/W ratio: 1.6; SB: present at pointed end, but inconspicuous; SSB, PSB: both absent; SR: composed of 2–3 granules, 1.6–2.4, scattered at equator of SP; SZ: curved, but do not fill SP and each has an RB, ~3.2 wide. Distinctive features of SP: they do not fill the volume of the space within the oocyst and they have a tiny, indistinct SB.

Prevalence: This species was found in 12/45 (27%) *P. assimilis*, and in 7/14 (50%) *P. inornata*.

Sporulation: Unknown. The feces were held dry, often for months or years, prior to immersion in 2.5% (w/v) potassium dichromate solution ($K_2Cr_2O_7$) in which they were later stored at 4°C for up to 3.5 years.

Prepatent and patent periods: Unknown.

Site of infection: Unknown, oocysts recovered only from the feces.

Endogenous stages: Unknown.

Cross-transmission: None to date.

Pathology: Not described.

Materials deposited: None.

Etymology: This species name was derived from the locality where a monospecific infection occurred in *P. assimilis*.

Remarks: Oocysts of *E. boonderooensis* were only measured from one animal in which a monospecific infection was found. Barker et al. (1988c) distinguished the sporulated oocysts of this species from those of the other six species they described as follows. They differed from those of *E. petrogale*, with which it often co-occurred in *P. assimilis* and in *P. inornata*, and with which both oocyst and sporocysts lengths overlap, based on the larger mean oocyst and sporocyst size, the more uniform shape of this species, and on comparisons of oocysts in monospecific infections with each. Barker et al. (1988c) said that combined infections were present in several *P. assimilis* and *P. inornata*, but their finding of many animals with oocysts only in the size range of *E. petrogale*, and a few with oocysts only in the range of *E. boonderooensis*, resulted in their interpretation that these are two distinct species. This species was common in *P. assimilis* and in *P. inornata*, but was noticeably absent in other *Petrogale* species examined by Barker et al. (1988c) suggesting to them that it may have evolved relatively recently.

EIMERIA GODMANI BARKER, O'CALLAGHAN, BEVERIDGE, AND CLOSE, 1988c

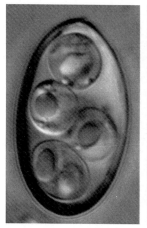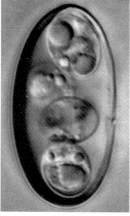

FIGURES 4.57, 4.58 Two photomicrographs of sporulated oocysts of *Eimeria godmani*, both originals from M. O'Callaghan.

Type host: *Petrogale godmani* Thomas, 1923, Godman's Rock-wallaby.

Type locality: AUSTRALIA: Queensland: Mount Carbine, "Curraghmore."

Other hosts: *Petrogale assimilis* Ramsay, 1877, Allied Rock-wallaby; *Petrogale lateralis pearsoni* Thomas, 1922, Black-flanked Rock-wallaby.

Geographic distribution: AUSTRALIA: Queensland; South Australia.

Description of sporulated oocyst: Oocyst shape: ellipsoidal–ovoidal; number of walls: 2; wall characteristics: outer layer is smooth, slightly pitted, brownish tint, 1.6 thick; inner layer is colorless, ~0.4 thick; L×W ($n=20$): 29.8×17.1 (26–32×14–18); L/W ratio: 1.7; M: present, 2–3 wide; OR: absent; PG: small, ~0.4 wide. Distinctive features of oocyst: slightly pitted outer wall, presence of an M, and having a very small PG, but lacking an OR.

Description of sporocyst and sporozoites: Sporocyst shape: ellipsoidal; L×W ($n=20$): 12.1×8.4 (10–13×8–9); L/W ratio: 1.4; SB, SSB, PSB: all apparently absent; SR: a few scattered granules, ~1.0–2.4 wide; SZ: do not fill SP and each has an RB, ~4.8 wide. Distinctive features of sporocyst: lacking SB, SSB, and PSB, and small size of SZ within SP.

Prevalence: Found in 3/24 (12.5%) *P. godmani*, and in only 1/45 (2%) *P. assimilis* from Queensland (Barker et al., 1988c), and O'Callaghan et al. (1998) found *E. godmani* in 3/34 (9%) *P. l. pearsoni*, rock-wallabies, on Pearson Island.

Sporulation: Unknown. The feces were held dry, often for months or years, prior to immersion in 2.5% (w/v) potassium dichromate solution ($K_2Cr_2O_7$) in which they were later stored at 4°C for up to 3.5 years (Barker et al., 1988c). Although O'Callaghan et al. (1998) collected fecal samples directly from each *P. l. pearsoni* on Pearson Island and immediately stored them in 2% (w/v) potassium dichromate ($K_2Cr_2O_7$) to allow them to sporulate, no mention was made of the time it took each of their four eimerians (*E. godmani*, *E. inornata*, *E. petrogale*, and *E. sharmani*) to complete this process.

Prepatent and patent periods: Unknown.

Site of infection: Unknown, oocysts recovered only from the feces.

Endogenous stages: Unknown.

Cross-transmission: None to date.

Pathology: Not described.

Materials deposited: None.

Etymology: This species name was derived from that of its type host.

Remarks: The measurements given above are from oocysts from the type host. Barker et al. (1988c) also measured 20 sporulated oocysts from *P. assimilis*; these oocysts were L×W: 32.8×17.8 (30–36×17–18); L/W ratio: 1.8, and their sporocysts were L×W: 11.7×8.6 (11–13×8–10); L/W ratio: 1.4. The authors distinguished this species from the other six eimerians they described from *Petrogale* species by the presence of an M on the oocyst and an apparent lack of an SB on the SP. A decade later, O'Callaghan et al. (1998) reported four of their previously described (1988c) eimerians, including *E. godmani*, in the Pearson Island Rock Wallaby from Pearson Island, South Australia; only three *P. l. pearsoni* were found to be shedding oocysts of this species, but two of them also had *E. petrogale* and *E. sharmani*. O'Callaghan et al. also measured 20 oocysts from the three infected wallabies and they were L×W: 29.2×19.2 (27–32×18–21); L/W ratio: 1.5, and their sporocysts were L×W: 11.4×8.2 (10–12×8–9); L/W ratio: 1.4. They (1998) again based their identification on the M, lack of an SB on the SP, and dimensions of both oocysts and sporocysts.

EIMERIA INORNATA BARKER, O'CALLAGHAN, BEVERIDGE, AND CLOSE, 1988c

Type host: *Petrogale inornata* Gould, 1842, Unadorned Rock-wallaby.

Type locality: AUSTRALIA: Queensland: Collinsville, Mount Johnnycake.

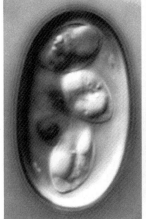
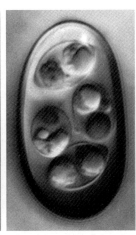

FIGURES 4.59, 4.60 Two photomicrographs of sporulated oocysts of *Eimeria inornata*, both originals from M. O'Callaghan.

Other hosts: *Petrogale lateralis pearsoni* Thomas, 1922, Black-flanked Rock-wallaby; *Petrogale penicillata* (Gray, 1827), Brush-tailed Rock-wallaby.

Geographic distribution: AUSTRALIA: Queensland; South Australia.

Description of sporulated oocyst: Oocyst shape: irregular ellipsoidal to cylindroidal; number of walls: 2; wall characteristics: outer layer is smooth, clear, brownish tint, 1.6 thick; inner layer is clear, colorless, ~0.4 thick; L×W ($n=13$): 34.9×20.2 (33–39×19–22); L/W ratio: 1.7; M, OR: both absent; PG: present, usually two to five. Distinctive features of oocyst: cylindroidal shape, lacking M, OR, and with multiple PG.

Description of sporocyst and sporozoites: Sporocyst shape: ellipsoidal, tapering at both ends; L×W ($n=13$): 13.2×8.0 (12–14×7–9); L/W ratio: 1.7; SB: present, but inconspicuous; SSB: present; PSB: absent; SR: a loose aggregate of fine granules at equator of SP; SZ: do not fill SP and each has a prominent RB, ~5.6 wide. Distinctive features of sporocyst: tapers at both ends, slightly, and the presence of both an SB and SSB.

Prevalence: Found in 1/14 (7%) *P. inornata*, and in 1/20 (5%) *P. penicillata* from Queensland (Barker et al., 1988c), and O'Callaghan et al.

(1998) found *E. inornata* in 1/34 (3%) *P. l. pearsoni*, rock-wallabies, on Pearson Island.

Sporulation: Unknown. The feces were held dry, often for months or years, prior to immersion in 2.5% (w/v) potassium dichromate solution ($K_2Cr_2O_7$) in which they were later stored at 4°C for up to 3.5 years (Barker et al., 1988c). Although O'Callaghan et al. (1998) collected fecal samples directly from each *P. l. pearsoni* on Pearson Island and immediately stored them in 2% (w/v) potassium dichromate ($K_2Cr_2O_7$) to allow sporulation, no mention was made of the time it took each of their four eimerians (*E. godmani, E. inornata, E. petrogale,* and *E. sharmani*) to complete this process.

Prepatent and patent periods: Unknown.

Site of infection: Unknown, oocysts recovered only from the feces.

Endogenous stages: Unknown.

Cross-transmission: None to date.

Pathology: Not described.

Materials deposited: None.

Etymology: This species was named for the type host.

Remarks: The measurements given above are from oocysts from the type host. Barker et al. (1988c) also measured 10 sporulated oocysts of *E. inornata* from *P. penicillata*; these oocysts were L×W: 33.9×19.1 (33–37×18–20); L/W ratio: 1.8, and their sporocysts were L×W: 13.4×8.2 (13–14×8–9); L/W ratio: 1.6. Barker et al. (1988c) distinguished this form from the other six they described from *Petrogale* species by the shape of the oocysts and sporocysts, the absence of an M, and the presence of both an SB and SSB. Later, O'Callaghan et al. (1998) reported four of their previously described seven (Barker et al., 1988c) eimerians, including *E. inornata*, in the Pearson Island Rock Wallaby from Pearson Island, South Australia; only one *P. l. pearsoni* was found to be shedding oocysts of this species. O'Callaghan et al. measured 22 oocysts from the infected wallaby and they were L×W: 37.1×25.9 (36–39×25–27); L/W ratio: 1.4, and their sporocysts were L×W: 15.5×10.0 (15–16×10); L/W ratio: 1.5. These

dimensions are a little larger than those of *E. inornata* from other rock wallabies, but their overall morphology is consistent, particularly the presence of an SSB, which seems to be unique among all eimerians now known from rock wallabies.

EIMERIA OCCIDENTALIS BARKER, O'CALLAGHAN, BEVERIDGE, AND CLOSE, 1988c

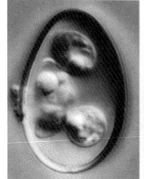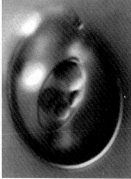

FIGURES 4.61, 4.62   Two photomicrographs of sporulated oocysts of *Eimeria occidentalis*, both originals from M. O'Callaghan.

Type host: *Petrogale lateralis* Gould, 1842, Black-flanked Rock-wallaby.

Type locality: AUSTRALIA: Western Australia: North West Cape, "Ningaloo."

Other hosts: *Petrogale brachyotis* (Gould, 1841), Short-eared Rock-wallaby; *Petrogale rothschildi* Thomas, 1904, Rothschild's Rock-wallaby.

Geographic distribution: AUSTRALIA: Northern Territory; Western Australia.

Description of sporulated oocyst: Oocyst shape: ovoidal, stout; number of walls: 2; wall characteristics: outer layer is smooth, clear, colorless, 0.8 thick; inner layer is colorless, ~0.4 thick; L×W (*n*=20): 23.4×18.1 (22–26×16–19); L/W ratio: 1.3; M, OR: both absent; PG: present. Distinctive features of oocyst: stout ovoidal shape with a thin, colorless wall.

Description of sporocyst and sporozoites: Sporocyst shape: ellipsoidal, tapering slightly toward one end; L×W ($n=20$): 11.2×6.2 (10–12×5–6.5); L/W ratio: 1.8; SB: present at pointed end, but inconspicuous; SSB, PSB: both absent; SR: one or two granules, ~2.0 wide, or very small granules at the equator of SP; SZ: do not fill SP and each SZ has an RB, ~4.0 wide. Distinctive features of sporocyst: tapering ellipsoidal shape with a very small SB.

Prevalence: Found in 2/18 (11%) *P. lateralis*, in 2/6 (33%) *P. rothschildi*, and in 2/8 (25%) *P. brachyotis*.

Sporulation: Unknown. The feces were held dry, often for months or years, prior to immersion in 2.5% (w/v) potassium dichromate solution ($K_2Cr_2O_7$) in which they were later stored at 4°C for up to 3.5 years.

Prepatent and patent periods: Unknown.

Site of infection: Unknown, oocysts recovered only from the feces.

Endogenous stages: Unknown.

Cross-transmission: None to date.

Pathology: Not described.

Materials deposited: None.

Etymology: The name of this species was based on the observation that it seemed to be limited to hosts found only in the western part of Australia (Barker et al., 1988c).

Remarks: The measurements given above are from oocysts from the type host. Barker et al. (1988c) also measured 10 sporulated oocysts of *E. occidentalis* from *P. rothschildi*; these oocysts were L×W: 24.2×18.2 (23–26×17–19), L/W ratio: 1.3, and their sporocysts were L×W: 9.7×6.2 (9–10×6–7), L/W ratio: 1.6; they also measured 16 sporulated oocysts from *P. brachyotis* and these oocysts were L×W: 24.6×16.0 (20–26×14–18), L/W ratio: 1.5, and their sporocysts were L×W: 9.8×5.8 (9–11×5–6), L/W ratio: 1.7. Barker et al. (1988c) distinguished the sporulated oocysts of *E. occidentalis* from those of *E. petrogale*, to which they are most similar, by "the combination of its uniformly ovoid shape and relatively high width:length ratio (≥2.3)."

However, Barker et al., (1988c) then qualified this statement by saying, "the assignment of oocysts from *P. brachyotis* to the former species, and those from *P. lateralis* to the latter, was arbitrary, based on the regular ovoid shape of the former and the variable shape of the latter." I am not quite sure how to interpret that statement.

EIMERIA PETROGALE BARKER, O'CALLAGHAN, BEVERIDGE, AND CLOSE, 1988c

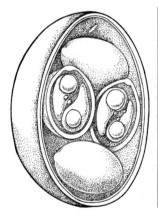 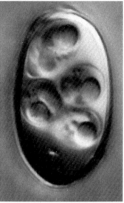

FIGURES 4.63, 4.64 **4.63.** Line drawing of a sporulated oocyst of *Eimeria petrogale*. **4.64.** Photomicrograph of a sporulated oocyst of *E. petrogale*; both figures are unpublished originals from M. O'Callaghan.

Type host: *Petrogale assimilis* Ramsay, 1877, Allied Rock-wallaby.

Type locality: AUSTRALIA: Queensland: Hughenden, "Boonderoo," Porcupine Gorge.

Other hosts: *Petrogale godmani* Thomas, 1923, Godman's Rock-wallaby; *Petrogale inornata* Gould, 1842, Unadorned Rock-wallaby; *Petrogale lateralis* Gould, 1842, Black-flanked Rock-wallaby; *Petrogale lateralis pearsoni* Thomas, 1922, Black-flanked Rock-wallaby; *Petrogale penicillata* (Gray, 1827), Brush-tailed Rock-wallaby; *Petrogale persephone* Maynes, 1982, Proserpine Rock-wallaby.

Geographic distribution: AUSTRALIA: New South Wales; Queensland; South Australia (Pearson Island, Great Australian Bight); Victoria; Western Australia (Mondrain and Wilson Islands, Recherche Archipelago).

Description of sporulated oocyst: Oocyst shape: highly variable, from ovoidal to irregularly ellipsoidal and slightly pointed at one end, often flattened on one side; number of walls: 2; wall characteristics: outer layer is smooth, clear, colorless, 1.0 thick; inner layer is clear, colorless, ~0.4 thick; L×W ($n=97$): 23.0×14.1 (20–26×11–17); L/W ratio: 1.6; M, OR, PG: all absent, but there is a "motile rod," ~2.0 long, at pointed end of oocyst. Distinctive features of oocyst: highly variable shape and the presence of a "motile rod" at one end.

Description of sporocyst and sporozoites: Sporocyst shape: ellipsoidal, slightly pointed at one end; L×W ($n=97$): 9.0×5.5 (8–10×4–6); L/W ratio: 1.6; SB: present at pointed end, but inconspicuous; SSB, PSB: both absent; SR: 2–3 granules, ~0.8 wide, scattered at equator; SZ: curved, but not filling SP, and each SZ has a prominent RB, 1.6×3.2–4.0, near one end. Distinctive features of sporocyst: smallest size of any eimerian from *Petrogale* species and presence of an inconspicuous SB.

Prevalence: Found in 40/45 (89%) *P. assimilis*, in 15/24 (62.5%) *P. godmani*, in 12/14 (86%) *P. inornata*, in 2/18 (11%) *P. lateralis*, in 19/20 (95%) *P. penicillata*, and in 1/3 (33%) *P. persephone* by Barker et al. (1988c). A decade later, O'Callaghan et al. (1998) found *E. petrogale* in 32/34 (94%) *P. l. pearsoni*, rock-wallabies, on Pearson Island.

Sporulation: Unknown. The feces were held dry, often for months or years, prior to immersion in 2.5% (w/v) potassium dichromate solution ($K_2Cr_2O_7$) in which they were later stored at 4°C for up to 3.5 years (Barker et al., 1988c). Although O'Callaghan et al. (1998) collected fecal samples directly from each *P. l. pearsoni* on Pearson Island, and immediately stored them in 2% (w/v) potassium dichromate ($K_2Cr_2O_7$) to allow them to sporulate, no mention was made

of the time it took each of their four eimerians (*E. godmani*, *E. inornata*, *E. petrogale*, and *E. sharmani*) to undergo the sporulation process.

Prepatent and patent periods: Unknown.

Site of infection: Unknown. Oocysts recovered only from the feces.

Endogenous stages: Unknown.

Cross-transmission: None to date.

Pathology: Not described.

Materials deposited: None.

Etymology: The specific name of this species was derived from the generic name of the host.

Remarks: The oocysts of *E. petrogale* are always the most prevalent in *Petrogale* species in which it is found, except in *P. lateralis*, for reasons that are currently unexplained. The measurements given above are for oocysts from the type host. Barker et al. (1988c) also measured sporulated oocysts of *E. petrogale* from four other *Petrogale* species. Those from *P. inornata* were L×W ($n=30$): 22.6×14.2 (20–24×13–15); L/W ratio: 1.6, and their sporocysts were L×W: 9.5×5.9 (9–10×5–6); L/W ratio: 1.6; those from *P. godmani* were L×W ($n=10$): 21.7×13.4 (19–26×12–14); L/W ratio: 1.6, and their sporocysts were L×W: 9.0×5.9 (8–10×5–6); L/W ratio: 1.5; those from *P. penicillata* were L×W ($n=20$): 22.2×12.8 (20–25×12–14); L/W ratio: 1.7, and their sporocysts were L×W: 9.0×5.8 (8–10×5–6); L/W ratio: 1.6; and those from *P. lateralis* were L×W ($n=20$): 23.1×14.8 (20–26×14–16); L/W ratio: 1.6, and their sporocysts were L×W: 9.7×5.5 (9–10×5–6); L/W ratio: 1.8. Barker et al. (1988c) distinguished this species from the other six they described from *Petrogale* species by the combination of dimensions of oocysts and sporocysts along with the suite of morphological characteristics they described. O'Callaghan et al. (1998) reported four of their previously described seven (Barker et al., 1988c) eimerians, including *E. petrogale*, in the Pearson Island Rock Wallaby from Pearson Island, South Australia; *E. petrogale* was found in 32/34 (94%) *P. l. pearsoni* they examined. O'Callaghan et al. (1998) also measured 40 oocysts from three *P. l. pearsoni* and these were L×W: 20.9×15.4 (17–23×13–17); L/W ratio: 1.4, and their sporocysts were L×W: 10.0×5.9 (8–11.5×5–7); L/W ratio: 1.7. The mean oocyst length may be slightly smaller, but the other dimensions mostly concur with those of *E. petrogale* given by Barker et al. (1988c).

EIMERIA SHARMANI BARKER, O'CALLAGHAN, BEVERIDGE, AND CLOSE, 1988c

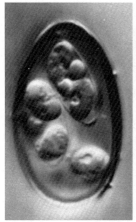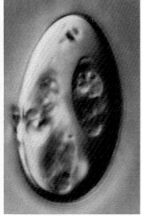

FIGURES 4.65, 4.66 Two photomicrographs of sporulated oocysts of *Eimeria sharmani*, both originals from M. O'Callaghan.

Type host: *Petrogale assimilis* Ramsay, 1877, Allied Rock-wallaby.

Type locality: AUSTRALIA: Queensland: Onion Bay, Great Palm Island.

Other hosts: *Petrogale godmani* Thomas, 1923, Godman's Rock-wallaby; *Petrogale inornata* Gould, 1842, Unadorned Rock-wallaby; *Petrogale lateralis* Gould, 1842, Black-flanked Rock-wallaby; *Petrogale lateralis pearsoni* Thomas, 1922, Black-flanked Rock-wallaby; *Petrogale penicillata* (Gray, 1827), Brush-tailed Rock-wallaby; *Petrogale persephone* Maynes, 1982, Proserpine Rock-wallaby; *Petrogale rothschildi* Thomas, 1904, Rothschild's Rock-wallaby.

Geographic distribution: AUSTRALIA: New South Wales; Queensland; Victoria; Western Australia (Recherche Archipelago: Mondrain, Salisbury, and Wilson Islands).

Description of sporulated oocyst: Oocyst shape: elongate ovoidal, occasionally nearly ellipsoidal; number of walls: 2; wall characteristics: outer layer is smooth, clear, slightly mammillated, light tan, 1.0 thick; inner layer is clear, ~0.4 thick; L×W (*n*=26): 27.5×16.9 (25–30×15–18); L/W ratio: 1.6; M: absent; OR and PG: one or two granules are present that may represent either a diffuse OR or multiple PGs. Distinctive features of oocyst: large size, slightly mammillated outer wall, and presence of one to two granules, that may represent either a diffuse OR or multiple PGs.

Description of sporocyst and sporozoites: Sporocyst shape: ellipsoidal, tapering slightly toward one end; L×W (*n*=26): 13.4×5.8 (12–14×5–7); L/W ratio: 2.3; SB: present at tapered end, but inconspicuous; SSB, PSB: both absent; SR: 3–5 granules, 0.8–2.0 wide, scattered or aggregated loosely about equator of SP; SZ: do not fill the space in the SP, but each SZ has a prominent round or elongate RB. Distinctive features of sporocyst: largest L/W ratio, >2.0, of any eimerian that infects *Petrogale* species.

Prevalence: Barker et al. (1988c) found *E. sharmani* in 14/45 (31%) *P. assimilis*, in 7/24 (29%) *P. godmani*, in 3/14 (21%) *P. inornata*, in 4/18 (22%) *P. lateralis*, in 10/20 (50%) *P. penicillata*, and in 1/6 (17%) *P. rotschildi*. O'Callaghan et al. (1998) found *E. sharmani* in 17/34 (50%) *P. l. pearsoni*, rock-wallabies, on Pearson Island.

Sporulation: Unknown. The feces were held dry, often for months or years, prior to immersion in 2.5% (w/v) potassium dichromate solution ($K_2Cr_2O_7$) in which they were later stored at 4°C for up to 3.5 years (Barker et al., 1988c). Although O'Callaghan et al. (1998) collected fecal samples directly from each *P. l. pearsoni* on Pearson Island and immediately stored them in 2% (w/v) potassium dichromate ($K_2Cr_2O_7$) to allow them to sporulate, no mention was made of the time it took each of their four eimerians

(*E. godmani, E. inornata, E. petrogale,* and *E. sharmani*) to achieve sporulation.

Prepatent and patent periods: Unknown.

Site of infection: Unknown, oocysts recovered only from the feces.

Endogenous stages: Unknown.

Cross-transmission: None to date.

Pathology: Not described.

Materials deposited: None.

Etymology: This species was named in recognition of Professor G.B. Sharman, a noted Australian mammalogist.

Remarks: The measurements given above are from oocysts from the type host. Barker et al. (1988c) also measured sporulated oocysts of *E. sharmani* from five other *Petrogale* species. Those from *P. inornata* were L×W (*n*=20): 26.4×16.1 (24–28×15–18); L/W ratio: 1.6, and their sporocysts were L×W: 13.4×6.1 (12–14×5–6.5); L/W ratio: 2.2; those from *P. godmani* were L×W (*n*=20): 26.5×15.6 (24–30×13–18); L/W ratio: 1.7, and their sporocysts were L×W: 13.4×5.8 (12–15×5–6); L/W ratio: 2.3; those from *P. penicillata* were L×W (*n*=10): 27.9×17.4 (25–30×16–18); L/W ratio: 1.6, and their sporocysts were L×W: 13.3×5.6 (11–14×5–6); L/W ratio: 2.4; those from *P. lateralis* were L×W (*n*=10): 27.0×17.6 (25–29×15–20); L/W ratio: 1.5, and their sporocysts were L×W: 13.6×5.6 (13–14×5.6); L/W ratio: 2.4; and those from *P. rothschildi* were L×W (*n*=10): 28.1×19.4 (26–30×18–20); L/W ratio: 1.4, and their sporocysts were L×W: 14.0×5.8 (13–14×5–6); L/W ratio: 2.4. Barker et al. (1988c) distinguished this species from the other six they described from *Petrogale* species by the long, narrow sporocysts, which always have an L/W ratio of >2.1. O'Callaghan et al. (1998) reported four of their previously described seven (Barker et al., 1988c) eimerians, including *E. sharmani*, in 50% of the *P. l. pearsoni* they examined from Pearson Island, South Australia. O'Callaghan et al. (1998) measured 15 sporulated oocysts of *E. sharmani* from three *P. l. pearsoni*, and they were L×W: 25.6×17.5 (23–28×15–20); L/W ratio: 1.5, and their sporocysts were L×W: 13.9×6.4 (13–15×6–7); L/W ratio: 2.2.

EIMERIA XANTHOPUS BARKER, O'CALLAGHAN, BEVERIDGE, AND CLOSE, 1988c

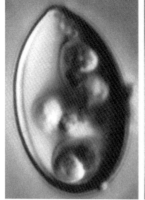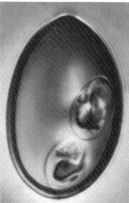

FIGURES 4.67, 4.68 Two photomicrographs of sporulated oocysts of *Eimeria xanthopus*, both originals from M. O'Callaghan.

Type host: *Petrogale xanthopus* Gray, 1855, Yellow-footed Rock-wallaby.

Type locality: AUSTRALIA: South Australia: north Flinders Ranges, "Arkaroola."

Other hosts: None to date.

Geographic distribution: AUSTRALIA: South Australia.

Description of sporulated oocyst: Oocyst shape: ellipsoidal to ovoidal, tapering to a slight protuberance at one end; number of walls: 2; wall characteristics: outer layer is smooth, clear, slightly mammillated, tan, 1.0 thick, but thinning at protuberant apex; inner layer is colorless, ~0.4 thick; L×W (*n*=20): 25.4×17.1 (23–29×15–19); L/W ratio: 1.5; M: the protuberance at one end does not present itself as a clear-cut M; OR: present as an irregular or filamentous structure at the protuberant apex; PG: absent. Distinctive features of oocyst: M-like protuberance at tapered end.

Description of sporocyst and sporozoites: Sporocyst shape: ellipsoidal, tapering slightly toward one end; L×W (*n*=20): 10.2×6.7 (9–11×6–7); L/W ratio: 1.5; SB: present at tapered end, but inconspicuous; SSB, PSB: both absent; SR: an aggregate of numerous, fine granules, ~3.2 wide; SZ: do not fill the space in the SP and each SZ has an RB, ~3.2–4.0 wide. Distinctive features of sporocyst: tapered ellipsoid with an SR of aggregated fine granules, ~3.2 wide.

Prevalence: Found in 6/7 (86%) of the type host.

Sporulation: Unknown. The feces were held dry, often for months or years, prior to immersion in 2.5% (w/v) potassium dichromate solution ($K_2Cr_2O_7$) in which they were later stored at 4 °C for up to 3.5 years.

Prepatent and patent periods: Unknown.

Site of infection: Unknown, oocysts recovered only from the feces.

Endogenous stages: Unknown.

Cross-transmission: None to date.

Pathology: Not described.

Materials deposited: None.

Etymology: The specific epithet is based on that of the type host.

Remarks: Barker et al. (1988c) distinguished the oocysts of this eimerian from *P. xanthopus* from the oocysts of the other six *Eimeria* species they described by the presence of the thin-walled protuberance at its tapered end. In many other aspects, the oocysts resemble those of *E. petrogale*. It would be useful to have some molecular signatures to distinguish these two forms from each other, or not.

GENUS *SETONIX* LESSON, 1842 (MONOTYPIC)

EIMERIA QUOKKA BARKER, O'CALLAGHAN, AND BEVERIDGE, 1988b

Type host: *Setonix brachyurus* (Quoy and Gaimard, 1830), Quokka.

Type locality: AUSTRALIA: Western Australia: Rottnest Island.

Other hosts: None to date.

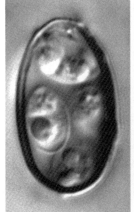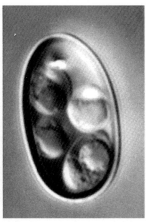

FIGURES 4.69, 4.70 Photomicrographs of two sporulated oocyst of *Eimeria quokka*, both originals from M. O'Callaghan. **4.69**. Shows a sporocyst in long section with its clearly visible SB. **4.70**. Shows the slightly pointed nature of the oocyst.

Geographic distribution: AUSTRALIA: Western Australia.

Description of sporulated oocyst: Oocyst shape: ellipsoidal with one end slightly pointed; number of walls: 2; wall characteristics: outer layer is smooth, colorless, ~1.0 thick; inner layer, ~0.4 thick; L×W: 18.0×10.8 (14–22×9–15); L/W ratio: 1.7; M, OR: both absent; PG: present. Distinctive features of oocyst: ellipsoidal shape that is slightly pointed at one end.

Description of sporocyst and sporozoites: Sporocyst shape: ellipsoidal to slightly ovoidal; L×W: 7.7×5.0 (6–10×4–6); L/W ratio: 1.5; SB: small, present at slightly pointed end of sporocyst; SSB, PSB: both absent; SR: present; SR characteristics: a tight, granular spheroidal mass, ~2.4 wide; SZ: completely fill the SP, have granular cytoplasm, and each has a large RB, 3.2×2.4. Distinctive features of sporocyst: small size with a tiny SB and the SZ completely pack the SP.

Prevalence: Barker et al. (1988b) reported this form in 6/19 (84%) *S. brachyurus* examined from the type locality.

Sporulation: Could not be determined because specimens in 2.5% (w/v) potassium dichromate

$(K_2Cr_2O_7)$ solution spent varying periods in transit before reaching the lab.

Prepatent and patent periods: Unknown.

Site of infection: Unknown.

Endogenous stages: Unknown.

Cross-transmission: None to date.

Pathology: Not described.

Materials deposited: None.

Remarks: Barker et al. (1988b) distinguished the oocysts of *E. quokka* from the other two eimerians named from *S. brachyurus*, "based on dimensions of oocysts and sporocysts, in combination with the suite of morphologic characteristics described." In particular, this species has the smallest sporocysts that distinguish it from the other two species found in quokkas to date. These are the only three eimerians described from the quokka, and they are different enough from each other, and from other eimerians of other genera in the family, that their (Barker et al., 1988b) reasoning to call them different species seems justified. Barker et al. (1988a,b) hypothesized that as eimerians coevolved with their Australian marsupial hosts, they would be relatively conservative in their morphology, and that such evidence (if it existed) could provide clues to phylogenetic relationships among Macropodoidea. Their earlier work (1988a) suggested there may be value in this hypothesis for rock wallabies (*Petrogale* spp.), but the evidence garnered from their limited examination of coccidia from the Potoroidae failed to show morphologic similarities to suggest relative relatedness of groups of hosts at the generic level. Overall, these studies were unable to demonstrate any obvious patterns of oocyst morphology that could suggest phylogenetic relationships among genera of Macropodidae they examined.

EIMERIA SETONICIS BARKER, O'CALLAGHAN, AND BEVERIDGE, 1988b

Type host: *Setonix brachyurus* (Quoy and Gaimard, 1830), Quokka.

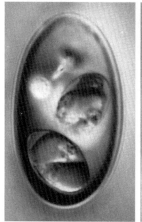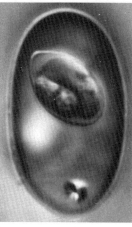

FIGURES 4.71, 4.72 Photomicrographs of two sporulated oocysts of *Eimeria setonicis*, both originals from M. O'Callaghan. **4.71.** Shows a single sporocyst with SB and the distinct, refractile PG. **4.72.** Shows a sporocyst and SZ.

Type locality: AUSTRALIA: Western Australia: Rottnest Island.

Other hosts: None to date.

Geographic distribution: AUSTRALIA: Western Australia.

Description of sporulated oocyst: Oocyst shape: ellipsoidal to cylindroidal; number of walls: 2; wall characteristics: outer layer is smooth, colorless, ~1.0 thick; inner layer, ~0.4; L × W: 29.9 × 17.9 (26–34 × 17–19); L/W ratio: 1.7; M, OR: both absent; PG: present. Distinctive features of oocyst: cylindroidal shape, smooth outer wall, presence of a highly refractile PG.

Description of sporocyst and sporozoites: Sporocyst shape: ellipsoidal, slightly pointed at one end; L × W: 12.0 × 7.7 (10–14 × 7–9); L/W ratio: 1.6; SB: present at pointed end of sporocyst; SSB: present, lenticulate, wider than SB; PSB: absent; SR: present; SR characteristics: a tight aggregate of fine granules, ~4.0 wide; SZ: described as "curved," with finely granular cytoplasm, each with one large RB, ~4.0 wide. Distinctive features of sporocyst: "typical" ovoidal/ellipsoidal shape with a small, knob-like SB and a lenticulate SSB.

Prevalence: Barker et al. (1988b) found this form in 14/19 (74%) *S. brachyurus* examined from the type locality.

Sporulation: Could not be determined because specimens in 2.5% (w/v) potassium dichromate (K$_2$Cr$_2$O$_7$) solution spent varying periods in transit before reaching the lab.

Prepatent and patent periods: Unknown.

Site of infection: Unknown.

Endogenous stages: Unknown.

Cross-transmission: None to date.

Pathology: Not described.

Materials deposited: None.

Remarks: Barker et al. (1988b) distinguished the oocysts of *E. setonicis* from the other two eimerians named from *S. brachyurus*, "based on oocyst and sporocyst dimensions, in combination with the suite of morphologic characteristics described." These are the only three eimerians known, to date, from the quokka, and they are different enough from each other, and from other eimerians from other genera in the family, that their (Barker et al., 1988b) reasoning to consider them different species seems justified. Barker et al. (1988a,b) hypothesized that as eimerians coevolved with their Australian marsupial hosts, they would be relatively conservative in their morphology, and that such evidence (if it existed) could provide clues to phylogenetic relationships among Macropodoidea. Their earlier work (Barker et al., 1988a) suggested there may be value in this hypothesis for rock wallabies (*Petrogale* spp.), but the evidence garnered from their limited examination of coccidia from the Potoroidae failed to show morphologic similarities to suggest relative relatedness of groups of hosts at the generic level.

EIMERIA VOLCKERTZOONI BARKER, O'CALLAGHAN, AND BEVERIDGE, 1988b

Type host: *Setonix brachyurus* (Quoy and Gaimard, 1830), Quokka.

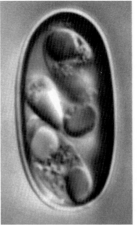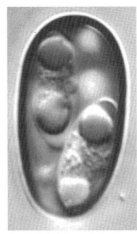

FIGURES 4.73, 4.74 Photomicrographs of two sporulated oocysts of *Eimeria volckertzooni*, both originals from M. O'Callaghan. **4.73.** Shows three of four sporocysts, smooth outer oocyst wall, and large RB in SZ. **4.74.** Shows a clear long-section of a sporocyst with its SB, two SZ, and large RB in each SZ.

Type locality: AUSTRALIA: Western Australia: Rottnest Island.

Other hosts: None to date.

Geographic distribution: AUSTRALIA: Western Australia.

Description of sporulated oocyst: Oocyst shape: bluntly ellipsoidal, sometimes flatter on one side; number of walls: 2; wall characteristics: outer layer is smooth, colorless, ~0.6 thick; inner layer is colorless, ~0.3 thick; L×W: 21.9×12.9 (20–24×12–14); L/W ratio: 1.7; M: absent; OR: reported as present in the form of scattered granules, but these also could be considered to be PG, which were also said to be present. Distinctive features of oocyst: bluntly ellipsoidal shape that is sometimes flattened on one side and possessing both OR (?) and/or PG.

Description of sporocyst and sporozoites: Sporocyst shape: elongate-ellipsoidal, slightly pointed at one end; L×W: 12.6×5.5 (11–15×5–6); L/W ratio: 2.3; SB: inconspicuous and present at pointed end of sporocyst; SSB, PSB: both absent; SR: present; SR characteristics: a tight, finely granular spheroidal mass, ~2.4 wide; SZ: described as "elongate," with finely granular cytoplasm, each with two RB, the larger is 3.2 wide, while the smaller is 2.4 wide. Distinctive features of sporocyst: each is very long, comprising 50–60% of the length of the oocyst, and they have a very high L/W ratio of 2.3.

Prevalence: Barker et al. (1988b) found this form in 5/19 (26%) *S. brachyurus* examined from the type locality.

Sporulation: Could not be determined because specimens in 2.5% (w/v) potassium dichromate ($K_2Cr_2O_7$) solution spent varying periods in transit before reaching the lab.

Prepatent and patent periods: Unknown.

Site of infection: Unknown.

Endogenous stages: Unknown.

Cross-transmission: None to date.

Pathology: Not described.

Materials deposited: None.

Etymology: This species was named in recognition of Samuel Volckertzoon, the Dutch navigator who made the first written description of the quokka in 1658 (Strahan, 1983).

Remarks: Barker et al. (1988b) distinguished the oocysts of this form from the other two eimerians named from *S. brachyurus*, "based on oocyst and sporocyst dimensions, in combination with the suite of morphologic characteristics described." In particular, the very long, narrow sporocysts (L/W = 2.3) distinguish this eimerian from the other two species found in the quokka. These three eimerians known from the quokka are different enough from each other, and from other eimerians of other genera in the family, that their (Barker et al., 1988b) reasoning to call them different species seems justified. Barker et al. (1988a,b) hypothesized that as eimerians coevolved with their Australian marsupial hosts, they would be relatively conservative in their morphology and that such evidence (if it existed) could provide clues to phylogenetic relationships among Macropodoidea. However, On the basis of the sum of all their observations describing oocysts from many Australian marsupials, there seems to be no obvious morphologic similarities among sporulated oocysts to suggest relatedness of groups of hosts at the generic level.

GENUS *THYLOGALE* GRAY, 1837 (7 SPECIES)

EIMERIA OBENDORFI BARKER, O'CALLAGHAN, AND BEVERIDGE, 1988b

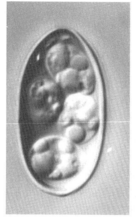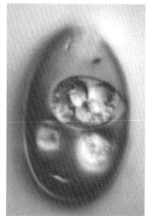

FIGURES 4.75, 4.76 Photomicrographs of two sporulated oocysts of *Eimeria obendorfi*, both originals from M. O'Callaghan.

Type host: *Thylogale billardierii* (Desmarest, 1822), Tasmanian Pademelon.

Type locality: AUSTRALIA: Tasmania: in the vicinity of Launceston.

Other hosts: None to date.

Geographic distribution: AUSTRALIA: Tasmania.

Description of sporulated oocyst: Oocyst shape: ellipsoidal with one end slightly pointed, occasionally flattened on one side; number of walls: 2; wall characteristics: outer layer is smooth, colorless, ~1.0 thick, thinning at apex of oocyst; inner layer, ~0.4 thick; L×W: 29.5×16.2 (26–32×15–18); L/W ratio: 1.8; M, OR, PG: all reported as absent, but there appear to be floating refractile rods within the oocyst (similar to those seen in *E. ringaroomaensis*, but less abundant). Distinctive features of oocyst: ellipsoidal shape that is slightly pointed at one end, and some floating fragments or refractile rods within the oocyst.

Description of sporocyst and sporozoites: Sporocyst shape: ellipsoidal; L×W: 10.6×7.7 (10–11×7–8); L/W ratio: 1.4; SB: reported as absent by Barker et al. (1988b), but I believe a small one is present at slightly pointed end of the SP; SSB, PSB: both absent; SR: present; SR characteristics: a loose aggregate of granules, 1.0–2.0 wide, scattered about equator of SP; SZ: stout, curved, do not completely fill SP, and each SZ has one RB, 3.2 wide. Distinctive features of sporocyst: small size, with a tiny SB, and the SZ do not fill the sporocyst.

Prevalence: Barker et al. (1988b) found this form in 3/5 (60%) *T. billardierii* examined from the type locality.

Sporulation: Could not be determined because specimens in 2.5% (w/v) potassium dichromate ($K_2Cr_2O_7$) solution spent varying periods in transit before reaching the lab.

Prepatent and patent periods: Unknown.

Site of infection: Unknown.

Endogenous stages: Unknown.

Cross-transmission: None to date.

Pathology: Not described.

Materials deposited: None.

Etymology: This species was named in recognition of Dr. David Obendorf, Mt. Pleasant Laboratories, Tasmanian Department of Agriculture.

Remarks: Barker et al. (1988b) distinguished the oocysts of this form from the other two eimerians named from *T. billardierii*, "based on oocyst and sporocyst dimensions, in combination with other morphologic characteristics described." In particular, this species has the smallest sporocysts of the three species from pademelons, which distinguishes it from the other two species. These are the only three eimerians yet described from *T. billardierii* and their sporulated oocysts are different enough from each other, and from those of other eimerians from other genera in

the family, that their (Barker et al., 1988b) reasoning seems justified. Barker et al. (1988a,b) hypothesized that as eimerians coevolved with their Australian marsupial hosts, they would be relatively conservative in their morphology and that such evidence (if it existed) could provide clues to phylogenetic relationships among Macropodoidea. Overall, however, their studies (Barker et al., 1988a,b,c; 1989) were unable to demonstrate to them any obvious patterns of oocyst morphology that could suggest phylogenetic relationships among genera of Macropodidae they examined.

EIMERIA RINGAROOMAENSIS BARKER, O'CALLAGHAN, AND BEVERIDGE, 1988b

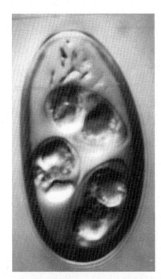

FIGURE 4.77   Photomicrograph of a sporulated oocyst of *E. ringaroomaensis*, from Barker et al. (1988b), with permission from all authors and with kind permission from Elsevier, publisher of the *International Journal for Parasitology*.

Type host: *Thylogale billardierii* (Desmarest, 1822), Tasmanian Pademelon.

Type locality: AUSTRALIA: Tasmania: in the vicinity of Launceston.

Other hosts: None to date.

Geographic distribution: AUSTRALIA: Tasmania.

Description of sporulated oocyst: Oocyst shape: ellipsoidal/ovoidal with one end slightly pointed; number of walls: 2; wall characteristics: outer layer is smooth, colorless, ~0.8 thick; inner layer is transparent, ~0.4 thick; L×W: 28.4×17.9 (25–32×16–20); L/W ratio: 1.6; M, OR, PG: all absent, but there seem to be a number of refractile, rodlike structures present at the slightly pointed end. Distinctive features of oocyst: refractile rods scattered at apex of oocyst.

Description of sporocyst and sporozoites: Sporocyst shape: ellipsoidal to slightly ovoidal; L×W: 12.3×8.0 (11–14×7–8); L/W ratio: 1.5; SB: small, inconspicuous, present at slightly pointed end of sporocyst; SSB: described only as lenticulate; PSB: absent; SR: present; SR characteristics: 3.2 wide, composed of a compact cluster of granules each ~1.2 wide; SZ: curved, do not completely fill the space in the SP, and each SZ has a large RB, 4.0 wide. Distinctive features of sporocyst: small size, with a tiny SB, and the SZ do not completely pack the SP.

Prevalence: Barker et al. (1988b) found this form in 4/5 (80%) *T. billardierii* examined from the type locality.

Sporulation: Could not be determined because specimens in 2.5% (w/v) potassium dichromate (K$_2$Cr$_2$O$_7$) solution spent varying periods in transit before reaching the lab.

Prepatent and patent periods: Unknown.

Site of infection: Unknown.

Endogenous stages: Unknown.

Cross-transmission: None to date.

Pathology: Not described.

Materials deposited: None.

Etymology: This species was named for Ringarooma, a town in the vicinity of the locality where infected pademelons were collected.

Remarks: Barker et al. (1988b) distinguished the oocysts of this form from the other two eimerians named from *T. billardierii*, "based on oocyst and sporocyst dimensions, in combination with other morphologic features." In particular, sporulated oocysts of this species differ from those of *E. thylogale* by a smooth oocyst wall and smaller sporocysts; they differ from those of *E. obendorfi* by sporocyst shape and size and the presence of an SSB. These are the only three eimerians yet described from *T. billardierii*, and they are different enough from each other, and from other eimerians from other genera in the family, that their separation into distinct species seems justified. Overall, the studies on eimerians from marsupials in Australia (Barker et al., 1988a,b,c; 1989) do not demonstrate any obvious patterns of oocyst morphology that could suggest phylogenetic relationships among genera of Macropodidae.

EIMERIA THYLOGALE BARKER, O'CALLAGHAN, AND BEVERIDGE, 1988b

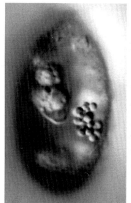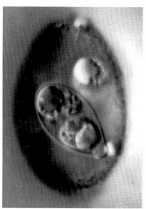

FIGURES 4.78, 4.79 Photomicrographs of two sporulated oocysts of *Eimeria thylogale*, both from Barker et al. (1988b), with permission from all authors and with kind permission from Elsevier, publisher of the *International Journal for Parasitology*.

Type host: *Thylogale billardierii* (Desmarest, 1822), Tasmanian Pademelon.

Type locality: AUSTRALIA: Tasmania: in the vicinity of Launceston.

Other hosts: None to date.

Geographic distribution: AUSTRALIA: Tasmania.

Description of sporulated oocyst: Oocyst shape: ellipsoidal or slightly elongate-ovoidal; number of walls: 2; wall characteristics: outer layer with small nodules on its surface, radial striations in optical section, and clear, but with a brown tint, ~1.6 thick and thinning at narrow apex of oocyst; inner layer, ~0.4 thick; L × W: 32.2 × 20.6 (30–35 × 19–22); L/W ratio: 1.6; M: absent; PG: thought to be absent, but numerous refractile rods seem to be present at one end of oocyst; OR: present as irregular aggregate, ~7–8 wide, comprising granules 0.8–1.6 wide. Distinctive features of oocyst: there are numerous refractile rods at apex of the oocyst, and the aggregate of granules forming the OR also make it unique.

Description of sporocyst and sporozoites: Sporocyst shape: ovoidal to slightly pyriform; L × W: 15.0 × 8.2 (14–16 × 7–10); L/W ratio: 1.8; SB: present as a caplike structure covering the SSB at the slightly pointed end of sporocyst; SSB: present, lenticulate; PSB: absent; SR: present; SR characteristics: a tight aggregate of fine granules, ~4.8 wide, at equator of SP; SZ: have granular cytoplasm and do not completely fill the SP; each SZ has an RB, 4.8 wide. Distinctive features of sporocyst: slightly pyriform shape and SZ do not fill the space within the SP.

Prevalence: Barker et al. (1988b) found this form in 4/5 (80%) *T. billardierii* examined from the type locality.

Sporulation: Could not be determined because specimens in 2.5% (w/v) potassium dichromate (K$_2$Cr$_2$O$_7$) solution spent varying periods in transit before reaching the lab.

Prepatent and patent periods: Unknown.

Site of infection: Unknown.

Endogenous stages: Unknown.

Cross-transmission: None to date.

Pathology: Not described.

Materials deposited: None.

Remarks: Barker et al. (1988b) distinguished the oocysts of this form from the other two eimerians named from *T. billardierii*, "based on oocyst and sporocyst dimensions, in combination with the suite of morphologic characteristics described." In particular, sporulated oocysts of *E. thylogale* have the largest oocysts and sporocysts of the three species from pademelons, which distinguishes them from the other two species known. These are the only three eimerians described from the *T. billardierii* and they are different enough from each other, to warrant separate species status.

GENUS *WALLABIA* TROUESSART, 1905 (MONOTYPIC)

EIMERIA BICOLOR BARKER, O'CALLAGHAN, AND BEVERIDGE, 1988b

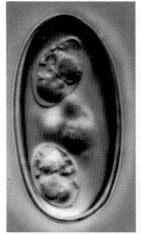 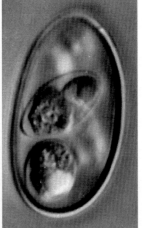

FIGURES 4.80, 4.81 Photomicrographs of two sporulated oocysts of *E. bicolor*, both originals from M. O'Callaghan.

Type host: *Wallabia bicolor* (Desmarest, 1804), Swamp Wallaby.

Type locality: AUSTRALIA: Victoria: Darthmouth and Mitta Mitta.

Other hosts: None to date.

Geographic distribution: AUSTRALIA: New South Wales (Sydney, Macquarie University); South Australia (Adelaide, Cleland Conservation Park), Victoria.

Description of sporulated oocyst: Oocyst shape: irregular ellipsoidal to cylindroidal, often slightly pointed at one end and flat on one side; number of walls: 2; wall characteristics: outer layer is smooth, colorless, ~0.8 thick, thinning at one apex, but no clear-cut MP; L×W: 22.6×13.4 (18.5–28×11–16); L/W ratio: 1.7; M, OR: both absent; PG: present. Distinctive features of oocyst: irregular ellipsoidal to cylindroidal shape, often pointed at one end and flat on one side.

Description of sporocyst and sporozoites: Sporocyst shape: ellipsoidal, slightly pointed at one end; L×W: 8.4×6.3 (7–11×5–8); L/W ratio: 1.3; SB: small and inconspicuous, present at slightly pointed end of sporocyst; SSB, PSB: both absent; SR: present; SR characteristics: a few granules scattered about equator of SP; SZ: with finely granular cytoplasm, not filling SP, and each with an RB, 2.4 wide. Distinctive features of sporocyst: nothing special.

Prevalence: Barker et al. (1988b) found this form in 8/13 (62%) *W. bicolor* examined from four localities, several of which were captive animals from Macquarie University and from the Cleland Conservation Park.

Sporulation: Could not be determined because specimens in 2.5% (w/v) potassium dichromate (K$_2$Cr$_2$O$_7$) solution spent varying periods in transit before reaching the lab.

Prepatent and patent periods: Unknown.

Site of infection: Unknown.

Endogenous stages: Unknown.

Cross-transmission: None to date.

Pathology: Not described.

Materials deposited: None.

Remarks: Barker et al. (1988b) distinguished the oocysts of this form from those of *E. wallabiae*, the only other eimerian named from *W. bicolor*, "based on oocyst and sporocyst dimensions in combination with other morphologic features." In particular, the sporulated oocysts of *E. bicolor* differ from those of *E. wallabiae* by having smaller oocysts and sporocysts accompanied by consistently smaller L/W ratios of both. These are the only two eimerians described from *W. bicolor*, and they are different enough from each other and from other eimerians from other genera in the family, that calling them different species seems justified.

EIMERIA WALLABIAE BARKER, O'CALLAGHAN AND BEVERIDGE, 1988b

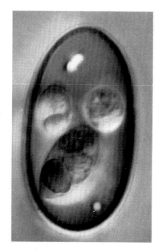

FIGURE 4.82 Photomicrograph of a sporulated oocyst of *E. wallabiae* from Barker et al. (Figure 9, 1988b), with permission from all authors and with kind permission from Elsevier, publisher of the *International Journal for Parasitology*.

Type host: *Wallabia bicolor* (Desmarest, 1804), Swamp Wallaby.

Type locality: AUSTRALIA: Victoria: Darthmouth and Mitta Mitta.

Other hosts: None to date.

Geographic distribution: AUSTRALIA: South Australia (Adelaide, Cleland Conservation Park); Victoria.

Description of sporulated oocyst: Oocyst shape: irregular ellipsoidal to cylindroidal, often slightly pointed at one end; number of walls: 2; wall characteristics: outer layer is smooth, colorless, ~1.2 thick; inner layer is transparent, ~0.4 thick; L×W: 32.9×20.1 (29–36×16–22); L/W ratio: 1.6; M, OR: both absent; PG: present, refractile. Distinctive features of oocyst: large size, high L/W ratio, and irregular ellipsoidal to cylindroidal shape.

Description of sporocyst and sporozoites: Sporocyst shape: ellipsoidal to slightly ovoidal; L×W: 12.9×8.5 (10–16×8–10); L/W ratio: 1.5; SB: small and inconspicuous, present at slightly pointed end of sporocyst; SSB: present, but inconspicuous; PSB: absent; SR: present; SR characteristics: 7.0 wide, composed of a dense aggregate of fine granules; SZ: not described, but said to each have a large RB, 4.8 wide. Distinctive features of sporocyst: compact, distinct SR.

Prevalence: Barker et al. (1988b) found this form in 3/13 (80%) *W. bicolor* examined from three localities, one of which was a captive animal in the Cleland Conservation Park.

Sporulation: Could not be determined because specimens in 2.5% (w/v) potassium dichromate ($K_2Cr_2O_7$) solution spent varying periods in transit before reaching the lab.

Prepatent and patent periods: Unknown.

Site of infection: Unknown.

Endogenous stages: Unknown.

Cross-transmission: None to date.

Pathology: Not described.

Materials deposited: None.

Remarks: Barker et al. (1988b) distinguished the oocysts of this form from *E. bicolor*, the only other eimerian named from *W. bicolor*, "based on oocyst and sporocyst dimensions, in combination with other morphologic features." The sporulated oocysts of this species differ from those of *E. bicolor* by having larger oocysts and sporocysts. These two eimerians described from *W. bicolor* are different enough from each other, and from other eimerians from other genera in the family, that they warrant separate species status.

DISCUSSION AND SUMMARY

The following **suborders** (-iformes), families (-idae), subfamilies (-inae), tribes (-ini), and genera (number) in this order of Australian marsupials either have no Apicomplexa parasites in the Eimeriidae described from them, or they have never been examined/surveyed for them: **Suborder** Vombatiformes: Phascolarctidae: *Phascolarctos* (1); **Suborder** Phalangeriformes: Burramyidae: *Burramys* (1), *Cercartetus* (4); Phalangeridae: Ailuropinae: *Ailurops* (2); Phalangerinae: Phalangerini: *Phalanger* (13), *Spilocuscus* (4); Trichosurini: *Strigocuscus* (2), *Wyulda* (1); Pseudocheiridae: Hemibelideinae: *Hemibelideus* (1), *Petauroides* (1); Pseudocheirinae: *Petropseudes* (1), *Pseudocheirus* (1), *Pseudochirulus* (8); Pseudochiropsinae: *Pseudochirops* (5); Petauridae: *Dactylopsila* (4), *Gymnobelideus* (1); Tarsipedidae: *Tarsipes* (1); Acrobatidae: *Acrobates* (1), *Distoechurus* (1), **Suborder** Macropodiformes: Potoroidae: *Caloprymnus* (1); Macropodidae: Sthenurinae: *Lagostrophus* (1); Macropodinae: *Dorcopsis* (4), *Dorcopsulus* (2), *Onychogalea* (3). In addition, in the Macropodidae, 7 of the 11 (64%) genera have been examined, but only 26/65 (40%) species have been examined. These include only 1/12 (8%) *Dendrolagus* species, only 1/4 (25%) *Lagorchestes* species, 12/14 (86%) *Macropus* species, 9/16 (56%) *Petrogale* species, and only 1/7 (14%) *Thylogale* species have been examined. In the Phalangeridae, only 1/6 genera (17%) have been examined for coccidia, and only 3/27 (11%) species; these include three of five *Trichosurus* species. In the Potoridae, 3/4 (75%) genera have been sampled, but only 3/10 (30%) species. In the Vombatidae, 2/3 species (67%) in the only two genera have been looked at for coccidia. The summation of these numbers tells us that 5/11 (45%) families, but only 14/39 (36%) genera and only 35/143 (24%) of all Diprotodontia species, in Australia have been examined for intestinal coccidians.

From this quite modest sampling, 44 *Eimeria*, but no *Isospora* species have been found. In addition, a wide variety of about 30 more apicomplexan forms found in the gastrointestinal tract, tubules of the kidneys, or in the muscles have been reported in Diprotodontia species, including *Coccidium, Cryptosporidium, Eimeria* or *Eimeria*-like, *Klossiella, Sarcocystis,* and *Tyzzeria*-like organisms. Unfortunately, so little information has been documented on these that they must remain of "uncertain status," and I have relegated them to *species inquirendae* (see Chapter 10, Tables 11.1 and 11.2).

Given the above information about the eimeriid coccidians found in Australian diprotodontid marsupials, I can only make the following sad conclusions: (1) We know even less about the *biology* of these species than we do about those from American didelphimorphids (Chapter 3); (2) the time it takes for oocysts to sporulate once they leave their host's intestinal tract is known (but not very precisely) for only three of the 44 (7%) known species (*E. macropodis, E. ursini,* and *E. wombati*); (3) we do not know the prepatent or the patent period for any of the 44 known eimerians; (4) we only know the relative site of infection in the intestine for three of the 44 (7%) species (*E. arundeli, E. macropodis,* and *E. wombati*); (5) we only know about one or two of the endogenous stages for the three above eimerians, but there have been *no studies* to delineate the complete endogenous life cycle for any of the 44 eimerians that infect diprotodontid marsupials; (6) there have been no cross-transmission studies on any of these 44 known eimerians; (7) we do know that at least three eimerians can cause pathology in their host marsupials; these include *E. wombati* (mild), *E. arundeli* (severe), and *E. macropodis* (severe); (8) type specimens have been deposited into accredited museums for only two of the 44 (4.5%) eimerians: *E. arundeli* (tissue sections) and *E. trichosuri* (phototype). But the good news is that we now have partial gene sequences, something desperately needed for every eimerian species, for two of the 44 eimerians, *E. macropodis,* and *E. trichosuri.*

Finally, in the late 1980s and early 1990s, it was still more or less presumed that *Eimeria* species were highly host specific, being restricted to a single host species or no more than a few closely related (congeneric) species. Barker et al. (1979, 1988a,b,c, 1989), who have discovered, described, and named most of the *Eimeria* species in the Diprotodontia, especially in the Macropodidae, began their survey work under two premises: (1) reasonably strict host specificity; and (2) that coccidia of macropodid marsupials may have trailed behind their hosts in terms of morphological divergence, while radiating with them. They were looking for oocyst similarities to serve as markers that might help support/refute established phylogenetic relationships of their hosts. That, of course, was long before the advent of molecular techniques. Basically, what they learned was that there were no strong morphological similarities among the oocysts of the five *Eimeria* species they found in the Hypsiprymnodontidae (1 species) and the 4 *Eimeria* species they found in the Potoridae (3 genera, 1 species each), but they were generalizing about the size and shape of oocysts and sporocysts from these hosts. Perhaps there are other, better, characters to suggest a phylogenetic signal. For example, if we look at some of the qualitative characters (presence/absence), we see in Table 11.3 that eight of the nine *Eimeria* species have sporocysts that have both an SB and SSB, eight of nine likely lack an OR, and eight of nine lack an M. The only species that has an M also has an OR (*E. potoroi*).

Others have looked at phylogenetic relationships of mammalian eimerians and have reported two different lineages, based partially on oocyst size and shape, but primarily on the presence or absence of the OR (Reduker et al., 1987; Hnida and Duszynski, 1999a,b; Zhao and Duszynski 2001a,b). Using plastid ORF 470, 23S rDNA, and nuclear 18S rDNA sequences, they showed distinct phylogenetic relationships among rodent eimerians in three families based on the presence/absence of the OR (Zhao et al., 2001b).

Kvičerová et al. (2008) examined the phylogenetic relationships among 11 *Eimeria* species infecting domestic rabbits in the Czech Republic. Sporulated oocysts of those species are comparatively heterogenous relative to their oocyst and sporocyst morphology and size, the location of their endogenous stages in the host, and the pathology they exhibit (low, moderate, high). Using partial sequences of 18S rDNA from these 11 rabbit species, when compared to all the *Eimeria* sequences available in GenBank at the time, they found what they described as a clear phylogenetic signal, indicating that the rabbit-specific *Eimeria* formed a monophyletic species group/cluster; and of all the morphological and biological characters used in their analysis, only the presence/absence of an OR strictly followed the phylogenetic division into two monophyletic sister lineages. Their conclusion was that the presence/absence of an OR seemed to be an evolutionarily conservative feature. It would be interesting to pursue this line of research with the *Eimeria* species of marsupials.

It is also interesting to see that only 7/44 (16%) of Diprotodontia eimerian oocysts, but none of the Didelphimorphia or Peramelemorphia eimerian oocysts, have an OR. About a third, 14/44 (32%), of the known diprotodontid eimerians have (or presumably have) an M,

but only four of those have both an M and an OR (*E. arundeli, E. potori, E. trichosuri,* and *E. xanthopus*), while three species (*E. aepyprymni, E. thylogale,* and *E. prionotemni*) have an OR, but no M. Demonstrating any obvious patterns of oocyst morphology that could suggest phylogenetic relationships among marsupial genera should be pursued with all the molecular tools now available.

Clearly, enormous amounts of research remain to be started and completed. This must include, but not be limited to, systematic surveys (all species, wide geographic ranges); detailed descriptive taxonomy (quantitative, qualitative, type specimens, etc.); life cycle studies (all endogenous stages, cross-transmission); veterinary investigations (pathology, immunology); ecological and epidemiological studies (especially in habitats where multiple species ranges overlap); and molecular sequencing and analyses (multiple genes including nuclear, mitochondrial, etc.). And this needs to be done sooner rather than later, before habitat loss and pollution eliminate most of the marsupials forever from the Earth. It would be gratifying to learn that this synopsis of what is not known will stimulate Australian parasitologists and mammalogists to work together.

Order Peramelemorphia—Eimeriidae

ORDER PERAMELEMORPHIA AMEGHINO, 1889

INTRODUCTION

The Peramelemorphia is an order of rodent-like marsupials that go by a variety of common names including bandicoot, bilby, and echymipera. These marsupials are characterized by a long, pointed nose, a short neck, a marsupium that opens to the rear, and a stocky body with short legs; some species have long, rabbit-like ears. Most are **nocturnal**, so they are equipped with eyes well adapted for night vision and a well-developed sense of smell. Individuals are about the size of a cottontail rabbit or smaller, but they can range in size from <100g to >5kg. They are **omnivorous**, with a diet consisting mainly of insects, but also some small vertebrates, and a variety of vegetable material; they are widespread throughout Australia, New Guinea, Tasmania, and the surrounding islands (Frens, 2011).

Within the marsupial lineage, the position of the Peramelemorphia has a long history of controversy because they all have two morphological features thought to show a clear evolutionary link with other marsupial groups. All species in the order have several pairs of lower front teeth, a character state called **polyprotodontia**, and the species in this order have three pairs. This suggests that they evolved with or within the Dasyuromorphia, an order of marsupial carnivores that includes the Tasmanian devil. However, the conundrum is that their second morphological character state seems to unite them with a different order of marsupials. The second and third toes on their hind foot are fused together (although they maintain separate claws), a feature called **syndactyly**, and an adaptation for climbing; it is also a condition characteristic of the order Diprotodontia, an order of marsupial herbivores (kangaroos, wombats, etc.). Several contradictory explanations have been offered as to which character state came first and which evolved secondarily, and each has serious proponents. Unfortunately, recent molecular evidence, to date, has not resolved this puzzle. Meredith et al. (2008) analyzed the sequences of five nuclear protein-coding genes (ApoB, BRCA1, IRBP, Rag1, and vWF) using maximum parsimony, maximum likelihood, and Bayesian methods to estimate times of divergence of each lineage within the Peramelemorphia. Their work did not resolve the question regarding which of the above morphological characters may have evolved first, but they did strongly suggest that whatever the relationship of the bandicoot group to the other marsupial orders may be, it is a distant one, with *Macrotis* being basal to the remaining living bandicoots (Meredith et al., 2008).

Peramelemorphids are important components of the ecosystems they inhabit. They are known to occupy a variety of habitats, from rainforests, to grasslands, to deserts, and some peramelemorphs can be found living as high as 2000 m in elevation (Frens, 2011). They play a vital role in their ecosystems as members of food chains (both predator and prey) and in control of insect pest populations. As omnivores, they consume a variety of invertebrates (arthropods, arachnids, annelids) and plants (grasses, seeds, bulbs), as well as occasional small vertebrates (mice, lizards, birds). They, in turn, are consumed by owls, dingoes, foxes, and feral or domestic dogs and cats. In addition to controlling some insect pests, they may play a role in seed dispersal; a few of the **semifossorial** bilbies help aerate the soil via their burrowing habits, and some species are still hunted for food and for their fur by humans (Frens, 2011).

This order is divided into 3 families, 8 genera, and 21 species, although 1 monotypic family is likely extinct, with the last known specimen collected about 110 years ago (Groves, 2005). This leaves only 2 extant families, with 7 genera and 20 species. One of these species, *Macrotis leucura* (Thomas, 1887), also likely is extinct, because what eventually became the type specimen was sent by the South Australia Museum's taxidermist to London; Thomas thought it might have originated near Adelaide or in the northern part of South Australia. No other specimens have been collected since then (Groves, 2005). The **IUCN** also lists this species as extinct, as does Groves (2005). Below, I list the only two genera, one species each in the Peramelemorphia, that have been examined for intestinal coccidia and from which two *Eimeria* species have been described.

SPECIES DESCRIPTIONS

FAMILY PERAMELIDAE GRAY, 1825 (6 GENERA, 18 SPECIES)

SUBFAMILY PERAMELINAE GRAY, 1825

GENUS ISOODON DESMAREST, 1817 (3 SPECIES)

EIMERIA QUENDA BENNETT AND HOBBS, 2011

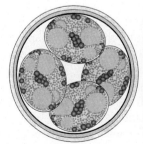 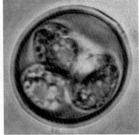

FIGURES 5.1, 5.2 **5.1.** Line drawing of the sporulated oocyst of *Eimeria quenda*. **5.2.** Photomicrograph of a sporulated oocyst of *E. quenda*. Both figures from Bennett and Hobbs, 2011, with permission from the Editor of the *Journal of Parasitology*.

Type host: *Isoodon obesulus urita* (Shaw, 1797), Southern Brown Bandicoot.

Type locality: AUSTRALIA: Western Australia: Forrestfield (31° 59' S, 116° 00' E).

Other hosts: None to date.

Geographic distribution: AUSTRALIA: Western Australia.

Description of sporulated oocyst: Oocyst shape: spheroidal to subspheroidal; number of walls: 3; wall characteristics: ~1.8 (1.6–2.0) thick; outer wall smooth, yellow; middle layer is brown; inner layer is black; L×W: 24.5×23.6 (22.5–26×22.5–25); L/W ratio: 1.0; M, OR, PG: all absent. Distinctive features of oocyst: trilaminate oocyst wall with inner two layers darker in color than clear outer layer.

Description of sporocyst and sporozoites: Sporocyst shape: subspheroidal to slightly ellipsoidal (line drawing); L×W: 12.6×9.2 (12–14×8.5–10); L/W ratio: 1.4; SB, SSB, PSB: all absent; SR: present; SR characteristics: composed of disbursed granules; SZ: comma-shaped, each with two RB, a larger one at the rounded end, and a smaller one at the pointed end; N: not visible. Distinctive features of sporocyst: subspheroidal to slightly ellipsoidal shape and lack of SB, SSB, and PSB.

Prevalence: Oocysts were found in 10/24 (42%) fecal samples from the type host, but only 3 of the 10 samples had viable oocysts that sporulated.

Sporulation: Oocysts sporulated in 1–3 days at 25 °C while in 2.5% (w/v) potassium dichromate solution (Bennett and Hobbs, 2011).

Prepatent and patent periods: Unknown.

Site of infection: Unknown, oocysts were recovered from the feces.

Endogenous stages: Unknown.

Cross-transmission: None to date.

Pathology: Unknown.

Materials deposited: Photomicrographs of sporulated oocysts are deposited in the United States National Parasite Collection, Beltsville, Maryland as USNPC No. 104697 and in the Australian Registry of Wildlife Health, Toronga Zoo, Mosman, New South Wales as ARWH No. 8015.1.

Etymology: The specific epithet *quenda* is the Nyoongar word (local Australian aboriginal) for *I. obesulus*.

Remarks: Oocysts of this species are about 30% larger than those of *Eimeria kanyana* (below), the only other eimerian described from peramelid marsupials; additionally, its oocysts lack a PG, and its sporocysts lack an SB, both present in *E. kanyana*. Bennett and Hobbs (2011) noted that the juvenile male *I. obesulus*, whose feces contained the oocysts described in their paper, had a male pouch-mate, whose feces also contained oocysts of *E. quenda*, as did the mother's feces.

GENUS *PERAMELES* É. GEOFFROY, 1804 (4 SPECIES)

EIMERIA KANYANA BENNETT, WOOLFORD, O'HARA, NICHOLLS, WARREN, AND HOBBS, 2006

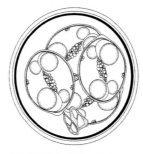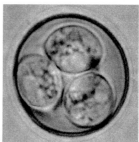

FIGURES 5.3, 5.4 **5.3.** Line drawing of the sporulated oocyst of *Eimeria kanyana*. **5.4.** Photomicrograph of a sporulated oocyst of *E. kanyana*. Both figures from Bennett et al., 2011, with permission from the Editor of the *Journal of Parasitology*.

Type host: *Perameles bougainville* Quoy and Gaimard, 1824, Western Barred Bandicoot.

Type locality: AUSTRALIA: Western Australia: Gooseberry Hill, Kanyana Wildlife Rehabilitation Center (31° 57' S, 116° 03' E).

Other hosts: None to date.

Geographic distribution: AUSTRALIA: Western Australia.

Description of sporulated oocyst: Oocyst shape: spheroidal to subspheroidal; number of walls: 3; wall characteristics: ~1.0 (0.7–1.3) thick; outer wall smooth, yellow; middle layer is brown; inner layer is black; L x W: 18.8 × 17.9 (17–21 × 16–20); L/W ratio: 1.05 (1.0–1.2); M, OR: both absent, PG: present, small, refractile. Distinctive features of oocyst: tri-laminate oocyst wall with inner two layers darker in color than the clear outer layer, plus the presence of a refractile PG.

Description of sporocyst and sporozoites: Sporocyst shape: slightly ovoidal; L x W: 9.1 × 7.0 (8–11 × 6–9); L/W ratio: 1.3; SB: present as a small knoblike structure at slightly pointed end of sporocyst; SSB, PSB: both absent; SR: present; SR characteristics: a cluster of granules between and around SZ; SZ: comma-shaped, each with two spheroidal RB, a larger one at the rounded end and a smaller one at the pointed end; N: not visible. Distinctive features of sporocyst: slightly ovoidal shape and the presence of a small SB.

Prevalence: Oocysts of this species were found in 10/17 (59%) bandicoots including 5/9 (55%) in a captive breeding colony at the Kanyana Wildlife Rehabilitation Center Inc.; in 1/1 in a captive breeding colony in the Dryandra Woodland (32° 46′ S, 116° 58′ E); in 1/3 (33%) in their natural range on Dorre Island (25° 03′ S, 113° 06′ E); and in 3/4 (75%) in a reintroduced colony in Heirisson Prong (26° 02′ S, 113° 22′ E).

Sporulation: Oocysts sporulated in 2–5 days at 25 °C while in 2.5% (w/v) potassium dichromate solution (Bennett et al., 2006).

Prepatent and patent periods: Unknown.

Site of infection: Unknown, oocysts were recovered from the feces.

Endogenous stages: Unknown.

Cross-transmission: None to date.

Pathology: Bennett et al. (2006) suggested that this eimerian parasite "is likely to be only mildly pathogenic."

Materials deposited: A series of three photomicrographs of sporulated oocysts (syntypes) is deposited in the United States National Parasite Collection, Beltsville, Maryland as USNPC

No. 097437.00 and in the Australian Registry of Wildlife Health, Taronga Zoo, Mosman, New South Wales, Australia as ARWH 5055.1.

Etymology: The specific epithet *kanyana* acknowledges Kanyana Wildlife Rehabilitation Center Inc. Kanyana means "gathering place" or "place of the waters" in an Australian aboriginal language.

Remarks: At the time, this was the first formal description of an *Eimeria* species from any member of the order Peramelemorphia. The Western Barred Bandicoot is an endangered Australian marsupial; it has persisted in natural populations only on Bernier and Dorre Islands, Shark Bay, Western Australia. Feces from routine monitoring of captive breeding colonies and wild populations were found to contain the oocysts described by Bennett et al. (2006).

DISCUSSION AND SUMMARY

Only 2 of the 19 extant (10.5%) species, in 2 of the 7 (28.5%) extant genera in this order have been checked for eimeriid coccidia, and these are noted above. Although both surveys had reasonable-to-modest sample sizes (24 and 17 animals, respectively), to my knowledge, this is the only work ever done on these widespread omnivorous marsupials. There are no eimeriid coccidia described from the following peramelemorphia families (-idae), subfamilies (-inae), and genera (species number): Thylacomyidae: *Macrotis* (1); Permelidae: Peramelinae: *Isoodon* (2 of 3), *Permeles* (3 of 4); Peroryctinae: *Peroryctes* (2); Echymiperinae: *Echymipera* (5), *Microperoryctes* (3), *Rhynchomeles* (1); and Chaeropodidae: *Chaeropus* (1); it should be noted that the only species in this family, *Chaeropus ecaudatus* (Ogilby, 1838), the Pig-footed Bandicoot, is likely extinct, with the last known specimen taken in 1907 (Groves, 2005). The **IUCN** also lists it as extinct.

This seems such a tractable group to work with because of the small number of species in this marsupial order, that it presents a wonderful opportunity for a young undergraduate or Masters student in parasitology to take on a survey of all species in the order to gain a better understanding of the true apicomplexan biodiversity that likely exists within these species. One of the beauties of working with the intestinal coccidia is that they are the ideal candidates for surveying a group with many threatened and endangered species, because they can be collected easily by noninvasive collections of fecal material. If the previous two surveys are any indication of prevalence (20/41 (49%)) of coccidia in the feces, there should be a plethora of new species and new information to be discovered!

MARSUPIAL ORDERS WITHOUT EIMERIIDAE

Four of the seven marsupial orders have no eimeriid coccidia described from them; this seems almost unbelievable to me.

Paucituberculata. This order comprises a small, homogeneous group of about six extant species (three genera) called shrew- or rat-opossums, or caenolestids, that are confined to the Andes Mountains of South America. Much like their placental shrew cousins, they are mostly carnivorous and active hunters known to consume insects, earthworms, and small mammals. They are thought to be an ancient group of small animals that live in the grasslands and forests of the high Andes, which is the main reason that so little is known about them. Even less is known about their parasites. To my knowledge, there are no reports that any of these species have been examined for any kind of apicomplexan (or other) parasites. It would take some effort to get to their rugged habitat(s) and to trap them, but what a great opportunity to be the first person to discover what new and exciting kinds of parasites they have, and most likely discover new species of shrew opossums!

Microbiotheria. This order is comprised of one vulnerable (IUCN) extant species called the Monito del Monte, that lives on Chiloe Island, Chile. It was once included in the Didelphimorphia along with the American opossums, but recent molecular work and older fossil evidence (from South America, Australia, western Antarctica) now indicate it is more closely related to the Australian marsupials (see Chapter 2). To my knowledge, the only time this species was examined for parasites was when blood samples of 77 specimens of this single species were collected and examined for DNA and blood parasites (Merino et al., 2009); 35/73 (48%) were found to harbor what was initially thought to be an intraerythrocytic *Hepatozoon* species. However, molecular analysis suggested this may be an, as yet, unnamed genus and species of parasite that is closely related to the Sarcocystidae (see Chapters 7, 10). Since 77 animals were collected, ear-tagged, and released, it is not clear to me why feces was not collected so the authors could look for intestinal coccidians of this very rare species.

Notoryctemorphia. This order consists of two rare, extant species of burrowing marsupials that are confined to the deserts of Western Australia. They provide a remarkable example of **convergent evolution** with placental moles (Insectivora), because they spend most of their time underground, as do the insectivorous moles. Like moles, they are blind, with only **vestigial** eyes and no external ears. These marsupial moles do not seem to be closely related to other extant marsupials, having followed their own developmental strategy for at least 50 **MY** (Chapter 2), but to my knowledge, they have never been surveyed for any apicomplexan parasites. We know that placental moles have many intestinal coccidians representing several different genera and many species (Duszynski and Upton, 2000), because their burrows are so conducive to preserve and concentrate oocysts. Thus, I suspect that if these two species could be sampled in their natural habitat, they also might be found to be parasite-rich. Another great project for an aspiring parasitology student!

Dasyuromorphia. This order includes the majority of Australia's carnivorous marsupials, with such forms as numbats, dunnarts, quolls, and the Tasmanian devil. The members of this order were divided into three families with 23 genera comprised of 71 species (Groves, 2005), but recently, Baker et al. (2015) combined morphological, biogeographical, ecological, behavioral, and DNA data, and concluded that the total evidence strongly supports the existence of 15 *Antechinus* species, rather the 10 listed in Groves (2005). Thus, there are now 76 extant dasyuromorph species. It may be of interest to some to note that the "sex-crazed" *Antechinus* species have received a lot of media attention since 2014, because of their two to three week, highly promiscuous, mating season, with coitus lasting for up to 14 hours and both males and females romping from mate to mate (see, www.dailymail.co.uk/sciencetech/ and www.cbsnews.com/news/newly-discovered-marsupials-mate-to-death/ for examples).

The dasyurid marsupials range in size from the narrow-nosed planigale (*Planigale tenuirostris* Troughton, 1928) at the small end (5–10 g), one of the world's smallest mammals, to the Tasmanian devil (*Sarcophilus harrisii* Boitard, 1841), which can weigh up to 10 kg (Obendorf, 1983). Dasyurids primarily eat invertebrates and small vertebrates, but some species also add fruits and vegetables to their diets. The smaller dasyurids like quolls (*Dasyurus* spp.), dunnarts (*Smithopsis* spp.), and antechinuses (*Antechinus* spp.) have only minor variations on a common morphological body theme when compared to their larger herbivorous relatives (e.g., kangaroos). Loss and alteration of habitat due to human colonization and agriculture and the introduction of numerous herbivores (e.g., rabbits, sheep, goats) and nonnative predators (cats, foxes) has severely influenced the quantity and quality of suitable habitats for dasyurids in Australia. Only in the last three decades have we begun to understand the role of their disease-causing apicomplexans.

At least five species in three genera of dasyuromorphids (see Table 11.2) have been documented to have sarcocysts of several unnamed *Sarcocystis* species in their muscles (Chapter 10), and oocysts of one or more unidentified *Cryptosporidium* species have been found in the feces of *Antechinus stuartii* (Barker et al., 1978) and another *Antechinus* sp. (O'Donoghue, 1985), but no eimeriid coccidia have ever been documented from any of the species in this order. *Toxoplasma gondii* or *T.* sp. has been documented from at least 9 genera, including 12 species: *Antechinomys laniger*, *Antechinus minimus*, *Antechinus swainsonii*, *Dasycercus cristicauda*, *Dasyuroides byrnei*, *Dasyurus viverrinus*, *Parantechinus apicalis*, *Phascogale tapoatafa*, *Pseudantechinus macdonnellensis*, *Sminthopsis crassicaudata*, *Sminthopsis leucopus*, and *Sminthopsis macroura*. I think it very unlikely that eimerian, and perhaps isosporan species, do not use these marsupials as host animals. A more likely explanation for the absence of these coccidians from the dasyuromorphids is simply that no one has looked for them in the members of this host lineage. There is still so very much to learn!

Adeleidae in Marsupials

EUCOCCIDIORIDA: ADELEIDAE MESNIL, 1903

INTRODUCTION

At the beginning of Chapter 1, I mentioned the two major suborders of eucoccidian apicomplexans covered in this book, Eimeriorina and Adeleorina, and the life cycle stages in the latter (syzygy, few microgametes) that separate them from members of the Eimeriorina (Upton, 2000). Chapters 3, 4, and 5 cover the *Eimeria* and *Isospora* species in the Eimeriidae (Eimeriorina) that have been reported from marsupials. Here, I detail what little we know about the 11 *Klossiella* species (Adeleorina: Klossiellidae) reported to date from marsupials.

The adeleorine coccidia are the most poorly understood group of parasites within the Apicomplexa, but they are united biologically by their use of **syzygy** during gamete formation (Barta, 2000). These parasites have the typical complex life cycle of other coccidian groups involving at least one (but often several) asexual cycle(s) of merogony followed by gamogony, **syngamy**, and then sporogony. There are about seven families within the Adeleorina, only one of which has species known to infect marsupials and other mammals, Klossiellidae Smith and Johnson, 1902. The family has but 1 genus, *Klossiella* Smith and Johnson, 1902, and it contains about 18 named species that infect primarily mammals, in which it invariably undergoes

asexual and sexual development in the kidneys. For example, *Klossiella muris* is found in the kidneys of *Mus musculus*, *Klossiella cobayae* in the capillaries of the guinea pig (*Cavia porcellus*) kidney, *Klossiella equi* in the kidney of horses and jackasses, and others (Levine, 1973; Levine and Ivens, 1965). Levine and Ivens (1965) reviewed the history of discovery and the known developmental stages of this unusual coccidian. The *Klossiella* species that infect marsupials are presented below via order, family, and genus of the marsupials they have been reported from.

SPECIES DESCRIPTIONS

KLOSSIELLA IN MARSUPIALS

ORDER DIDELPHIMORPHIA GILL, 1872

FAMILY DIDELPHIDAE GRAY, 1821 (17 GENERA, 87 SPECIES)

GENUS DIDELPHIS L., 1758 (6 SPECIES)

KLOSSIELLA TEJERAI SCORZA, TORREALBA, AND DAGERT, 1957

Synonym: *Klossiella* sp. Edgcomb, Walker, and Johnson, 1976.

Type host: *Didelphis marsupialis* (L., 1758), Common Opossum.

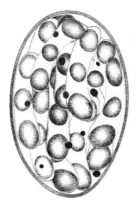
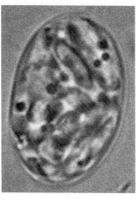

FIGURES 6.1, 6.2   **6.1.** Line drawing of the sporulated sporocyst of *Klossiella tejerai*. **6.2.** Photomicrograph of a sporulated sporocyst of *K. tejerai*. Both figures from Spitz dos Santos et al., 2014, with kind permission from Springer Science + Business Media, publishers of *Systematic Parasitology*.

Type locality: SOUTH AMERICA: Venezuela: Estado Guárico, San Juan de los Morros.

Other hosts: *Didelphis aurita* (Wied-Neuwied, 1826), Big-eared Opossum; *Marmosa murina* (L., 1758) (syns. *Marmosa cinerea demararae*, *Marmosa demerarae*), Linnaeus's Mouse Opossum.

Geographic distribution: CENTRAL AMERICA: Panama; SOUTH AMERICA: French Guiana (?); Venezuela.

Description of sporulated oocyst: Oocyst shape: irregular as it develops endogenously; number of walls: unknown; L × W in situ: 71.6 × 47.2 (57–103 × 36–57) (Spitz dos Santos et al., 2014); L/W ratio: 1.5; M, OR, PG: all absent. Distinctive features of oocyst: very large size as it develops within the epithelial cells of the renal tubules.

Description of sporocyst and sporozoites: Sporocyst shape: ellipsoidal; L × W: 12 × 9; L/W ratio: 1.3 (Scorza et al., 1957) or 20.4 × 12.7 (19–22 × 12–14); L/W ratio 1.6 (1.5–1.8) (Spitz dos Santos et al., 2014); SB, SSB, PSB: all absent; SR: present; SR characteristics: composed of scattered spherules/granules; SZ: 12 (Scorza et al., 1957) or 13 (12–14) (Spitz dos Santos et al., 2014) in each SP; SZs are sausage-shaped, each ~6 × 1, with anterior and posterior RBs, and a central N. Distinctive

features of sporocyst: found in the urine, each has numerous SR spherules with 8–20 SZ, each with two RB and a central N.

Prevalence: Found in 1/1 *D. marsupialis* in Venezuela (Scorza et al., 1957), 4/10 (40%) *D. marsupialis* in Panama (Edgcomb et al., 1975), and in 1/20 (5%) *D. aurita* from Brazil (Spitz dos Santos, 2014).

Sporulation: Endogenous, within a parasitophorous vacuole (PV) inside renal epithelial cells.

Prepatent and patent periods: Unknown.

Site of infection: Merogony, sporogony, and gamogony all take place inside a **PV**, within epithelial cells of renal tubules. Meronts and merozoites occur in the tufts of some glomeruli, and in the proximal convoluted tubules (Boulard, 1975), while gamogony and gamonts are found near the corticomedullary junction of the proximal convoluted tubules and the descending portion of the loop of Henle of the kidney (Spitz dos Santos et al., 2014).

Endogenous stages: Boulard (1975) outlined the endogenous development in the kidney as follows. Merogony occurred in the internal border of Bowman's capsule; the capsule was not deformed, and he presented two clear photomicrographs of developing meronts. Gametogony and sporogony took place in the proximal convoluted tubules, but not in Henle's loop. The meronts were ovoidal, 12–30 × 6–23 in tissue sections and 42–47 × 30–38 in tissue smears. They contained 40–56 merozoites around a central residuum. In tissue smears, the merozoites were 14 × 3, rounded at one end and pointed at the other, with an N nearer the pointed end than the rounded one. The macrogamonts were spheroidal or slightly ovoidal, with a mean diameter of 12, in tissue smears. The microgamonts were ovoidal, 9 × 6, and formed four spheroidal microgametes, ~3 wide, and a residual body. Boulard (1975) saw no flagella on the microgametes. The young oocysts were slightly ovoidal, 8 × 6 in tissue sections and contained in a large PV. The mature oocysts were 80×40 in sections and contained 16–22 sporocysts that measured 17×14 in smears and 14×9 in tissue sections. Each sporocyst contained 14–22 SZ and an SR. SZs were "elongate" with rounded ends and measured 8×15 (sic?) (Likely this was a typographical error for 1.5 as all of his other measurements gave the larger figure first.). Macrogamonts and microgamonts are in syzygy.

Cross-transmission: None to date.

Pathology: Edgcomb et al. (1976) said that "passage of schizonts and merozoites through the glomerular membranes occurs without inflammation and hemorrhage. These forms of the parasites evidently have membranes that permit their passage through the entire glomerular wall with restoration of the wall to an intact functional state after passage." This seems an odd interpretation from observing just a few tissue sections. I can envision how merozoites can penetrate cell membranes, but not "schizonts" (=meronts). They went on to say, "The invasion of tubular epithelial cells by gametes, particularly by macrogametes, is associated with ballooning necrosis of the invaded cells." Spitz dos Santos et al. (2014) cautioned that Edgcomb et al. (1976) may have misinterpreted their photomicrographs.

Materials deposited: Samples of preserved sporocysts (in 10% aqueous buffered formalin and in 70% ethanol) and renal tissue slides are deposited in the Parasitology Collection of the Laboratório de Coccídios e Coccidioses, Universidade Federal Rural do Rio de Janeiro, Municipality of Seropedica, Rio de Janerio, Brazil; photovouchers and line drawings are deposited and available (http://rl.ufrrj.br/lcc) all with the repository number 53/2014 (Spitz dos Santos et al., 2014).

Etymology: The species name was proposed in honor of Doctor Enrique Tejera (Scorza et al., 1957).

Remarks: Edgcomb et al. (1976) found what was presumably *Klossiella tejerai* in *D. marsupialis* in Panama.

GENUS MARMOSA GRAY, 1821 (9 SPECIES)

KLOSSIELLA TEJERAI SCORZA, TORREALBA, AND DAGERT, 1957

Type host: *Didelphis marsupialis* L., 1758, Common Opossum.

Remarks: Boulard (1975) said he found this species in the "Mouse Opossum," which he identified as *Marmosa cinerea demararae*, from French Guiana. I cannot find this species listed in any form in Wilson and Reeder (2005, vol. 1, or in their online updates: http://www.vertebrates.si.edu/msw/mswcfapp/msw/index.cfm); however, the species likely was *M. murina*, the only Mouse Opossum currently documented in French Guiana. Other information from Boulard (1975) on the endogenous development is included in the description details, above.

ORDER DIPROTODONTIA OWEN, 1866

FAMILY MACROPODIDAE GRAY, 1821 (11 GENERA, 65 SPECIES)

GENUS LAGORCHESTES GOULD, 1841 (4 SPECIES)

KLOSSIELLA BEVERIDGEI BARKER, MUNDAY, AND HARTLEY, 1985

Figures: For LM photomicrographs of gametes, sporoblasts, and sporocysts of *Klossiella beveridgei* within the loop of Henle in the kidney, see Barker et al. (1985; their Figure 4).

Type host: *Lagorchestes conspicillatus* (Gould, 1842), Spectacled Hare-Wallaby.

Type locality: AUSTRALIA: Queensland: Rubyvale.

Other hosts: None to date.

Geographic distribution: AUSTRALIA: Queensland.

Description of sporulated oocyst: No oocysts were seen.

Description of sporocyst and sporozoites: Sporocysts (or sporoblasts) in tissue sections were 10×4.

Prevalence: Barker et al. (1985) did not mention the number of wallabies examined nor the number infected.

Sporulation: Endogenous, within the host cells.

Prepatent and patent periods: Unknown.

Site of infection: In the cells of thin tubules, the loop of Henle, in the inner renal cortex.

Endogenous stages: Macrogametes were 6 wide, had a prominent, pinpoint, basophilic N (in tissue section), and were found in a PV up to 14 wide. Early sporonts were 14 wide. Up to 24 sporoblasts (sporocysts) were found in a single tissue section of a vacuole in a host cell.

Cross-transmission: None to date.

Pathology: The authors said that no inflammatory host reaction was evident (Barker et al., 1985).

Materials deposited: None.

Etymology: This species was named for Dr Ian Beveridge, who first recognized it (Barker et al., 1985).

Remarks: Only the descriptive parameters detailed above, and one photomicrograph (their Figure 4) of gametes, sporoblasts, and sporocysts in a loop of Henle, led Barker et al. (1985) to call this form a new species. Their argument was similar to the one they used a decade earlier (Barker et al., 1975), that "morphologic variations, differences in location within the host, and taxonomic and ecologic separation of hosts are considered, in combination, to justify erection of new species, in the absence of information that cross-infection between hosts may occur." Following this justification, they addressed the issue of *Klossiella* infecting several families of marsupials in Australia, and being found in American opossums. They suggested that the association of *Klossiella* species with many host species may be ancient, antedating the break up of Gondwonaland, and showing that the genus has undergone a wide range of radiation among marsupials paralleling the evolution of their hosts.

GENUS MACROPUS SHAW, 1790 (14 SPECIES)

KLOSSIELLA CALLITRIS BARKER, MUNDAY, AND HARRIGAN, 1975

Figures: For LM photomicrographs of micro- and macrogametes of *Klossiella callitris* within the loop of Henle in the kidney, see Barker et al. (1975; their Figure 7).

Type host: *Macropus fuliginosus melanops* (Desmarest, 1817), Western Grey Kangaroo.

Type locality: AUSTRALIA: Victoria: Pine Plains Station, via Patchewollock.

Other hosts: None to date.

Geographic distribution: AUSTRALIA: Victoria.

Description of sporulated oocyst: No oocysts were seen.

Description of sporocyst and sporozoites: Mature sporocysts were seen in a single host kidney cell, the PV of which was distended, ~14×6, and contained SZs. No other structural information was given.

Prevalence: Barker et al. (1975) found this species in 5/6 (83%) *Macropus fuliginosus* from Victoria.

Sporulation: Endogenous, within the host cells.

Prepatent and patent periods: Unknown.

Site of infection: All stages, from gametocytes to sporocysts, were found in cells of the thin loop of Henle in the medulla, but not extending into the papilla of the kidney.

Endogenous stages: Single macrogametes were 7×5.5 wide; frequently, one to three macrogametes, ~3 wide, were seen in the same PV. Sporonts were ~35×25 wide, and sporogony occurred by budding from their periphery. Often up to 20–25 sporoblasts or mature sporocysts with SZs were seen in a single host cell.

Cross-transmission: None to date.

Pathology: Unknown.

Materials deposited: None.

Etymology: The authors proposed this species name after *Callitris* sp., the Murray Pine, "the local prevalence of which suggested the name of the type locality" (Barker et al., 1975).

Remarks: Barker et al. (1975) examined the kidney tissues of 137 marsupials representing 18 species in 16 genera of 6 families and found 14 animals (10%) representing 6 species, each in a separate genus, to harbor a *Klossiella* species. They decided to name the stages seen in four of the six host genus/species as new, based on the level of nephron infected, number of sporocysts produced per sporont, and on the relative ecologic or phylogenetic isolation of these hosts from one another. Only the stages in *Potorous apicalis*, the Southern Potoroo from Winkleigh, Tasmania, lacked sufficient distinction to be given a name.

KLOSSIELLA RUFI BARKER, MUNDAY, AND HARTLEY, 1985

Figures: For LM photomicrographs of macrogametes of *Klossiella rufi* within the loop of Henle in the kidney, see Barker et al. (1985; their Figure 2).

Type host: *Macropus rufus* (Desmarest, 1822), Red Kangaroo.

Type locality: AUSTRALIA: New South Wales: Olive Downs, near Tibooburra.

Other hosts: None to date.

Geographic distribution: AUSTRALIA: New South Wales.

Description of sporulated oocyst: No oocysts were seen.

Description of sporocyst and sporozoites: Mature sporocysts were not seen.

Prevalence: Barker et al. (1985) made no mention of how many *M. rufus* they examined from New South Wales nor how many were infected.

Sporulation: Endogenous, within the host cells.

Prepatent and patent periods: Unknown.

Site of infection: Cells lining the thin tubules of the loops of Henle in the medullary rays of the inner and outer cortex.

Endogenous stages: Numerous gametes and sporogonous stages were seen in the inner and outer cortex of the kidney. Macrogametes were 6–8 wide and located in PVs, ~30 wide. Sporonts with early sporoblast development at the periphery were 18 wide. About 20 sporoblasts, 12 × 4, were in a single PV within a host cell.

Cross-transmission: None to date.

Pathology: Barker et al. (1985) saw scattered mild infiltrates of plasma cells and eosinophils in the renal cortical interstitium.

Materials deposited: None.

Remarks: With only the descriptive parameters noted above, and one photomicrograph (their Figure 2) of macrogametes in PVs, Barker et al. (1985) called this form a new species. Their argument was similar to the one they used earlier (Barker et al., 1975), that "morphologic variations, differences in location within the host, and taxonomic and ecologic separation of hosts are considered, in combination, to justify erection of new species, in the absence of information that cross-infection between hosts may occur." Following this justification, they addressed the issue of *Klossiella* infecting several families of marsupials in Australia and being found in American opossums. This tie to the Americas led them to suggest that the association of *Klossiella* species with many marsupial species may be ancient, antedating the break up of Gondwanaland and showing that the genus has undergone a wide range of radiation among marsupials paralleling the evolution of their hosts.

KLOSSIELLA RUFOGRISEI BARKER, MUNDAY, AND HARTLEY, 1985

Figures: For LM photomicrographs of microgametes and macrogametes of *Klossiella rufogrisei* within a tubule of the kidney, see Barker et al. (1985; their Figure 1).

Type host: *Macropus rufogriseus* (Desmarest, 1817), Bennett's or Red-necked Wallaby.

Type locality: AUSTRALIA: Tasmania: Blackwood Creek.

Other hosts: None to date.

Geographic distribution: AUSTRALIA: Tasmania.

Description of sporulated oocyst: No oocysts were seen.

Description of sporocyst and sporozoites: Mature sporocysts were not seen.

Prevalence: Barker et al. (1985) made no mention of how many *M. rufogriseus* they examined from Tasmania, nor how many were infected.

Sporulation: Endogenous, within the host cells.

Prepatent and patent periods: Unknown.

Site of infection: Endothelium of interstitial capillaries in the renal cortex and in the epithelium of the thin loop of Henle in the inner cortical and outer medullary areas of the kidney.

Endogenous stages: A single meront in an endothelial cell of an interstitial capillary was 16×6. Numerous gametes were seen in the epithelium of the thin loop of Henle. Macrogametes in vacuoles, ~12 across in the host cell cytoplasm, were ~8 wide with an eccentrically placed N. Microgametes were up to 2.5 wide, and usually two or four were in the PV containing a macrogamete. Immature sporonts were ~18 wide, while those budding peripheral sporoblasts were up to 26 wide. More than 20 sporoblasts, 8×2, were seen in a single PV.

Cross-transmission: None to date.

Pathology: No inflammatory reaction was noted by the authors.

Materials deposited: None.

Remarks: With only the descriptive parameters detailed above and one photomicrograph (their Figure 1) of several microgametes along with one macrogamete in a PV led Barker et al. (1985) to call this form a new species. Their argument was similar to the one noted previously, that "morphologic variations, differences in location within the host, and taxonomic and ecologic separation of hosts are considered, in combination, to justify erection of new species, in the absence of information that cross-infection between hosts

may occur." And, again, they suggested that the association of *Klossiella* species within marsupials in both America and Australia is ancient, antedating the break up of Gondwonaland, and showing that the genus has undergone a wide range of radiation among marsupials paralleling the evolution of their hosts.

GENUS *THYLOGALE* GRAY, 1837 (7 SPECIES)

KLOSSIELLA THYLOGALE BARKER, MUNDAY, AND HARTLEY, 1985

Figures: For LM photomicrographs of sporonts, sporoblasts, sporocysts, and macrogametes of *Klossiella thylogale* within the kidney, see Barker et al. (1985; their Figure 3).

Type host: *Thylogale billardierii* (Desmarest, 1822), Red-bellied or Tasmanian Pademelon.

Type locality: AUSTRALIA: Tasmania: Woodsdale.

Other hosts: None to date.

Geographic distribution: AUSTRALIA: Tasmania.

Description of sporulated oocyst: No oocysts were seen.

Description of sporocyst and sporozoites: Mature sporocysts in tissue sections were 16×8, and contained >20 small, thin SZ nuclei.

Prevalence: Barker et al. (1985) mentioned neither how many animals were examined, nor how many were infected.

Sporulation: Endogenous, within the host cells.

Prepatent and patent periods: Unknown.

Site of infection: Within the tubular epithelium of the inner cortex at the corticomedullary junction of the kidney.

Endogenous stages: Macrogametes were 8 wide, and were present in PVs, ~12–14, along with one or two microgametes. Sporonts had sporoblasts that were budded peripherally and measured ~34 wide. Up to 16 sporoblasts, 14×6, were observed to develop in a single infected host cell.

Cross-transmission: None to date.

Pathology: No inflammatory response was evident to Barker et al. (1985).

Materials deposited: None.

Remarks: Only the descriptive parameters detailed above, and one photomicrograph (their Figure 3) of macrogametes, a sporont, sporoblasts, and a sporocyst in a PV, led Barker et al. (1985) to call this form a new species. Their argument for doing so, along with the issue of *Klossiella* being found in both American and Australian marsupials in different orders has been presented several times (above).

GENUS *WALLABIA* TROUESSART, 1905 (MONOTYPIC)

KLOSSIELLA SERENDIPENSIS BARKER, MUNDAY, AND HARRIGAN, 1975

Figures: For LM photomicrographs of early sporont, micro- and macrogamete of *Klossiella serendipensis* within cells in the proximal convoluted tubule of the kidney, see Barker et al. (1975; their Figure 6).

Type host: *Wallabia bicolor* (Desmarest, 1804), Swamp Wallaby.

Type locality: AUSTRALIA: Victoria: Lara, at the Serendip Research Station of the Victoria Department of Fisheries and Wildlife.

Other hosts: None to date.

Geographic distribution: AUSTRALIA: Victoria.

Description of sporulated oocyst: No oocysts were seen.

Description of sporocyst and sporozoites: No sporocysts were seen in the tissues.

Prevalence: Barker et al. (1975) found this species in 1/2 (50%) *W. bicolor* from Lara, Victoria.

Sporulation: Endogenous, within the host cells.

Prepatent and patent periods: Unknown.

Site of infection: Epithelial cells of proximal convoluted tubules of the kidney of one animal.

Endogenous stages: Macrogametes were the only endogenous stage observed; they were ~7 wide in the PVs that measured 25 × 15. No other structural information was given by the authors concerning this form.

Cross-transmission: None to date.

Pathology: Unknown.

Materials deposited: None.

Etymology: The authors derived the specific epitaph of this species from the research station where the infected Swamp Wallaby had been maintained for several years (Barker et al., 1975).

Remarks: Barker et al. (1975) examined the kidney tissues of 137 marsupials representing 18 species, in 16 genera, of 6 families, and found 14 animals (10%) representing 6 species, each in a separate genus, to harbor a *Klossiella* species. They decided to name the stages seen in four of the six host genus/species as new based on the level of nephron infected, number of sporocysts produced per sporont, and on the relative ecologic or phylogenetic isolation of these hosts from one another. Only the endogenous stages in the kidney of *P. apicalis*, the Southern Potoroo from Tasmania, lacked sufficient distinction to be given a name.

FAMILY POTOROIDAE GRAY, 1821 (4 GENERA, 10 SPECIES)

GENUS *BETTONGIA* GRAY, 1837 (4 SPECIES)

KLOSSIELLA BETTONGIAE BARKER, MUNDAY, AND HARTLEY, 1985

Figures: For LM photomicrographs of macrogametes of *Klossiella bettongiae* within epithelial cells of convoluted tubules throughout the renal cortex of the kidney, see Barker et al. (1985; their Figures 5 and 6).

Type host: *Bettongia gaimardi* (Desmarest, 1822), Tasmanian or Eastern Bettong.

Type locality: AUSTRALIA: Tasmania: Blessington.

Other hosts: None to date.

Geographic distribution: AUSTRALIA: Tasmania.

Description of sporulated oocyst: No oocysts were seen.

Description of sporocyst and sporozoites: Sporocysts in one tissue section were 16 × 4, and each contained >20 SZ nuclei within a vacuole up to 60 across.

Prevalence: Barker et al. (1985) neglected to mention the number of Bettongs examined and the number found to be infected.

Sporulation: Endogenous, within the host cells.

Prepatent and patent periods: Unknown.

Site of infection: In the epithelium of convoluted tubules throughout the renal cortex.

Endogenous stages: Macrogametes were 8–10 wide, found in PVs up to 20 across. Other than sections of sporocysts (above), no other parasite stages were seen.

Cross-transmission: None to date.

Pathology: No host reaction was noted by Barker et al. (1985).

Materials deposited: None.

Remarks: Only the descriptive parameters detailed above, and two photomicrographs (their Figures 5 and 6) of macrogametes and sporocysts in convoluted tubules, led Barker et al. (1985) to call this form a new species.

FAMILY PSEUDOCHEIRIDAE WINGE, 1893 (6 GENERA, 17 SPECIES)

GENUS *PETAUROIDES* THOMAS, 1888 (MONOTYPIC)

KLOSSIELLA SCHOINOBATIS BARKER, MUNDAY, AND HARTLEY, 1985

Figures: For LM photomicrographs of gametes of *Klossiella schoinobatis* within the loop of Henle in the kidney, see Barker et al. (1985; their Figure 7).

Type host: *Petauroides volans* (Kerr, 1792), Greater Glider.

Type locality: AUSTRALIA: New South Wales: near Wee Jasper.

Other hosts: None to date.

Geographic distribution: AUSTRALIA: New South Wales.

Description of sporulated oocyst: No oocysts were seen.

Description of sporocyst and sporozoites: Sporocysts in tissue sections were 12 × 4 and contained >12 SZ nuclei per tissue section.

Prevalence: Barker et al. (1985) did not mention the number of gliders examined nor the number infected with this form.

Sporulation: Endogenous, within the host cells.

Prepatent and patent periods: Unknown.

Site of infection: Within cells of the loop of Henle in the medullary rays of the renal cortex and near the cortiomedullary junction.

Endogenous stages: Gametes and sporogonous stages were sparsely scattered in host cells. Macrogametes were ~6 wide, and accompanying microgametes were in vacuoles, ~8–12 across. Early sporonts were 16–18 wide and up to 16 sporocysts were seen in a single host cell.

Cross-transmission: None to date.

Pathology: Barker et al. (1985) said that a host reaction to the parasite was not evident.

Materials deposited: None.

Remarks: The descriptive parameters detailed above, and one photomicrograph (their Figure 7) of only gametes in a loop of Henle, led Barker et al. (1985) to call this form a new species. Their argument was similar to the one already mentioned above.

GENUS *PSEUDOCHEIRUS* OGILBY, 1837 (MONOTYPIC)

KLOSSIELLA CONVOLUTOR BARKER, MUNDAY, AND HARRIGAN, 1975

Figures: For LM photomicrographs of a sporont and a macrogamete of *Klossiella convolutor* developing in a secondary tubule of the kidney, see Barker et al. (1975; their Figure 4).

Type host: *Pseudocheirus peregrinus* (Boddaert, 1785), Common Ringtail.

Type locality: AUSTRALIA: Tasmania: Prospect.

Other hosts: None to date.

Geographic distribution: AUSTRALIA: Tasmania; Victoria.

Description of sporulated oocyst: No oocysts were seen.

Description of sporocyst and sporozoites: Undeveloped sporocysts (sporoblasts), sometimes up to seven, were seen in PVs in the tissue of the kidneys and measured 11×7. No other structural information was given.

Prevalence: Barker et al. (1975) found this species in 2/6 (33%) *P. peregrinus* from Tasmania and Victoria.

Sporulation: Unknown.

Prepatent and patent periods: Unknown.

Site of infection: Found in cells lining the loop of Henle near the corticomedullary junction of the kidneys.

Endogenous stages: Macrogametes, ~6 wide, were contained in a PV, ~16 wide. Occasionally, a microgamete was seen in the same vacuole. Early sporonts, ~12–13 wide, contained four to six peripheral N. No other developmental information was given.

Cross-transmission: None to date.

Pathology: Barker et al. (1975) saw no host reaction around the stages they found in the loop of Henle kidney cells.

Materials deposited: None.

Etymology: The authors gave the specific epitaph of this species after the subspecific name of the Tasmanian ringtail opossum (Barker et al., 1975).

Remarks: Baker et al. (1975) examined the kidney tissues of 137 marsupials representing 18 species in 16 genera of 6 families and found 14 animals (10%) representing 6 species, each in a separate genus, to harbor a *Klossiella* species. They decided to name the stages seen in four of the six host genus/species as new based on the level of nephron infected, number of sporocysts produced per sporont, and on the relative ecologic or phylogenetic isolation of these hosts from one another. The stages they saw in *P. apicalis*, the Southern Potoroo from Winkleigh, Tasmania, lacked sufficient distinction to be given a name.

ORDER PERAMELEMORPHIA AMEGHINO, 1889

FAMILY PERAMELIDAE GRAY, 1825 (6 GENERA, 18 SPECIES)

GENUS *ISOODON* DESMAREST, 1817 (3 SPECIES)

KLOSSIELLA QUIMRENSIS BARKER, MUNDAY, AND HARRIGAN, 1975

Figures: For LM photomicrographs of sporonts, sporoblasts, sporocysts, microgametes, and macrogametes of *Klossiella quimrensis* within the kidney tissue, see Barker et al. (1975; their Figures 1–3) and Bennett et al. (2007; their Figures 1–3).

Synonym: *Klossiella* sp. of Derrick and Smith in Mackerras et al. (1953).

Type host: *Isoodon obesulus* (Shaw, 1797), Southern Brown Bandicoot.

Type locality: AUSTRALIA: Tasmania: Maria Island.

Other hosts: *Perameles gunnii* Gray, 1838, Eastern Barred Bandicoot; *Perameles bougainville* Quoy and Gaimard, 1824, Western Barred Bandicoot.

Geographic distribution: AUSTRALIA: Tasmania; Western Australia.

Description of sporulated oocyst: No oocysts have been described to date.

Description of sporocyst and sporozoites: Bennett et al. (2007) reported seeing only one unsporulated sporocyst in the urine of *P. bougainville*, and described it as ellipsoidal, 17 × 11, with a rough, dark outer wall and an MP at the more acutely tapered pole. Mature sporocysts have only been seen and reported in tissue sections by Barker et al. (1975, see below).

Prevalence: Barker et al. (1975) found this species in 1/2 (50%) *I. obesulus*, and in 3/14 (21%) *P. gunnii* on Maria Island, Tasmania; Bennett et al. (2007) found tissue stages in the kidneys of 6/20 (30%) *P. bougainville* in Western Australia.

Sporulation: Occurs endogenously, within the host.

Prepatent and patent periods: Unknown.

Site of infection: Found in cells lining the thin tubules of the loop of Henle in the kidneys by Barker et al. (1975) and within PVs of epithelial cells located near the renal corticomedullary junction by Bennett et al. (2007).

Endogenous stages: Barker et al. (1975) found stages, from gametocytes to mature sporocysts, in PVs in pedunculated cells of the thin loops of Henle, especially in the papillary border of the medulla in the kidneys. Frequently, >20 sporoblasts or crenated sporocysts, 11 × 5.5, were seen in a large PV. Mature sporocysts contained numerous elongate, closely packed SZs. Macrogametes, ~7 wide, with a single basophilic N, and found in a PV ~four times larger, sometimes contained a microgamete, ~1.5 wide. Mature sporonts were ~30 wide. The sporonts formed many sporoblasts, which were initially 7 × 3, and developed many N from which SZs developed. Meronts and merogony apparently were not observed.

Bennett et al. (2007) found only sporonts, sporoblasts, and macrogametes in the tissues they examined. Sporonts were round to ovoidal, ~25 wide, and had 12–16 deeply basophilic N around the circumference. These N apparently bud from the sporont, producing ovoidal sporoblasts, 5 × 7.5, arranged around a residual body of amorphous cytoplasm. Mature sporoblasts were ovoidal, 10 × 7.5, with multiple basophilic N. Mature sporoblasts within PVs ranged from 7 to 24. Macrogametes were round to ovoidal, 8.5 wide, and were contained within round-to-irregular PVs up to 23 wide. Bennett et al. (2007) never saw microgametes in the tissues they examined.

Cross-transmission: None to date.

Pathology: Barker et al. (1975) saw no host reaction around the gamonts, zygotes, or oocysts. Bennett et al. (2007) confirmed the observation (Barker et al., 1975) stating that PVs containing developmental stages were not associated with any adjacent host inflammatory response, and that the focally moderate parasite burden they observed would not, of themselves, severely compromise renal function in these bandicoots.

Materials deposited: None by the original authors (Barker et al., 1975), but Bennett et al. (2007) deposited renal tissue slides of *P. bougainville* infected with *K. quimrensis* with the Australian Registry of Wildlife Health, Taronga Zoo, Mosman, New South Wales, Australia as ARWH 5055.2.

Etymology: Barker et al. (1975) gave the specific epitaph of this species based on the acronym QIMB for Queensland Institute of Medical Research where Derek and Smith (presumably) first observed it.

Remarks: Baker et al. (1975) examined the kidney tissues of 137 marsupials representing 18 species in 16 genera of 6 families and found 14 animals representing 6 species, each in a separate genus, to harbor a *Klossiella* species. They decided to name the stages seen in four of the six host genus/species as new based on the level of the nephron infected, number of sporocysts produced per sporont, and on the relative ecologic or phylogenetic isolation of these hosts from one another.

GENUS PERAMELES GEOFFROY, 1804 (4 SPECIES)

KLOSSIELLA QUIMRENSIS BARKER, MUNDAY, AND HARRIGAN, 1975

Type host: *Isoodon obesulus* (Shaw, 1797), Southern Brown Bandicoot.

Remarks: Baker et al. (1975) also identified what they believed to be stages of *K. quimrensis* in *P. gunnii*. They said that the morphology and development of the organism in *P. gunnii* resembled that seen in *I. obesulus*, and since the hosts are closely related and, in some areas sympatric, they proposed to consider that both hosts harbored the same species of *Klossiella*.

KLOSSIELLA QUIMRENSIS BARKER, MUNDAY, AND HARRIGAN, 1975

Type host: *Isoodon obesulus* (Shaw, 1797), Southern Brown Bandicoot.

Remarks: Bennett et al. (2007) said they observed *K. quimrensis* in 6/20 (30%) Western Barred Bandicoots, *P. bougainville*, from Western Australia, because their observations were so similar to those of Barker et al. (1975). They described sporonts, sporoblasts, and macrogametes in kidney tissue sections and noted one unsporulated sporocyst in the urine, and all of these are noted in the full description for *K. quimrensis*, above. They reasoned that *P. bougainville* once occurred across much of mainland Australia, but that its range declined severely because of habitat destruction and introduced predators. Thus, it was likely sympatric with *I. obesulus* in New South Wales, Victoria, South Australia, and Western Australia. The similarities in morphology of life cycle stages in the kidney and the historic overlap of natural ranges led them (Bennett et al., 2007) to propose that *K. quimrensis* was the etiological agent they found in the kidneys of *P. bougainville*.

DISCUSSION AND SUMMARY

To date, there are about 18 named species of *Klossiella* that have been reported in three eutherian orders, Perissodactyla, Rodentia, and Chiroptera (Levine, 1988), and in three marsupial orders, Didelphimorphia, Diprotodontia, and Peramelemorphia (Tables 11.1 and 11.2). Eleven of the 18 (61%) named *Klossiella* species are found in marsupials, 10 of which occur in Australian marsupials; and there are three other references to unnamed *Klossiella* species being reported in the long-nosed or Southern Potoroo, *Potorous tridactylus*, by Barker et al. (1975), in the Long-nosed Bandicoot, *Perameles nasuta*, by Mackerras (1958), and in the Herbert River Ringtail, *Pseudochirulus herbertensis*, by Speare et al. (1984), but these were never described in any detail, or named, so they must be relegated to *species inquirendae* (see Chapter 10, Tables 11.1 and 11.2).

Given what is presented in this chapter, it is evident that studying *Klossiella* in marsupials, whether in Australia or the Americas, is an area ripe with potential rewards for new information. Parasitologists should begin to incorporate collecting urine into their field protocols so that we can gain a sense of what oocysts and sporocysts of *Klossiella* really look like, and what variation can exist among the various species. Collecting kidney and related tissue samples for squash preparations/smears to be stained, and blocks of kidney to be fixed, embedded, sectioned, and prepared for histological examination will be critical. It will be an innovative milestone when someone can infect several specimens of a marsupial species with oocysts/sporocysts, and then trace the sequential development over time of a complete life cycle within their kidneys. And, of course, it is imperative that DNA be collected and sequenced in the future, so that we gain an exact sense of the nature and affinity of these very interesting parasites—about which we know so little—to other species groups of the Apicomplexa: Eucoccidiorida. There are certainly a vast number of potential and obvious research projects available within this system to explore and problems to solve. This presents a wonderful opportunity, especially for graduate students who are teaching, to recruit and interest undergraduates to help them with both field and lab work.

Sarcocystidae: Sarcocystinae (*Sarcocystis*) in Marsupials

The Biology and Identification of the Coccidia (Apicomplexa) of Marsupials of the World
http://dx.doi.org/10.1016/B978-0-12-802709-7.00007-2

EUCOCCIDIORIDA: EIMERIORINA: SARCOCYSTIDAE

INTRODUCTION

A second major family within the Eimeriorina, Sarcocystidae Poche, 1913, has two subfamilies, Sarcocystinae Poche, 1913 (*Sarcocystis, Frankelia*) and Toxoplasmatinae Biocca, 1957 (*Besnoitia, Hammondia, Neospora, Toxoplasma*). Members of the Sarcocystinae reported from marsupials are given in this chapter; as far as I know, there are no *Frankelia* species known in marsupials so all of the organisms covered here are *Sarcocystis* species. Members of the Toxoplasmatinae reported from marsupials—there are no *Hammondia* or *Neospora* species yet described from marsupials—are covered in Chapter 8.

Sarcocystis species have been reported and described in a wide variety of mammals, birds, and reptiles throughout the temperate and tropical countries of the world. They also have been described on many occasions from marsupials, as both definitive and intermediate hosts, but many are not well studied, and their species status is often difficult to determine unless molecular gene sequences can be compared.

SARCOCYSTINAE: *SARCOCYSTIS* IN MARSUPIALS

The history of discovery, and the two-host life cycle for *Sarcocystis* species, has been reviewed many times (Levine, 1982; Dubey et al., 1989, 2015; Duszynski and Couch, 2013; others) and need not be repeated. As far as we now know, all *Sarcocystis* species require an intermediate host, which have within them viable tissue cysts (sarcocysts) that result from multiple asexual developmental processes (merogony); the intermediate host then must be eaten by a definitive (carnivore, omnivore) host in which only sexual reproduction (gamogony) occurs, only in the gut, and that process results in the formation, and sporulation, of thin-walled oocysts that release

their sporocysts. The sporocysts of all known *Sarcocystis* species are only found in the feces of their definitive host, and all sporocysts are very nearly identical in both quantitative and qualitative features. Thus, it is imperative for those who study these species to employ molecular techniques to help distinguish between them. We also have learned that some *Sarcocystis* species can infect certain intermediate hosts, but not others, so that experimental cross-transmission work also is necessary to help researchers be able to distinguish between closely related, but different, *Sarcocystis* species. There now are ~180 named species in this genus, of which 10 infect marsupials; the full life cycles are known for only ~26/180 (14%) *Sarcocystis* species (Dubey et al., 2015), but none of these are in the marsupialia. In addition to the 10 valid species covered in this chapter, there are another 23+ *Sarcocystis*-like organisms reported from marsupials (Chapter 10, Tables 11.1 and 11.2).

In **homoxenous** eimeriid species, the sporulated oocyst has a relatively thick wall that keeps the sporocysts together, and both oocyst and its sporocysts have a combination and variety of structures and sizes that often can play an important role in helping distinguish between species. In *Sarcocystis* species, however, the oocysts sporulate within the host's intestinal epithelial cells, and the *very* thin wall almost always tears when leaving its host cell, or in its transit down the intestine. Thus, only sporocysts are found in the fecal material of definitive hosts and they mostly all look alike, being similar in size, and all having the same structural features. Thus, I've included only a few line drawings and photomicrographs of sporocysts; once you've seen one *Sarcocystis* sporocyst, you've basically seen them all. Sarcocysts in muscle tissues also can look similar when they are young, but as they grow, their size and shape can vary with age. It is only when "mature" sarcocysts are studied with the electron microscope that their cyst walls can begin to help distinguish *some* species from others, but this is a less than satisfying pursuit. For example, Dubey et al. (2015) distinguished 42

Sarcocystis-wall types, many of which had from 2 to 15 subtypes!

SPECIES DESCRIPTIONS

ORDER DIDELPHIMORPHIA GILL, 1872

FAMILY DIDELPHIDAE GRAY, 1821 (17 GENERA, 87 SPECIES)

GENUS *DIDELPHIS* L., 1758 (6 SPECIES)

SARCOCYSTIS DIDELPHIDIS SCORZA, TORREALBA, AND DAGERT, 1957

Figures: For a line drawing of a group of sporocyst zoites see Scorza et al. (1957; their Figure 10); this is the only figure provided in the original description.

Definitive type host: Unknown.

Type locality: SOUTH AMERICA: Venezuela.

Other definitive hosts: Unknown.

Intermediate type host: *Didelphis marsupialis* L., 1758, Common Opossum.

Other intermediate hosts: Unknown.

Geographic distribution: SOUTH AMERICA: Venezuela.

Description of sporulated oocyst: Unknown.

Description of sporocyst and sporozoites: Unknown.

Prevalence: Unknown.

Sporulation: Unknown, but likely endogenous with infective sporocysts shed in the feces of the definitive host.

Prepatent and patent periods: Unknown.

Site of infection, definitive host: Unknown.

Site of infection, intermediate host: Sarcocysts are found in the tongue.

Endogenous stages, definitive host: Unknown.

Endogenous stages, intermediate host: Only sarcocysts in the tongue are known. These are small, compartmented, 935 × 345, with a finely striated wall, ~5.2 thick. Merozoites in sarcocysts are ~6.5 × 1.5, rounded at one end, and attenuated at the other.

Cross-transmission: None to date.

Pathology: Unknown.

Materials deposited: None.

Remarks: Scorza et al. (1957) provided only a sketchy description of a sarcocyst from the tongue and the only illustration they provided was a line drawing of several "spores" (probably bradyzoites). Kalyakin and Zasukhin (1975) said that this species was probably *Besnoitia*, but I am unaware of the evidence on which this remark was based. For the time being I list this as a valid species, but it would be useful for some investigators to examine more *D. marsupialis* in Venezuela, to verify that this species is real by doing cross-transmission and molecular sequencing work with it.

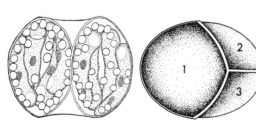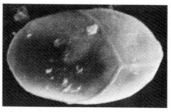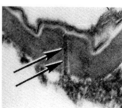

FIGURES 7.1–7.4. **7.1.** Line drawing of the sporulated oocyst of *Sarcocystis falcatula* (originally described as *Isospora boughtoni*). **7.2.** Line drawing of a sporocyst of *S. falcatula* showing three of the four plates that separate to release sporozoites. **7.3.** Scanning electron micrograph (SEM) of a sporocyst of *S. falcatula* showing three of the four plates. **7.4.** Transmission electron micrograph (TEM) of the ridgelike site of apposition between two plates (double arrows) of the sporocyst wall. **7.1** from Volk, 1938; **7.2–7.4** from Box et al., 1980, with permission of the authors, and from the Editor of the *Journal of Parasitology*.

SARCOCYSTIS FALCATULA
STILES, 1893

Synonym: *Isospora boughtoni* Volk, 1938; *Sarcocystis debonei* Vogelsang, 1929.

Definitive type host: *Didelphis virginiana* Kerr, 1792, Virginia Opossum.

Type locality: SOUTH AMERICA: Uruguay.

Other definitive hosts: *Didelphis albiventris* Lund, 1840, White-eared Opossum (Dubey et al., 2000c); *Didelphis aurita* (Wied-Neuwied, 1826), Big-eared Opossum (Monteiro et al., 2013); *Didelphis marsupialis* L., 1758, Common Opossum (Dubey et al., 2001e; Monteiro et al., 2013).

Intermediate type host: *Molothrus bonarensis* (Gmelin, 1788), Shiny Cowbird.

Other intermediate hosts: Box and Duszynski (1978), Box and Smith (1982), and others investigated the intermediate host spectrum of this species by feeding sporocysts from opossums to birds in four orders and found they were susceptible to infection: **Colubriformes**: *Columba livia* (Gmelin, 1789), Domestic Pigeon; **Passeriformes**: *Molothrus ater* (Boddaert, 1783), Brown-headed Cowbird; *Passer domesticus* L., 1758, House Sparrow; *Quiscalus* (syn. *Cassidix*) *mexicanus* (Gmelin, 1788), Great-tailed Grackle; *Quiscalus quiscula* (L., 1758), Common Grackle; *Serinus canarius* (L., 1758), Island Canary; *Taeniopygia* (syn. *Poephilia*) *guttata* Reichenbach, 1862, Zebra Finch; **Psittaciformes**: *Melopsittacus undulatus* (Shaw, 1805), Budgerigar; *Rhynchopsitta pachyrhyncha* Swainson, 1827, Thick-billed Parrot; and **Galliformes**: *Numida meleagris* (L., 1758), Helmeted Guinea Fowl (but *Gallus gallus* (L., 1758), Red Junglefowl, was not susceptible to infection). Clubb et al. (1988) and Clubb and Frenkel (1992) greatly expanded the list of susceptible psittacine birds to include both New and Old World species. Bolon et al. (1989) added yet another psittacine species, the Patagonian Conure, to be infected with this species. Hillyer et al. (1991) further extended the psittacine list when they reported the deaths of 37 Old World psittacines at the San Diego Zoo; they were able

to transmit this parasite, and the disease, to budgerigars and a Cockatiel (*Nymphicus hollandicus* (Kerr, 1792)), with gut scrapings from the opossum. These provided them enough circumstantial evidence to conclude the infective agent was *Sarcocystis falcatula*.

Geographic distribution: NORTH AMERICA: USA: Alabama, Florida, Georgia, Maryland, Louisiana, Pennsylvania, Texas, Virginia; SOUTH AMERICA: Argentina; Brazil, Uruguay.

Description of sporulated oocyst: Oocyst shape: dumbbell-shaped; number of walls: 1; wall characteristics: very thin, stretched between the sporocysts; L×W: 17–20×11–12; L/W ratio: unknown; M, OR, PG: all absent. Distinctive features of oocyst: none, a typical sarcocystid oocyst of a very thin wall stretched by, and between, the sporocysts to give a dumbbell shape. It most often disintegrates in transit down the gut lumen releasing its sporocysts.

Description of sporocyst and sporozoites: Sporocyst shape: ellipsoidal with the side next to its neighbor somewhat flattened; L×W: 12×9 (12–13×8–10); L/W ratio: 1.3 (Volk, 1938) or, 11×7 (10–12×6–8); L/W ratio 1.6 (Ernst et al., 1969) or, 11.4×7.8 (11–12×7–8); L/W ratio: 1.5 (Duszynski and Box, 1978); SB, SSB, PSB: all absent; SR: present; SR characteristics: composed of scattered, large, hyaline granules; SZ: sausage-shaped, tapering at one end, 8×2 (Volk, 1938), often with a clear RB at one end. Distinctive features of sporocyst: none, this is a typical *Sarcocystis*-type sporocyst.

Prevalence: Box and Duszynski (1977) found this form macroscopically in the musculature of 53/253 (21%) *M. ater* in Texas; they then looked at the remaining 200 "negative" birds and found an additional 11 infected animals via microscopic examination of pressed abdominal muscle (4) or by pepsin digestion (7), which was the most sensitive technique for macroscopically negative birds. Smith et al. (1990b) reported *S. falcatula* in 4/4 (100%) Thick-billed Parrots that were in respiratory distress at the Gladys Porter Zoo in Brownsville, Texas.

Dubey (2000) took intestinal scrapings from 44 wild-caught *D. virginiana* from six US states; he found 24/44 (54.5%) infected with sporocysts of *Sarcocystis* species. Using bioassays of these sporocysts in birds (*M. undulatus*), and genetically engineered nude mice (C57BL/6JHfH11-Nu) and/or γ-interferon knockout (KO) mice (BALB/c^lfng), Dubey determined that sporocysts of *S. falcatula* were present in 21/44 (48%) opossums. Dubey et al. (2000c) found sporocysts of this species in 2/2 (100%) *D. albiventris* in Argentina, and confirmed their identification by inoculating budgerigars with these sporocysts; endogenous stages were isolated from the lungs of the budgerigars in which the infection was fatal. Similarly, Dubey et al. (2000d) took sporocysts from intestinal scrapings of one *D. marsupialis* and from eight *D. albiventris*, collected in/near São Paulo, Brazil, and fed them to captive budgerigars, and all became ill; they collected meronts from the lungs, and studied them in cell culture to confirm their identity as *S. falcatula*.

Sporulation: Oocysts sporulated in the intestine of the definitive host (Volk, 1938; Box and Duszynski, 1980).

Prepatent and patent periods: One opossum discharged sporocysts in its feces 10 days after ingesting six cowbirds (*M. ater*) infected with numerous sarcocysts in their muscles and a second opossum became patent 5 days after eating seven infected cowbirds. The second opossum continued to pass large numbers of sporocysts for at least 105 days (Duszynski and Box, 1978). In additional experimental infections, Box and Duszynski (1980) found sporocysts in the feces of one opossum that had been fed infected *Q. mexicanus* (great-tailed grackles) on day 10 postinoculation (PI), and in another opossum fed infected *M. ater* (brown-headed cowbirds) on day 11 PI. They said that all available evidence suggested the grackle and cowbird *Sarcocystis* are the same species, and no evidence has been presented since then to dispute their claim.

Site of infection, definitive host: Gamonts were abundant as early as 36 h after infection, and could be found throughout the length of the small intestine, although they were most plentiful in sections numbered 2–5 (of 1–10, Box and Duszynski, 1980), and least plentiful in its anterior and posterior tenths. Macrogamonts aligned at the base of the enterocytes, above the basement membrane, and in the lamina propria of the villi.

Site of infection, intermediate host: Sarcocysts found in the skeletal muscles of many bird species, in at least four orders and multiple families.

Endogenous stages, definitive host: Box and Duszynski (1980) described the gamonts, sporocysts, and sporozoites in the small intestine of opossums, *D. virginiana*, infected by feeding them sarcocyst-infected tissues from either the brown-headed cowbird, *M. ater*, or the boat-tailed grackle, *Q. mexicanus*. The intestinal stages looked alike, so they combined the descriptions from opossums infected from the two intermediate host species.

Macrogamonts were round to ovoidal, 5.9×5.5 ($4.5–8 \times 4.5–7$) in stained sections, with an N about 2–3 wide, but a nucleolus was not seen. In Giemsa-stained tissue smears, the macrogamonts were larger, 9.6×8.4 ($7–12 \times 7–11$). Most microgamonts were above the N in the villar epithelial cells, and as many as five were found in the same host cell. In stained sections, the microgamonts were 5.5×5.1 ($5–6 \times 4–6$) and contained 4–10 microgametes. In smears, the microgamonts were larger, about $7–10 \times 3–10$ and contained 13–17 microgametes. Individual microgametes in smears were $\sim 6 \times 0.75$, and had two flagella, ~8 long.

Sporulation occurred in the host intestinal tissues. Sporocysts were mature at 13.5 days PI, and their distribution in the intestine was similar to that of the gamonts. Some were in pairs within a thin oocyst wall, but most appeared to be single, having already separated from their thin walls. They were in the villar core, but more were seen at the tips of the villi. In tissue smears, the oocysts were 13.9×10.7 ($13–15 \times 10–12$) and the sporocysts were 10.7×7.6 ($9-12 \times 6-9$). Box and Duszynski (1980) saw no SR in the sporocysts in tissue sections or smears, but they clearly saw the SR in the sporocysts in opossum feces. The SZs were 5.5×1.1 ($5-6 \times 1-1.5$) in tissue sections and 5.8×1.1 ($5-6 \times 1-1.5$) in smears. They said that the N was at the posterior (larger) end. Upon reexamining their work (Figures 8 and 9), the N was central in the SZ, and rather indistinct, while an RB appears to stain heavily at the posterior end.

Endogenous stages, intermediate host: In *M. bonarensis*, the sarcocysts were $860-960 \times 250-350$, compartmentalized, with a thick wall composed of two layers; the outer is thicker and the inner much thinner (Vogelsang, 1929). Merozoites in the sarcocysts are banana-shaped, $80-90 \times 30-40$ (sic?), according to Vogelsang (1929), but this must be a typographical error and their size, more likely, is $8-9 \times 3-4$.

Duszynski and Box (1978) looked at early development in canaries fed 10^6 sporocysts of grackle or cowbird origin that were discharged by opossums. Many extracellular SZs were found in the small intestine with a few in mononuclear phagocytes, from 2 to 24 h PI. Of the internal organs they examined, the lungs were the most heavily parasitized. Only occasional SZs were found in the liver and/or the spleen; SZs were 2.4×5.7 ($2-3.5 \times 5-7$). They (Duszynski and Box, 1978) also infected sparrows with sporocysts, and surviving canaries and sparrows were necropsied 12–20 weeks PI, and examined for sarcocysts in their tissues. Most of the sparrows had heavy infections and cysts were visible on gross inspection, especially in abdominal musculature preparations. Their infected canaries, on the other hand, would have been evaluated as negative because no cysts were seen grossly; however, infections were detected in all canaries via tissue digestion (Box and Duszynski, 1977).

Clubb et al. (1988) outlined the sequence of infection soon after sporocysts were ingested. Sporozoites released from sporocysts in the intestine of the bird invade many tissues, but especially the lungs. Meronts pass through two asexual replicative events in the blood vessels; the first in endothelial cells of arterioles, and the second in endothelial cells of capillaries or venules in organs of the infected bird. Early lung stages are in the endothelium of pulmonary capillaries, then in the venules and veins. Finally, released merozoites eventually develop into typical muscle cysts (sarcocysts).

Cross-transmission: Box and Duszynski (1978) transmitted this species from *M. ater* and *Q. mexicanus* (both Icteridae) via the opossum (*D. virginiana*) to the house sparrow (*P. domesticus*) (Ploceidae) and the canary (*S. canarius*) (Fringillidae), but were not able to transmit it to ducks (*Anas platyrhynchos* L., 1758, Mallard) (Anatidae). Later, Box and Smith (1982) attempted to transmit this same *Sarcocystis*, via sporocysts from opossums, to six avian species including canaries (*S. canarius*), zebra finches (*T. guttata*), budgerigars (*M. undulatus*), pigeons (*C. livia*), chickens (*G. gallus* (L., 1758), red junglefowl), and guinea fowl (*N. meleagris*). All species, except *G. gallus*, were susceptible to merogony. Pigeons (Columbiformes) were susceptible to early merogony, but did not develop sarcocysts in their muscles. Passeriformes and Psittaciformes were completely susceptible to infection and the parasite developed sarcocysts in them. Such studies indicate that the intermediate host range for this (and perhaps other) *Sarcocystis* species is broader than had been previously thought at that time for most *Sarcocystis* species.

Pathology: Most of the work on the pathology due to this species has been done in bird intermediate hosts. Only Volk (1938), looked at the opossum which he found infected, and noted that it had a bloody mass containing numerous sporulated oocysts in the first 4 inches of the small intestine, and the outer cells of the villi were sloughed off into the lumen.

Studies that have examined changes in avian hosts experimentally infected with *S. falcatula* are much more extensive. For example, Duszynski and Box (1978) found that three of six canaries given 200×10^3 sporocysts from opossums became moribund and were killed 7–12 days PI. Breathing was labored, the lungs were gray and consolidated, and the spleens were enlarged. In tissue sections, lung capillaries were found outlined by the meronts and extracellular merozoites, and meronts were found in lung smears. Merozoites in smears were 5.5×1.9 (4–7×1.5–2). Four of 12 sparrows (*P. domesticus*) given 100–500×10^3 sporocysts died on days 11–16 PI; two sparrows had received sporocysts of cowbird origin and two had received sporocysts of grackle origin. The sparrows were not observed to be sick, but a certain proportion of these wild birds often die of stress after being confined in cages (Box and Duszynski, 1978). Asexual stages, similar to those seen in canaries, were seen in tissue smears and sections. Most meronts and merozoites were found in the lungs, a few in the spleen and liver, and several were found in the brain. Merozoites found in tissue smears were 6×2 (4–8×2).

In the late 1980s, Dr Edith Box and her colleagues at the University of Texas Medical Branch, Galveston, published a series of detailed papers on the pathogenesis of *S. falcatula* infections in the budgerigar (*M. undulatus*) at both the light microscope and ultrastructural levels. Their first paper in the series detailed the ultrastructural pathogenesis of early pulmonary SZs, merogony, and merozoites (Smith et al., 1987a) and followed the progression of early merogony in pulmonary capillaries and in venous endothelial cells. Their second contribution outlined lung epithelial cell hypertrophy and destruction, capillary obstruction preceding endothelial lysis, acute endophlebitis, and chronic periphlebitis that all impeded the outflow of the pulmonary vascular system resulting in interstitial, subpneumocytic, and airspace edema (Smith et al., 1987b). Their third paper was a quantitative analysis of the pathology of extrapulmonary disease due to merogony in the lamina propria of the small

intestine, liver, kidney, and lungs; sarcocysts, however, only formed in cardiac and skeletal muscles (Smith et al., 1989). The fourth paper used the transmission electron microscope to detail the ultrastructure of developing, mature, and degenerating muscle sarcocysts (Neill et al., 1989). In 1990a, Smith et al. compared the pathology previously documented in budgerigars to that seen in both canaries (*S. canarius*) and pigeons (*C. livia*) due to *S. falcatula*. Smith et al. (1990b) also reported *S. falcatula* in thick-billed parrots that died of respiratory distress at the Gladys Porter Zoo in Brownsville, Texas; the cause of their interstitial pneumonitis was attributed to this species. About the same time, Clubb et al. (1988) and Clubb and Frenkel (1992) reported that the early lung stages are in the endothelium of pulmonary capillaries, then in the venules and veins, where they obstruct blood outflow by stenosis or occlusion of vessels by endothelial hypertrophy, meronts, and endophlebitis. The subsequent edema is associated with displacement of the myelinoid surfactant layer, and retraction and degeneration of squamous pneumocytes.

Materials deposited: None.

Remarks: The oocysts were described by Volk (1938) and by Ernst et al. (1969). This life cycle was worked out by Duszynski and Box (1978), who called this form *S. debonei*, which was named and originally described in the cowbird, *M. bonarensis* in Uruguay, by Vogelsang (1929). The oocysts in *D. virginiana* were described under the name *I. boughtoni* by Volk (1938). Duszynski and Box (1978) put the two together. In a later paper, Box et al. (1984) redescribed and synonymized *S. debonei* to be a junior synonym of *S. falcatula*. Box et al. (1980) studied the fine structure of the sporocyst wall of this species. It is composed of four plates which often separated in pairs at the center of the sporocyst. The wall is composed of four layers, all of which are apparently found in each plate. Box and Smith (1982) commented on the cyst wall of sarcocysts in birds they had experimentally infected (see *Cross-transmission*, above). All cyst walls had small protrusions (villi) that varied in length from ~1 to 5. Zoites (bradyzoites) within the sarcocysts were similar in size in all birds that developed sarcocysts: 6.9 × 1.9 (canaries), 7.5 × 1.9 (zebra finches), 7.2 × 2.3 (budgerigars); their combined mean measurements were 7 × 2 (4.8–9.3 × 1.2–2.9).

The demonstrated infectivity of birds in diverse taxonomic orders deserves comment. Clearly, this *Sarcocystis* species is not as rigidly host-specific as in previously reported (at that time) mammalian sarcocystids. One interesting facet discussed in the study by Box and Smith (1982) is that this parasite can develop to different degrees in different intermediate host species. Box and Duszynski (1978) found that ducks (Anatidae) did not get infected by sporocysts of opossum–passerine origin; thus Anseriformes and most Galliformes (Box and Smith, 1982) are refractory to the infection, while birds in the Passeriformes are susceptible to all stages. The Columbiformes (pigeons) are intermediate in susceptibility in that they seem to be susceptible to premuscle merogony, but refractory to muscle meronts (sarcocysts). Their argument (Box and Smith, 1982) was that, "In nature, intensification of a predator–prey relationship between such a partially susceptible prey (with an occasional muscle cyst) and the predatory host could select for parasites more fully adapted to the prey in question and could widen the spectrum of intermediate hosts."

Psittaciformes also are intermediate in susceptibility, but in another way. Non-American psittacines, especially cockatoos, cockatiels, and African parrots, are all susceptible to infection and acute fatal illness, but American psittacine species seem to be resistant to the disease as adults, although nestlings can be infected with only brief illness and minor mortality (Clubb and Frenkel, 1992). To support their point, Clubb and Frenkel (1992) listed 45 American psittacine species in 12 genera that were exposed to the parasite on a farm and did not develop illness.

The relative resistance of American psittacines to this infection is thought to be the result of natural selection of these bird species in environments where opossums infected with *S. falcatula* are prevalent, whereas non-American psittacines evolved in an environment free of opossums, and have not been selected for resistance (Clubb and Frenkel, 1992).

Clubb and Frenkel (1992) demonstrated that the American cockroach, *Periplaneta americana* L., 1758, acted as a transport host for *S. falcatula* in a psittacine breeding colony in Florida. They fed starved cockroaches on opossum feces that contained sporocysts of *S. falcatula*, and then liquefied the roaches in a blender and fed two cockatoo species the suspension by gavage. The birds died on days 10 and 14 PI, and *S. falcatula* was identified as the causative agent when the birds were necropsied and its meronts were found in the lungs. Interestingly, the breeding facility used flightless (silky) chickens as a biological agent to control cockroach population. These chickens could not fly onto the tops of the cages of the psittacines to soil them with feces and they effectively reduced the cockroach population and thereby limited infections of the birds. Cool stuff.

Dubey et al. (2001b) reported on an acute *S. falcatula*-like infection in a carmine bee-eater (*Merops nubicus*) that died in a zoo in Florida, USA. They found meronts in the bird's lungs and immature sarcocysts in its skeletal muscles. Using electron microscopy and immunohistochemical tests, they found that the parasite did not conform to the parameters of *S. falcatula*, and offered an important caution. As detailed above, *S. falcatula* has a very broad range of avian hosts, and this has now led many investigators to suspect that it is, or may be, a mixture of more than one species because genetic variations suggest heterogenicity in this group (Marsh et al., 1999; Tanhauser et al., 1999).

Finally, Monteiro et al. (2013) reported DNA of *S. falcatula*-like sporocysts in *D. aurita* and *D. albiventris* from Brazil.

SARCOCYSTIS GARNHAMI MANDOUR, 1965

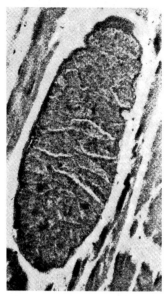

FIGURE 7.5   LM of a tissue section through a muscle sarcocyst of *Sarcocystis garnhami* in *Didelphis marsupialis*, from Mandour, 1965, with permission from John Wiley & Sons, publishers of the *Journal of Eukaryotic Microbiology* (formerly the *Journal of Protozoology*).

Definitive type host: Unknown.

Type locality: CENTRAL AMERICA: Belize (former British Honduras), Tela.

Other definitive hosts: Unknown.

Intermediate type host: *Didelphis marsupialis* L., 1758, Common Opossum.

Other intermediate hosts: *Philander mcilhennyi* Gardner and Patton, 1972, McIlhenny's Four-eyed Opossum.

Geographic distribution: CENTRAL AMERICA: Belize (former British Honduras); SOUTH AMERICA: Brazil.

Description of sporulated oocyst: Unknown.

Description of sporocyst and sporozoites: Unknown.

Prevalence: Unknown.

Sporulation: Unknown, but likely endogenous with infective sporocysts shed in the feces of the definitive host.

Prepatent and patent periods: Unknown.

Site of infection, definitive host: Unknown.

Site of infection, intermediate host: Striated muscles.

Endogenous stages, definitive host: Unknown.

Endogenous stages, intermediate host: Sarcocysts are compartmented, and varied greatly from 310 to 3.3 mm wide × 110–250 thick, with a wall, ~6–8 thick, containing cytophaneres (spines) 6–8 × 1.5–2. Trabeculae are present, and the cyst wall is not invaginated (Shaw and Lainson, 1969). Bradyzoites are curved, with one end pointed and the other rounded, ~5–7 × 1–2 (Mandour, 1965) or, they are 8.4 × 3.1 (6.5–10 × 2–4), with an N ~2.5 (2–3) wide, and located at the rounded end of the zoite (Shaw and Lainson, 1969).

Cross-transmission: None to date.

Pathology: Unknown.

Materials deposited: None.

Remarks: Mandour (1965) differentiated this species from *Sarcocystis didelphidis* because of the presence of cytophaneres in its sarcocyst wall; the wall of the sarcocyst of *S. didelphidis* is striated, but does not have spiny cytophaneres. In addition, Scorza et al. (1957), according to Mandour (1965), examined Mandour's material, and said that it was definitely not *S. didelphidis*. Mandour (1965), unfortunately, had only preserved (Bouin's fluid) and paraffin-embedded material to work with so he was only able to provide a photomicrograph of a sarcocyst in long section to support his species description.

Shaw and Lainson (1969) reported this species from the muscles of McIlhenny's four-eyed opossum, *P. mcilhennyi*, in Brazil; perhaps it was the same species, but there is no way to verify their observation. They said that it was **clearly** *S. garnhami*, its structure agreeing exactly with Mandour's description. Its sarcocysts were compartmented, 553–142, with a wall 1.3–2 thick containing rose-thorn-like cytophaneres, 6–8 × 1.3 in sections, or 10–11.5 × 2 in smears. Its merozoites ("spores") were 8 × 3 (6.5–10 × 2–4), with an N ~2.5 (2–3) in diameter.

SARCOCYSTIS GREINERI CHEADLE, 2001

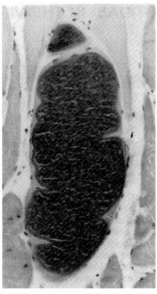

FIGURE 7.6 Photomicrograph (LM) of a sarcocyst of *Sarcocystis greineri* in skeletal muscle of *Didelphis virginiana*, from Cheadle, 2001 (his Figure 1), with permission from the Editor of the *Journal of Parasitology*.

Definitive type host: Unknown.

Type locality: NORTH AMERICA: USA: Florida, North-Central (29°–30° N, 82°–83° W).

Other definitive hosts: Unknown.

Intermediate type host: *Didelphis virginiana* Kerr, 1792, Virginia Opossum.

Other intermediate hosts: Unknown.

Geographic distribution: NORTH AMERICA: USA: Florida.

Description of sporulated oocyst: Unknown.

Description of sporocyst and sporozoites: Unknown.

Prevalence: Sarcocysts were found in the skeletal muscles of 2/20 (10%) *D. virginiana* (Cheadle, 2001); Baird et al. (2002) found 24/240 (10%) Virginia opossums infected with this species.

Sporulation: Unknown, but likely endogenous with infective sporocysts shed in the feces of the definitive host.

Prepatent and patent periods: Unknown.

Site of infection, definitive host: Unknown.

Site of infection, intermediate host: Sarcocysts have been found in the striated skeletal muscles of the tongue, thigh, and abdomen (Cheadle, 2001), and in the muscles of the diaphragm, leg, breast, tongue, back, and esophagus (Baird et al., 2002).

Endogenous stages, definitive host: Unknown.

Endogenous stages, intermediate host: Sarcocysts were 3.8 mm × 155 (2–6 mm × 108–189) as measured by Cheadle (2001), but Baird et al. (2002) said they ranged in size from 119–681 × 52–131 (means not given). In tissue sections (LM), the outer cyst wall was moderately to deeply invaginated throughout the entire length of the sarcocyst, and this appeared to completely bisect the cyst in some instances. Bradyzoites or metrocytes freed from the cyst wall were 11 × 4.4. Mature sarcocysts had a wall with stumpy, digit-like protrusions (villi), some of which were pedunculate near the cyst wall. By transmission electron microscopy, these protrusions were 3.4 × 1.5 (3–4 × 1–2); the interior-most portion of sarcocysts had thick septa, 0.2 × 4.5, that separated pockets of bradyzoites, which were 6–9 × 2–3 (Dubey et al., 2015).

Cross-transmission: Cheadle (2001) served 112 g of muscle from one infected opossum to a greyhound dog (*Canis familiaris*) and a domestic cat (*Felis catus*), but neither shed *Sarcocystis* sporocysts in its feces up to 30 days PI. Tissue samples from the dog were unavailable to Cheadle (2001) for examination, but the intestine, liver, lung, kidney, brain, heart, spleen, and muscle from the cat were all negative for sarcocysts. He also infected a wild-caught opossum that was negative for *Sarcocystis* via fecal flotation; it was fed tongue and skeletal muscle from 76 different opossums, seven of which contained sarcocysts that were confirmed with the LM. Fecal samples collected from this opossum from −30 to +74 days PI, and intestinal scrapings were negative for sporocysts; likewise, tissue sections of liver, lung, kidney, brain, heart, spleen, and muscle tissues all were negative for sarcocysts.

Pathology: No pathology was mentioned by Cheadle (2001).

Materials deposited: Histologic sections of sarcocysts are in the U.S. National Parasite Collection, Beltsville, Maryland, as UNMPC Nos. 90685, 90686.

Etymology: This species was named to honor Ellis C. Greiner, Department of Pathobiology, College of Veterinary Medicine, University of Florida, Gainesville, Florida, who has made major contributions to the diagnosis and study of coccidia and other parasites of veterinary importance.

Remarks: Cheadle (2001) used Odening's (1998) comprehensive review of *Sarcocystis* species to state that there were only three valid species of *Sarcocystis*, described from sarcocysts in the skeletal muscles of opossums, for him to compare to the muscle sarcocysts he found in Florida opossums: *S. didelphidis*, *S. garnhami*, and *S. marmosae*. Odening (1998) also emphasized that the ultrastructure of the sarcocyst wall was a reliable character in mature sarcocysts to help distinguish *Sarcocystis* species. Thus, using both structural features of the sarcocysts, and bradyzoites and host and geographic differences, Cheadle (2001) determined that this should be a valid species in *D. virginiana*, the Virginia opossum.

Of the 240 opossums studied by Baird et al. (2002), 24 were infected. From these the authors selected 11 positive opossums to determine which muscles were most likely to contain sarcocysts and found that the diaphragms had the highest specificity with 8/11 (73%) harboring sarcocysts, significantly more than any other muscle groups they examined.

SARCOCYSTIS INGHAMI ELSHEIKHA, FITZGERALD, MANSFIELD, AND SAEED, 2003

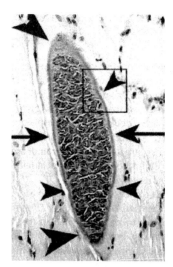

FIGURE 7.7 Photomicrograph (LM) of a sarcocyst in abdominal muscle of *Sarcocystis inghami*, from Elsheikha et al., 2003 (their Figure 3), with kind permission from Springer Science + Business Media, publisher of *Systematic Parasitology*.

Definitive type host: Unknown.

Type locality: NORTH AMERICA: USA: Michigan, South-Central (42° 43–79′ N, 84° 18–86′ W).

Other definitive hosts: Unknown.

Intermediate type host: *Didelphis virginiana* Kerr, 1792, Virginia Opossum.

Other intermediate hosts: Unknown.

Geographic distribution: NORTH AMERICA: USA: Michigan.

Description of sporulated oocyst: Unknown.

Description of sporocyst and sporozoites: Unknown.

Prevalence: Sarcocysts were found in 2/17 (12%) *D. virginiana* (Elsheikha et al., 2003); a year later, Elsheikha et al. (2004a) found *Sarcocystis inghami* in at least 3/137 (2%) *D. virginiana* which were coinfected with sarcocysts of *S. inghami*, sporocysts of *Sarcocystis neurona*, and tissue cysts of *Besnoitia darlingi*, but the overall preva-lence rate was not clear (Dubey et al., 2015).

Sporulation: Unknown, but likely endogenous with infective sporocysts shed in the feces of the definitive host.

Prepatent and patent periods: Unknown.

Site of infection, definitive host: Unknown.

Site of infection, intermediate host: Sarcocysts were found in skeletal muscles and the tongue.

Endogenous stages, definitive host: Unknown.

Endogenous stages, intermediate host: Sarco-cysts were studied with both the light (LM) and transmission electron microscopes (TEM). Under the LM, fusiform sarcocysts were micro-scopic, 493.4 × 91.4 (335–700 × 79–110). The cyst wall varied in thickness due to variation in the length of villar protrusions (VP), depending on the region of the cyst; it was generally thicker at the more pointed ends and relatively thin in the middle. The VP at the terminal ends of the sarco-cyst were hairlike, unequal in length, and longer than those in the mid-sarcocyst (Elsheikha et al., 2003). Longitudinally cut bradyzoites were banana-shaped, 10.7 × 4.4 (10–12 × 4–5), with a posterior N. Using TEM, Elsheikha et al., (2003) documented numerous, slender, longitudinally arranged microfilaments (microtubules), which ran from the tips of the VP to the granular layer. In cross section, each VP was noted to have hundreds of microtubules scattered throughout the entire filament core. Sarcocysts were sur-rounded by a PV membrane and its underlying electron-dense layer was 40 nm thick. The PV was ornamented with bump- or knob-like struc-tures, interrupted at regular intervals, giving the appearance of beadlike in-pocketing on the periphery of the PV.

Cross-transmission: None to date.

Pathology: Unknown.

Materials deposited: Syntype tissue sections on slides are deposited in the U.S. National Para-site Collection, Beltsville, Maryland, as USNPC No. 092429 and in the Natural History museum, London, UK, as Reg. No. 2003:31:3:1.

Etymology: The specific appellation *inghami* refers to Ingham County of Lansing, Michigan, USA, the locality from which the opossums were collected.

Remarks: Elsheikha et al. (2003) compared the measurements of sarcocysts, bradyzoites, and VP of their species to those of the other *Sarcocystis* species known at the time that used opossums as intermediate hosts. They noted that sarcocysts of *S. inghami* could be read-ily differentiated from the others (*S. didelphis*, *S. garnhami*, *S. marmosae*, *S. greineri*, *S.* sp. of Scholtyseck et al., 1982) by the characteristic morphology of the VP and their unique bifur-cations, along with their cyst wall that was highly variable in thickness.

Elsheikha et al. (2003, 2004a) found that both of their infected opossums had concurrent infec-tions with *B. darlingi* Brumpt, 1913 cysts in their muscles, and with *S. neurona* oocysts and spo-rocysts in their intestinal tissues. The identity of *B. darlingi* was based on the morphology of a cyst in a tissue section under LM, and their identification of *S. neurona* was done by geno-typing sporocysts recovered from the feces by polymerase chain reaction–restriction fragment length polymorphism (PCR-RFLP).

SARCOCYSTIS LINDSAYI DUBEY, ROSENTHAL AND SPEER, 2001G

Figures: For LM and TEMs of tissue cysts and of merogonous stages in the life cycle of *Sar-cocystis lindsayi*, see Dubey et al. (2001g, their Figures 1–4).

Definitive type host: *Didelphis albiventris* Lund, 1840, White-eared Opossum.

Type locality: SOUTH AMERICA: Brazil: Jabo-ticabal, University Campus.

Other definitive hosts: *Didelphis aurita* (Wied-Neuwied, 1826), Big-eared Opossum.

Intermediate type host: *Melopsittacus undulatus* (Shaw, 1805), Budgerigar (experimental).

Other intermediate hosts: Unknown.

Geographic distribution: SOUTH AMERICA: Brazil.

Description of sporulated oocyst: Unknown.

Description of sporocyst and sporozoites: Sporocyst shape: ellipsoidal; L × W: 12 × 7; L/W ratio: 1.7; SB, SSB, PSB: all absent; SR: present; SR characteristics: composed of large, hyaline granules that are either scattered or condensed at one end of the sporocyst even within the same oocyst; SZ: 6 long (Dubey et al., 2001g). Distinctive features of sporocyst: none, this is a typical *Sarcocystis*-type sporocyst.

Prevalence: Found in 1/3 (33%) adult specimens of the definitive type host and in 1/9 (11%) *D. aurita* by da Silva Stabenow et al. (2012).

Sporulation: Unknown, but likely endogenous with infective sporocysts shed in the feces of the definitive host.

Prepatent and patent periods: Unknown.

Site of infection, definitive host: Unknown, but likely in the intestinal epithelium.

Site of infection, intermediate host: Lungs, where division was by **endopolygeny**.

Endogenous stages, definitive host: Unknown.

Endogenous stages, intermediate host: Sarcocysts were not found in any of the budgerigars, but meronts were seen in sections of the lungs, and these reacted with anti-*S. falcatula* rabbit serum. Meronts and merozoites were observed in cultures inoculated with budgerigar lung tissue.

In vitro development: Isolates from budgerigar lungs were homogenized in RPMI 1640 cell culture medium and inoculated into equine kidney cell cultures. Early merozoites at 1–2 days PI were 5.1 × 1.7 (4–6 × 1.6–2.4) without a prominent nucleolus in the N, whereas (perhaps) slightly older merozoites were 6.9 × 2.9 (6–10 × 2–6) and had a prominent nucleolus. At day 2 PI merozoites began to develop into meronts; they still had one N and a prominent nucleolus, and were 9.3 × 6.0 (8–12 × 4–8), while early meronts (also day 2) had a single N with four or more prominent nucleoli and were 15.5 × 10.8 (10–22 × 8–16); by day 3 PI they were 22.2 × 15.6 (16–27 × 10–22). Mature meronts were seen on day 3 PI and had merozoites arranged peripherally around a residual body and measured 36.0 × 22.8 (29–43 × 20–26); merozoites from these mature meronts on day 3 PI were 5.8 × 1.6 (5–6 × 1.6). The number of merozoites per meront ranged from 14 to >100. On day 4 PI meronts were 31.0 × 22.2 (24–34 × 17–26), with merozoites 5.4 × 1.6 (5–6 × 1.6–2.4), and day 5 merozoites were 5.2 × 1.9 (4–6 × 1.6–2.4) (Dubey et al., 2001g).

Cross-transmission: Dubey et al. (2001g) took sporocysts from opossum feces and inoculated these into budgerigars that had been raised in captivity. da Silva Stabenow et al. (2012) found that 3/9 (33%) *D. aurita*, collected in the city of Seropédica, were passing sporocysts in their feces. Mucosal scrapings and sporocysts from each of the three were fed to five budgerigars, but only one developed tissue parasites of *Sarcocystis*. The morphology of all tissue stages was identical to those of *S. lindsayi*.

Pathology: Lungs from all infected Budgerigars were hemorrhagic and congested (Dubey et al., 2001g). All six budgerigars injected with culture-derived merozoites died, or became clinically ill by 22 days PI.

Materials deposited: Hepantotypes as histologic sections of sarcocysts from experimentally infected budgerigars are deposited in the U.S. National Parasite Collection, Beltsville, Maryland as USNPC Nos. 91269 and 91270, and an unstained phototype of a sporocyst from *D. albiventris* as USNPC No. 91272.

Etymology: This species was named in honor of Dr. David S. Lindsay, Virginia–Maryland Regional College of Veterinary Medicine, Virginia Tech, Blacksburg, Virginia, USA, who has made valuable contributions to the biology of coccidia.

Remarks: Antigenically, the *S. falcatula*-like organism isolated from *D. albiventris* was similar to *S. falcatula* isolated from *D. virginiana* because anti-*S. falcatula* serum reacted with the *S. falcatula*-like parasite in histological sections (Dubey et al., 2001e). However, TEM studies indicated that the merozoites of the "*S. falcatula*-like" parasite from Brazil had more micronemes than the merozoites of the Cornell isolate of *S. falcatula* (Lindsay et al., 1999; Dubey et al., 2001e). The *S. falcatula*-like parasite derived from *D. albiventris* from Brazil shared characters with both *S. falcatula* and *S. neurona*; it resembled the former because of its infectivity to budgerigars, and its reactivity with anti-*S. falcatula* serum, and it resembled the latter in molecular features and its development in cell culture. These features led Dubey et al. (2001e) to conclude, "The parasite...derived from *D. albiventris* from Brazil is a distinct species," but they did not name it at that time. However, after studying this organism in more detail, Dubey et al. (2001f) felt confident enough to name it a distinct species, *S. lindsayi*, because meront morphology and genetic variation at both the nuclear large subunit ribosomal RNA gene, and the internal transcribed spacer (ITS-1) gene, and each of two other genetic loci, make them genetically distinct from *S. falcatula*, *S. speeri*, and *S. neurona* (Dubey et al., 2000b).

SARCOCYSTIS NEURONA DUBEY, DAVIS, SPEER, BOWMAN, DE LAHUNTA, GRANSTROM, TOPPER, HAMIR, CUMMINGS, AND SUTER, 1991A

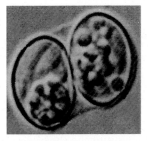

FIGURE 7.8 Photomicrograph of a sporulated oocyst of *Sarcocystis neurona* from Dubey et al., 2000d (their Figure F), with permission from the senior author and from the Editor of the *Journal of Parasitology*.

Definitive type host: *Didelphis virginiana* Kerr, 1792, Virginia Opossum.

Type locality: NORTH AMERICA: USA: Illinois.

Other definitive hosts: *Didelphis albiventris* Lund, 1840, White-eared Opossum (Dubey et al., 2001d,f); *Didelphis marsupialis* L., 1758, Common Opossum (Dubey et al., 2001d, 2015).

Intermediate type host: *Equus caballus* L., 1758, Horse.

Other intermediate hosts: *Dasypus novemcinctus* L., 1758, Nine-banded Armadillo (natural); *Enhydra lutris nereis* (Merriam, 1904), Sea Otter (natural); *Felis catus* L., 1758, Domestic Cat (experimental); *Mephitis mephitis* (Schreber, 1776), Striped Skunk (experimental); *Neovison vison* (Schreber, 1777), American Mink; *Phoca vitulina richardii* (Gray, 1864), Harbor Seal; *Procyon lotor* (L., 1758), Raccoon (natural); *Threskiornis* (syn. *Carphibis*) *spinicollis* Jameson, 1835, Straw-necked Ibis (natural?).

Geographic distribution: NORTH AMERICA: USA: California, Florida, Georgia, Illinois, Kansas (?), Louisiana, Maryland, Massachusetts, Michigan, Mississippi, New York, Ohio, Oregon, Pennsylvania, Virginia; CANADA: Saskatchewan.

Description of sporulated oocyst: Unknown.

Description of sporocyst and sporozoites: Sporocyst shape: ellipsoidal; L×W: 10.5–12×6.5–8; L/W ratio: unknown; SB, SSB, PSB: all absent; SR: present; SR characteristics: composed of large, hyaline granules that either are scattered or condensed at one end of the sporocyst even within the same oocyst (Figure 7.8, left); SZ: banana-shaped, without distinct RB or N visible (Dubey et al., 2000d). Distinctive features of sporocyst: none, this is a typical *Sarcocystis*-type sporocyst.

Prevalence: Dubey et al. (2000d) took intestinal scrapings from 44 wild-caught *D. virginiana* from six US states; they found 24/44 (54.5%) infected with sporocysts of *Sarcocystis* species. Using bioassays of these sporocysts in birds (*M. undulatus*), and genetically engineered nude mice (C57BL/6JHfH11-Nu) and/or γ-interferon KO mice (BALB/c[lfng]), they determined that sporocysts of *S. neurona* were present in 8/44 (18%) opossums. Dubey et al. (2001a) found sporocysts of *Sarcocystis* in intestinal scrapings from 24/72 (33%) *D. virginiana* from Mississippi; these were bioassayed by feeding sporocysts to γ-interferon KO mice. *Sarcocystis neurona* was detected in the brains of KO mice fed sporocysts, from 19/24 (79%) opossums, by immunohistochemical staining with anti-*S. neurona*-specific polyclonal rabbit serum, and by in vitro culture. Dubey et al. (2001h) found sarcocysts in 2/2 (100%) naturally infected sea otters, *Enhydra lutris*. The sarcocysts were characterized biologically (KO mice with γ-interferon gene), ultrastructurally, and genetically by PCR amplification followed by RFLP analysis and sequencing. Their (Dubey et al., 2001h) conclusion was that sea otters exposed to *S. neurona* sporocysts can support the development of mature sarcocysts that are infectious to competent definitive hosts (opossums). Houk et al. (2010) examined blood of *D. virginiana* for antibodies to six protozoan parasites including *S. neurona*; they found that 5/30 (17%) demonstrated antibodies against *S. neurona* using an indirect immunofluorescent antibody test against in vitro-produced antigens.

Sporulation: Endogenous with infective sporocysts shed in the feces of the definitive host (Dubey et al., 2000d).

Prepatent and patent periods: Two opossums fed sarcocyst-infected cat meat shed sporocysts at 11 and 13 days PI (Dubey et al., 2000d).

Site of infection, definitive host: Unknown, but likely the intestinal epithelium in opossums.

Site of infection, intermediate host: Brain and spinal cord in horses. In cats fed sporocysts from the opossum, sarcocysts were found in muscles of the tongue, diaphragm, abdomen, legs, spine, and head (Dubey et al., 2000d). Two raccoons (*P. lotor*) fed sporocysts of *S. neurona* from opossums developed clinical illness, and *S. neurona*-associated encephalomyelitis; they were killed 14 and 22 days postinfection, and meronts and merozoites were seen in encephalitic lesions (Dubey et al., 2001i).

Endogenous stages, definitive host: Unknown.

Endogenous stages, intermediate host: Meronts and merozoites are located in the cytoplasm of neural cells, leukocytes, and giant cells in gray and white matter of brain and spinal cord in the horse. Early uninucleated meronts are 4–7 × 4–5

with a large N and a nucleolus. As the meront grows the N becomes lobulated, but N division was not seen until the meronts were 15 long. Merozoites bud from the periphery of multilobed N, occasionally arranged in a rosette around a residual body. Mature meronts measured 5–35 × 5–20, and contain 4–40 merozoites. Mature merozoites are 2–4 × 1–2, with a centrally located N. Ultrastructurally, parasites in horse tissues and cell culture were found to be free in the cytoplasm, and not within a PV. Merozoites develop exclusively by endopolygeny, with two merozoite **anlagen** that appear in close proximity to a spindle apparatus associated with each lobe of a highly irregularly shaped N. Each merozoite anlagen was seen to elongate by posterior extension of its inner membrane complex and subpellicular microtubules, and eventually incorporate within each one a part of the meront N and cytoplasm (Dubey et al., 1991a). Merozoites measured in TEM were 4.1 × 1.2 (4–6 × 1–2), lacked rhoptries, but contained micronemes and usually a large, empty vacuole between the N and their anterior tip.

In cats fed sporocysts from opossums, sarcocysts found as early as 57 days PI contained only metrocytes, and even at 144 days, not all sarcocysts were mature. This suggested to Dubey et al. (2000d) a slow rate of maturation for *S. neurona* sarcocysts. The longest sarcocyst seen in tissue section was 700 and the widest one was 50. The sarcocyst wall was relatively thin with slender VP up to 2.5 long. Ultrastructurally, VP were seen to contain microtubules, and bradyzoites were slender, about 5–7 long (Dubey et al., 2000d). KO mice fed sporocysts from opossums had meronts, merozoites, or sporozoites in their tissues, mainly in visceral tissues during the first 10 days of infection. At 8 days PI, *S. neurona* organisms were seen consistently in the brain (Dubey et al., 2000d).

Cross-transmission: Sporocysts from eight naturally infected opossums were fed to budgerigars (*M. undulatus*) and γ-interferon KO mice (BALB/c^{lfng}). Budgerigars did not become infected, but the mice did, and meronts could be found in their brain and lung tissues (Dubey, 2000d). In an earlier study, Dubey et al. (1998) found that sporocysts of *S. neurona* induced encephalitis in KO and nude mice, and only meronts and merozoites were found in their tissues.

Pathology: Highly pathogenic, often fatal, in the horse intermediate host.

Materials deposited: Syntypes from horse no. 1 of Dubey et al. (1974) are deposited in the U.S. National Museum Helminthological Collection, USDA, Beltsville, Maryland as USNM Helminthological Collection No. 18450. Paratypes from a horse from Cornell University from which the organism was cultured in vitro were deposited as USNM Helminthological Collection No. 18451.

Etymology: The species name was derived from *neural* (Gk) and refers to the location of the parasite in the intermediate host.

Remarks: A fatal protozoan encephalomyelitis (EPM), thought to be *Toxoplasma gondii*, was first reported by Cusick et al. (1974) in two horses from Illinois, USA. At nearly the same time it was reported in horses in Ohio (Dubey et al., 1974) and Pennsylvania (Beech, 1974; Beech and Dodd, 1974), again as a *Toxoplasma*-like pathogen. Clark et al. (1981) were the first to report EPM from horses in Canada (Saskatchewan). Since then, EPM has been reported from horses throughout North America (see Dubey et al., 1991a, p. 212 and Dubey et al., 2015, for references). Mayhew et al. (1978) were among the first to notice that sera from many horses with EPM reacted with antigens of *Sarcocystis cruzi*, in the indirect hemagglutination test, suggesting to them that the EPM organism may be related to *Sarcocystis*. Dubey and Miller (1986) found EPM in a pony in Maryland and suggested the causative agent may be "related to *Sarcocystis*." However, it wasn't until more than a decade later, when Dubey et al. (1991a) described the structure of the

EPM organism, and named it *S. neurona*, from naturally infected horses. They examined specimens of brains and spinal cords from numerous horses including those from previously published reports, and from their own collections, and they cultured an EPM-like organism from a naturally infected horse in New York. Fenger et al. (1995) compared the small subunit ribosomal RNA (SSU rRNA) gene of *S. neurona* to those of *S. muris, S. cruzi, T. gondii,* and *Cryptosporidium parvum* to identify a unique region suitable for a species-specific amplification primer. They then used this *S. neurona* primer in a PCR assay to try to identify this organism in feces and intestinal digest of various wildlife specimens (raccoons, opossums, skunks, cats, a hawk (*Accipiter* sp.), and one coyote). They were the first to determine that the SSU rRNA gene of *S. neurona* had a 99.89% similarity with the sporocysts found in two opossums (*D. virginiana*); this led them to identify the opossum as the putative definitive host of *S. neurona*. Dubey et al. (1996) reported an *S. neurona* organism associated with encephalitis in a striped skunk (*M. mephitis*) in Massachusetts. Finally, Dubey et al. (2000d) completed the life cycle of *S. neurona* experimentally in the lab and described sarcocysts in an experimental intermediate host (*F. catus*, domestic cat), and sporocysts from the definitive host (*D. virginiana*). Dubey and Hamir (2000) reported producing a high-titer *S. neurona*-specific serum in a rabbit using cultured merozoites; then, using that serum's specificity, they were able to confirm *S. neurona* infections in two raccoons, two mink, two skunks, a cat, and a pony. They also mentioned that other *S. neurona*-like infections were found in California harbor seals (*Phoca vitulina richardsi*, Lapointe et al., 1998), and in sea otters (*E. lutris*, Lindsay et al., 2000; Rosonke et al., 1999; Dubey et al., 2001h). Cheadle et al. (2001b) and Tanhauser et al. (2001) also reported that armadillos (*D. novemcinctus*) can serve as intermediate hosts, and Dubey et al. (2001c) found a four-month-old, captive born, straw-necked ibis (*T. spinicollis*) in the Kansas City Zoological Park to be infected with an *S. neurona*-like organism. Numerous meronts and merozoites were found extravascularly in the bird in encephalitic lesions and the meronts reacted positively with anti-*S. neurona* polyclonal antibodies in an immunohistochemical test. Prior to their report, *S. neurona* had never been identified in tissues of any naturally infected birds. The meronts and merozoites in the brain of the ibis resembled *S. neurona* in structure, location, and antigenicity. Dubey et al. (2001c) cautioned that because the polyclonal anti-*Sarcocystis* sera they used wasn't species specific, "diagnosis should not be made at species level solely on immunohistochemistry." However, they did not mention the validity (or not) of earlier studies that reported "*S. neurona*-like organisms" in marine mammals and birds. Thus, *S. neurona* may have one of the widest known host ranges of all other *Sarcocystis* species (also see *S. falcatula*). Both *D. virginiana* in North America and *D. albiventris* in South America are known definitive hosts, but it is not known whether *S. neurona* can infect other species of South American opossums.

Structurally, meronts of *S. neurona* closely resemble those of other *Sarcocystis* species; however, the merozoites of *S. neurona* lack rhoptries, are located free in the host cell cytoplasm of cells in the brain and spinal cord, and divide by endopolygeny. This suite of characters helps distinguish *S. neurona* from other species of *Sarcocystis* found to date in other domestic animals.

Sarcocystis neurona is the etiological agent of protozoal myeloencephalitis, an often fatal disease of horses (Dubey et al., 1991a). Dame et al. (1995) hypothesized that *S. neurona* should be a junior synonym of *S. falcatula* based on some gene sequence similarities. However, Dubey and Lindsay (1998) and Dubey et al. (1998) distinguished the two species from each other, both structurally and antigenically, as well as from yet a third species (*S. speeri*) found in one

opossum. In addition, Lindsay et al. (1999) were able to grow *S. falcatula* in bovine turbinate cell cultures, and demonstrated that it is different from *S. neurona*. Because of such similarities, Speer and Dubey (1999) thought it is imperative to document structures of these parasites in detail so they undertook an ultrastructural study of the meronts and merozoites of *S. falcatula* to supplement the work of Smith et al. (1987a,b) with further details. Lindsay et al. (1999) grew merozoites of *S. falcatula* in bovine turbinate cell cultures and provided in vitro evidence of its development to further distinguish it from *S. neurona*. Monteiro et al. (2013) reported DNA of *S. neurona*-like and *S. falcatula*-like sporocysts in *D. albiventris* and *D. aurita* from Brazil.

Finally, Spitz dos Santos et al. (2014) pointed out how a wild animal like the opossum, that most people would never give a second thought to, can become epidemiologically relevant when they are identified as definitive hosts of a disease organism that impacts humans and their domestic animals with as much physical devastation as *S. neurona* does. Interestingly, more than a decade earlier, Rickard et al. (2001) addressed the same issue stating that despite the importance of this parasite, its epidemiology in the definitive host was poorly understood. They tried to examine certain "risk factors" that may be associated with the presence of *S. neurona* in the gut of opossums. They identified potential risk factors, such as locality, trap date, age, gender, the presence of young in the pouch of females, and body condition. Then they examined 72 *D. virginiana* that were live-trapped in March, 1999, and from November, 1999 to May, 2000. They detected sporocysts in 19/72 (26%) opossums and, using logistic regression analysis, only the season and body condition score were associated with increased odds of an opossum harboring sporocysts. Certainly, much more needs to be done to understand the epidemiology of this important parasite.

SARCOCYSTIS SPEERI DUBEY AND LINDSAY, 1999

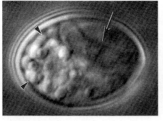 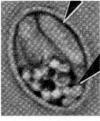

FIGURES 7.9, 7.10   **7.9.** Photomicrograph of a sporocyst of *Sarcocystis speeri* in intestinal scraping from *Didelphis virginiana*, in Dubey and Lindsay, 1999 (their Figure 1), with permission from both authors and from the Editor of the *Journal of Parasitology*. **7.10.** Photomicrograph of a sporocyst of *S. speeri* from feces of *D. virginiana*, in Dubey et al., 2000e (their Figure 1), with permission from the senior author and from the Editor of the *Journal of Parasitology*.

Definitive type host: *Didelphis virginiana* Kerr, 1792, Virginia Opossum.

Type locality: NORTH AMERICA: USA: Florida, Miami, trapped in a zoo.

Other definitive hosts: *Didelphis albiventris* Lund, 1840, White-eared Opossum; *Didelphis marsupialis* L., 1758, Common Opossum (Dubey et al., 2000a, 2015).

Intermediate type host: *Mus musculus* L., 1758 (experimental), Laboratory nude mice (C57BL/6JHFH11-Nu) (Jackson Laboratories, Bar Harbor, Maine).

Other intermediate hosts: *Mus musculus* L., 1758 (experimental), Laboratory γ-interferon KO mice (Jackson Laboratories, Bar Harbor, Maine).

Geographic distribution: NORTH AMERICA: USA: Florida, Louisiana, Maryland, Virginia; SOUTH AMERICA: Argentina: La Plata; Brazil (Dubey et al., 2000a,g).

Description of sporulated oocyst: Unknown.

Description of sporocyst and sporozoites: Sporocyst shape: ellipsoidal; L×W: 12–15×8–10 (Dubey and Lindsay, 1999) or, 12–14.5×9–11 (Dubey et al., 2000e); L/W ratio: unknown; SB, SSB, PSB: all absent; SR: present; SR characteristics: composed of large, hyaline granules that

are either scattered or condensed at one end of the sporocyst; SZ: sausage-shaped, without distinct RB or N visible (Dubey and Lindsay, 1999, their Figures 1 and 2) and one SZ measured 9 long (Dubey et al., 2000e, Figure 1, arrow). Distinctive features of sporocyst: none, this is a typical *Sarcocystis*-type sporocyst.

Prevalence: Sporocysts found in 2/2 (100%) *D. virginiana* by Dubey and Lindsay (1999). Dubey (2000) took intestinal scrapings from 44 wild-caught *D. virginiana* from six US states; he found 24/44 (54.5%) infected with sporocysts of *Sarcocystis* species. Using bioassays of these sporocysts in birds (*M. undulatus*), and genetically engineered nude mice (C57BL/6JHfH11-Nu) and/or γ-interferon KO mice (BALB/c^lfng), he determined that sporocysts of *S. speeri* were present in 8/44 (18%) opossums. Dubey et al. (2000e) found sporocysts of this species in 1/1 *D. albiventris* from Argentina.

Sporulation: Endogenous with infective sporocysts shed in the feces of the definitive host.

Prepatent and patent periods: Sporocysts were recovered from two experimentally infected opossums 11 and 12 days PI after ingesting infective sarcocysts in KO mice (Dubey et al., 2000e).

Site of infection, definitive host: Unknown, but likely the intestinal epithelium.

Site of infection, intermediate host: Merozoites were found in the liver, lung, and spleen of both nude and KO laboratory mice, and meronts also were found in the brain and uterus 34–72 days PI. Sarcocysts were found in KO mice 33–80 days PI, but only in the tongue of one mouse (Dubey and Lindsay, 1999). Meronts also have been grown in cell cultures seeded with merozoites from the liver of a KO mouse infected with an isolate from *D. albiventris* from Argentina. Merozoites from cell culture are not infective to KO mice, showing that *S. speeri* has an obligatory two-host life cycle (Dubey et al., 2000f, 2015).

Endogenous stages, definitive host: Unknown.

Endogenous stages, intermediate host: Sarcocysts in the leg muscles of KO mice were up to 1 mm long at 41 days PI, and up to 5 mm long 72 days PI; they are filiform in shape. Under the light microscope, the sarcocyst wall is <1 thick, but ultrastructurally it is up to 1.8 thick and has characteristic protrusions surmounted by a spire, type 38 (Dubey et al., 2015). No sarcocysts were seen in the heart of any experimentally infected mice (Dubey and Lindsay, 1999).

Cross-transmission: Budgerigars (*M. undulatus*) fed ~500,000 sporocysts of this species from infected opossums did not become infected, even though KO mice given the same inoculum did become infected (Dubey and Lindsay, 1999). Later, Dubey et al. (2000e) fed sporocysts of *S. speeri* to four budgerigars, which did not become infected.

Pathology: Unknown.

Materials deposited: Histologic sections of meronts and sarcocysts are in the U.S. National Parasite Collection, Beltsville, Maryland, as USNPC No. 89057.

Etymology: The authors named this species in honor of Professor C.A. Speer, Veterinary Molecular Biology, Montana State University, Bozeman, Montana, for his "valuable contributions to the understanding of the biology of *Sarcocystis* and other coccidia."

Remarks: Dubey et al. (1998) first isolated a third species of *Sarcocystis* from the feces of a road-kill opossum, that they were able to distinguish as different from *S. falcatula* and *S. neurona* in immunodeficient mice fed sporocysts. That prompted Dubey and Lindsay (1999) to name this form *S. speeri*. Later, Dubey et al. (2000e) found a similar form from *D. albiventris* in Argentina. They (Dubey et al., 2000e) were able to successfully transmit sporocysts of the Argentinian form to KO mice in which the parasite successfully developed sarcocysts, and these muscle sarcocysts were fed to a captive *D. virginiana*, which shed sporocysts 11 days later. These sporocysts from *D. virginiana* were then infective to nine KO mice, but not to four budgerigars. Meronts and sarcocysts of *S. speeri* were found in the tissues of the KO mice.

Sporocysts of this species from opossums are not infective to budgerigars and, therefore, can be distinguished from *S. falcatula*. This species was named as distinct also based on the structure of its sarcocysts, which is still thought to be a reliable taxonomic criterion for the genus (Dubey et al., 1989). The natural intermediate host for *S. speeri* remains unknown.

GENUS MARMOSA GRAY, 1821 (9 SPECIES)

SARCOCYSTIS MARMOSAE SHAW AND LAINSON, 1969

Figures: For an LM photomicrograph of a sarcocyst of *S. marmosae* in the thigh muscle of *Marmosa murina*, see Shaw and Lainson, 1969 (their Figure 4).

Definitive type host: Unknown.

Type locality: SOUTH AMERICA: Brazil: Pará state, Belém, Utinga Forest.

Other definitive hosts: Unknown.

Intermediate type host: *Marmosa murina* (L., 1758), Linnaeus's Mouse Opossum.

Other intermediate hosts: None to date.

Geographic distribution: SOUTH AMERICA: Brazil.

Description of sporulated oocyst: Unknown.

Description of sporocyst and sporozoites: Unknown.

Prevalence: Found in 1/1 *M. murina*.

Sporulation: Unknown, but likely endogenous with infective sporocysts shed in the feces of the definitive host.

Prepatent and patent periods: Unknown.

Site of infection, definitive host: Unknown, but likely in the epithelium of the intestine.

Site of infection, intermediate host: Sarcocysts were found only in the skeletal muscle of the thigh and cysts were "very scanty."

Endogenous stages, definitive host: Unknown.

Endogenous stages, intermediate host: Only sarcocysts in the muscle were observed. These are small, ovoidal, 2000 × 800, with a wall containing conspicuous fingerlike villi with rounded tips, measuring 11.5–13 × 3 in smears of crushed sporocysts. Bradyzoites (which they called "spores") in smears were 7.5 × 2 (6–9 × 2–3), tapering to a fine point at one end, with an area of delicate vacuolation in the cytoplasm toward the pointed end. The N of these zoites was located at their rounded end and measured 2.5 (2–3) wide.

Cross-transmission: None to date.

Pathology: Unknown.

Materials deposited: Syntypes are deposited within the Department of Parasitology, the London School of Hygiene and Tropical Medicine.

Remarks: During their early studies on the epidemiology of leishmaniasis in Brazil, Shaw and Lainson (1969) had the opportunity to examine a single specimen of two different opossums from Belém, Brazil, namely, one *Philander opossum* and one *M. murina*. Unfortunately, their study was limited to a macroscopic search of superficial muscles of skinned animals with only the ability to use low-power examination of muscle squash preparations looking for tissue cysts.

GENUS *PHILANDER* BRISSON, 1762 (4 SPECIES)

SARCOCYSTIS GARNHAMI MANDOUR, 1965

Intermediate type host: *Didelphis marsupialis* L., 1758, Common Opossum.

Remarks: Mandour (1965) descried this species from *D. marsupialis* from Belize (former British Honduras). Shaw and Lainson (1969) reported this species from the muscles of McIlhenny's four-eyed opossum, *P. mcilhennyi* (syn. *P. opossum*), in Belém, Brazil, and argued that it was **clearly** *S. garnhami*, its structure agreeing exactly with Mandour's description (see *Remarks* under *Didelphis*, above).

ORDER DIPROTODONTIA OWEN, 1866

FAMILY MACROPODIDAE GRAY, 1821 (11 GENERA, 65 SPECIES)

GENUS *PETROGALE* GRAY, 1837 (16 SPECIES)

SARCOCYSTIS MUCOSA (BLANCHARD 1885A,B) LABBÉ, 1889

Figures: For LM and TEM photomicrographs of gastrointestinal cysts and cystozoites see O'Donoghue et al. (1987, their Figures 1–12).

Synonyms: *Balbiania mucosa* Blanchard, 1885a,b; *Globidium mucosa* Nöller, 1920; *Sarcocystis macropodis* Gilruth and Bull, 1912; *Globidium mucosum* Zwart and Strik, 1964; *Eimeria mucosa* Levine, 1979.

Definitive type host: Unknown.

Type locality: EUROPE: France: Paris Garden of Acclimatation.

Other definitive hosts: Unknown.

Intermediate type host: *Petrogale penicillata* (Gray, 1827), Brush-tailed Rock Wallaby.

Other intermediate hosts: *Macropus rufogriseus* (Desmarest, 1817) (syn. *Macropus bennetti* Waterhouse, 1838), Red-necked or Bennett's Wallaby; *Petrogale assimilis* Ramsay, 1877, Allied Rock Wallaby; *Thylogale billardierii* (Desmarest, 1822), Tasmanian Pademelon.

Geographic distribution: AUSTRALIA.

Description of sporulated oocyst: Unknown.

Description of sporocyst and sporozoites: Unknown.

Prevalence: O'Donoghue et al. (1987) found macroscopic cysts of this species in the gastrointestinal walls of 2/23 (9%) *P. assimilis* and in 20/24 (83%) *M. rufogriseus*. Jakes (1998) found macroscopic sarcocysts of *S. mucosa* in 13% of Bennett's wallabies (*M. rufogriseus*) and in 16% of Tasmanian pademelons (*T. gillardierii*) surveyed (Dubey et al., 2015).

Sporulation: Unknown.

Prepatent and patent periods: Unknown.

Site of infection, definitive host: Unknown, but likely the intestinal epithelium in a carnivore that eats wallabies.

Site of infection, intermediate host: Cysts are visible from the serosal surface and appeared as small, white bumps, ~0.2–2.0 mm wide, in the gastrointestinal walls, predominantly in the fore-stomach, small intestine, colon, and sometimes the cecum and esophagus (O'Donoghue et al., 1987).

Endogenous stages, definitive host: Unknown.

Endogenous stages, intermediate host: Tissue cysts were located within the muscularis externa of infected organs, usually between the outer longitudinal and the inner circular smooth muscle layers. Via light microscopy, cysts were divided into numerous internal compartments by thin septa that radiated inward from their perimeter. Compartments near the periphery of each cyst were filled with numerous banana-shaped cystozoites, while those toward the center of the cyst either were completely empty or they contained small aggregates of granular material. Mean size of cystozoites was 10×2, and each had prominent PAS granules. Each cyst was composed of a thick wall, 1–2 wide, with numerous small knoblike protrusions surrounded by host cell N. Ultrastructural examination of the cysts showed they were surrounded by a primary cyst wall, which was repeatedly folded into bulbous-like protrusions that were perpendicular to the axis of the wall. These protrusions were 1.5–1.8 high, and consisted of a stalk, 0.5–0.8 thick, supporting a broader bulb, 1.2–1.8 wide. The stalks were filled with numerous microfibrils arranged perpendicular to the cyst wall axis. Cysts were not located within individual host cells or muscle fibers, but were surrounded by consecutive layers of amorphous material, collagen fibers, and connective tissue cells. O'Donoghue et al. (1987) identified two cell types within cyst compartments, cystozoites and metrocytes. Cystozoites were banana-shaped, $8.5–12 \times 1.5–2.8$, and

contained numerous apicomplexan organelles, whereas metrocytes were large undifferentiated cells bounded by a three-layered pellicle, contained a large diffuse N, but relatively few organelles, and were $10–20 \times 8–15$.

Cross-transmission: None to date; however, O'Donoghue et al. (1987) found that none of 25 Tasmanian pademelons (*T. billardierii*), four unadorned rock wallaby (*Petrogale inornata*), and seven Godman's rock wallaby (*Petrogale godmani*) were infected with this parasite during their survey.

Pathology: Tissue cysts were surrounded by loose strands of fibrous connective tissue and several host cell N, but no marked inflammatory reactions or cellular aggregations were seen by O'Donoghue et al. (1987).

Materials deposited: None.

Remarks: O'Donoghue et al. (1987) said the cysts they found in both *P. assimilis* and *M. rufogriseus* were similar in size, shape, and appearance to those originally described in *P. penicillata* by Blanchard (1885a,b) and later redescribed by Coutelen (1933). They also were compartmentalized by septa and contained numerous zoites similar in morphology to those previously described.

In comparison, the larger cysts found by Gilruth and Bull (1912) in the small intestinal submucosa of three *Petrogale* sp. were described as clusters of cysts surrounded by thick double-layered envelopes and accumulations of inflammatory cells. Similarly, the 1 mm wide macroscopic cysts found by Zwart and Strik (1964), in the small intestinal mucosa of one *M. rufogriseus*, were described as "conglomerates of schizonts" surrounded by an inflammatory zone. Thus, the cysts in both of these reports were different than those documented by Blanchard (1885a,b) and O'Donoghue et al. (1987).

The large and small cysts first found in the small intestinal mucosa of a *Macropus* sp. by Gilruth and Bull (1912) also need clarification; respectively, these were named *Ileocystis macropodis* and *Lymphocystis macropodis*. Later, Wenyon and Scott (1925) found similar cysts in the small intestinal mucosa of one *M. rufogriseus*, and these were described in more detail by Triffit (1926). These organisms were subsequently reassigned to *Globodium* by other authors, but they are now thought to represent different developmental stages of one or more *Eimeria* species (Pellérdy, 1974; O'Donoghue et al., 1987).

Given the obligate two-host (heteroxenous) life cycle of *Sarcocystis* species, O'Donoghue et al. (1987) speculated on what might be the definitive host for this species, the sporocysts of which are found in marsupial species in both Australia and Tasmania. Two introduced canids, the dingo, *Canis familiaris*, and the European red fox, *Vulpes vulpes*, are confined to mainland Australia and neither is found in Tasmania. Feral domestic cats, *F. catus*, are well established throughout Australia, but they are known to prey primarily on small animals and birds. Marsupial "native cats" (quolls), *Dasyurus* spp., occur in many areas of both Australia and Tasmania, but they are small opportunistic carnivores and scavengers, with insects as their most important dietary intake. Large reptiles (e.g., crocodiles, pythons) have limited distribution on mainland Australia, and birds of prey (e.g., eagles, owls, etc.) are known generally to feast on small animals, birds or fish, but not kangaroos. They concluded (1987) that the "determination of the definitive host for *S. mucosa* will therefore be difficult to ascertain because few candidate species are available and none exhibit a close predator–prey relationship with wallabies which could satisfactorily account for the prevalence and distribution of the parasite."

DISCUSSION AND SUMMARY

As a family, it could be argued that the Sarcocystidae may be the most successful protist clade in nature because virtually all vertebrate species can be infected by at least one species of its two most ubiquitous genera, *Sarcocystis*

and/or *Toxoplasma*. In this chapter, we see that *Sarcocystis* species can infect vertebrates, including marsupials, either as their intermediate, or as their definitive host, or both (e.g., American opossums, Tables 11.1 and 11.2), and in the next chapter, we will see that *Toxoplasma* is quite common, and pathogenic, in dozens of marsupial hosts.

Within the Marsupialia, at least four, and perhaps five (Microbiotheria?), of their seven orders, including eight (or nine?) families, 18 (or 19?) genera, and 32 (or 33) species have been reported to have *Sarcocystis* or sarcocystis-like species either as intermediate (muscle sarcocysts) or definitive (fecal sporocysts) hosts (Chapter 10, Tables 11.1 and 11.2). For example, opossums (Family Didelphidae: *Didelphis* spp.) are the definitive hosts for *S. falcatula*, *S. lindsayi*, *S. neurona*, and *S. speeri*, and very large numbers of sporocysts can be excreted in their feces (Box et al., 1984; Dubey and Lindsay, 1999; Dubey et al., 2001f; Tanhauser et al., 1999); in addition, *Lutreolina crassicaudata*, the Lutrine opossum, may be a definitive host for a *Sarcocystis* sp., the sporocysts of which were first seen by Carini (1939) (Chapter 10). Unfortunately, however, sporocysts are all nearly identical in the few structural features they possess, so although measurements can be gathered and presented, the actual identity of sporocysts of each species from naturally infected opossums is not definitive. For example, Cheadle et al. (2001a) provided measurements of at least four *Sarcocystis*-like sporocysts in feces of 17 naturally infected opossums: sporocysts of *S. neurona* were $10.7 \times 7.0\,\mu m$, *S. speeri* were $12.2 \times 8.8\,\mu m$, *Sarcocystis* species strain-1085 were $10.9 \times 6.8\,\mu m$, and those of *S. falcatula* were $11.0 \times 7.1\,\mu m$; these differences were all within 2-μm of each other so absolute identifications could not be determined or substantiated.

Marsupials also act as intermediate hosts for known *Sarcocystis* species. Within the Didelphidae (Didelphimorphia), *D. marsupialis*, *D. virginiana*, *M. murina*, and *P. mcilhennyi* are intermediate hosts for *S. didelphidis*, *S. garnhami*, *S. greineri*, *S. inghami*, and *S. marmosae*, and within the Macropodidae (Diprotodontia), *M. rufogriseus*, *P. assimilis*, *P. penicillata*, and *T. billardierii* act as intermediate hosts for *S. mucosa* (Tables 11.1 and 11.2). At least 15 genera and 23 species act as intermediate hosts for more than 20 *Sarcocystis*-like sarcocysts found in muscles (Chapter 10 and Tables 11.1 and 11.2).

Of the 10 *Sarcocystis* species known, to date, to infect marsupials, only *S. mucosa* has been recorded from Australian marsupials (*M. rufogriseus*, *P. assimilis*, *P. penicillata*, *T. billardierii*). The remaining nine *Sarcocystis* species, from which we know the most biology, and more accurate and reliable species identifications, are known from six opossums in the Americas: *D. albiventris*, *D. surita*, *D. mardupialis*, *D. virginiana*, *M. murina*, and *P. mcilhennyi*. It seems almost incredulous to me that only 32/336 (9.5%) marsupial species worldwide have been found to harbor *Sarcocystis* species either as intermediate or as definitive hosts.

In American marsupials, sarcocysts have been found in the muscles of individuals in four species from one family in one order: **Didelphimorphia**: Didelphidae: *D. marsupialis*, *D. virginiana*, *M. murina*, *P. mcilhennyi*. However, in Australian marsupials, sarcocysts in the muscles are known in 24 species from 7 families, in 3 orders: **Dasyumorphia**: Dasyuridae: *A. stuartii*, *A. swainsonii*, *A.* sp., *D. hallucatus*, *D. maculatus*, and *S. harrisii*. **Diprotodontia**: Macropodidae: *M. agilis*, *M. giganteus*, *M. rufogriseus*, *M. rufus*, *P. assimilis*, *P. brachyotis*, *P. concinna*, *P. penicillata*, *T. billardierii*, *W. bicolor*; Petauridae: *P. australis*; Phalangeridae: *T. caninus*, *T. vulpecula*; Potoridae: *B. lesueur*; Pseudocheiridae: *P. archeri*. **Peramelemorphia**: Peramelidae: *I. macrourus*, *I. obesulus*, *P. gunnii*, *P. nasuta*.

In recent years, bioassay and molecular methods have begun to help distinguish the sporocysts of different *Sarcocystis* species in opossum feces. One of the more reliable bioassays is the use of KO mice and budgerigars in cross-transmission studies to help differentiate between *Sarcocystis* sporocysts in opossum feces; *S. neurona* and *S. speeri* are not infective to budgerigars, and *S. falcatula* is not infective to KO mice (Dubey and Lindsay, 1998), while *S. speeri* and *S. neurona* in KO mice can be distinguished immunohistochemically (Dubey, 2000). In addition, molecular methods are now in place to distinguish *S. falcatula* and *S. neurona*, (Tanhauser et al., 1999). Early molecular characterizations used 18S rRNA markers on *Sarcocystis* strains isolated from horses (*S. neurona*), that placed them firmly within the Sarcocystidae and *showed* a close relationship with *S. muris* (Tanhauser et al., 1999). Later work at the 18S locus indicated that *S. neurona* might be synonymous with *S. falcatula* (Dame et al., 1995), but phylogenetic resolution between the two occurred when the ITS-1 locus, within the 18S rRNA gene array, was sequenced and distinct nucleotide differences between the two parasites were determined (Marsh et al., 1999). Later, panels of random amplified polymorphic DNA markers were developed to differentiate *S. neurona* isolates from other closely related coccidians (Elsheikha and Mansfield, 2007; Granstrom et al., 1994; Fenger et al., 1995; Tanhauser et al., 1999; Dubey et al., 2015). Using these markers, *S. neurona* was identified in 138/610 (23%) *D. virginiana* in about 15 states in the USA either by bioassay in KO mice and/ or by various molecular methods including RFLP and ITA-1 gene sequences (Dubey, 2000; Dubey et al., 2001a; Elsheikha et al., 2004a; Rejmanek et al., 2009, 2010; Dubey et al., 2015). These studies suggest that season, body condition, and presence of young in the pouch all are associated with the presence of sporocysts in the feces.

8

Sarcocystidae: Toxoplasmatinae (*Besnoitia, Toxoplasma*) in Marsupials

EUCOCCIDIORIDA: EIMERIORINA: SARCOCYSTIDAE

INTRODUCTION

In Chapter 7, I covered the Apicomplexans (*Sarcocystis* species) within the first subfamily, Sarcocystinae, of the Sarcocystidae that parasitize marsupials. In this chapter, there are two genera (*Besnoitia, Toxoplasma* species) within the second subfamily, Toxoplasmatinae, that infect marsupials. Each is covered below.

TOXOPLASMATINAE: *BESNOITIA* IN MARSUPIALS

Marsupials played a prominent role in the discovery of, and the narrative that has followed on *Besnoitia*. The story of finding the first *Besnoitia* species was nicely summarized by Schneider (1967a). Briefly, Dr. S.T. Darling, working in the Panama Canal Zone, found a cystic parasite in the common opossum, *Didelphis marsupialis*, and he placed it, taxonomically, into the genus *Sarcocystis*, even though he was troubled by some of the features he observed that separated it from the defining characteristics of the genus (Darling, 1910). Darling (1910) considered emending the biological characters applied to *Sarcocystis* to include parasites capable of developing in nonmuscular sites of their hosts, as did the cysts he observed (vs striated and heart muscle sites of *Sarcocystis*). He also noted that the cysts he found in the opossum lacked internal septa and divisions into compartments, also common characters of *Sarcocystis* cysts, but he did not propose a name for his parasite. Brumpt (1913, p. 109) chose to name Darling's parasite after him, *Sarcocystis darlingi*, using Darling's descriptive material, but disregarding Darling's reservations about the differences in tissue stages. Babudieri (1932) later placed *S. darlingi* into the genus *Fibrocystis* Hadwen, 1922, but Levine (1973) correctly pointed out that *Fibrocystis* is a synonym of *Besnoitia*. Levine also said (1973, p. 507), "The name *Globidium* has often been used instead of *Besnoitia* for members of this genus, but this in incorrect, since *Globidium* is a synonym of *Eimeria*." Finally, Mandour (1965) stated that the proper name for the parasite first seen by Darling should be *B. darlingi*.

The life cycles of *Besnoitia* species are obligatorily heteroxenous, similar to that of *Sarcocystis* species, but they differ from *Sarcocystis* in three unique ways: (1) oocysts shed by definitive hosts are unsporulated, and have relatively thick walls; (2) the completion of the sexual cycle in the definitive host is dependent upon ingestion of tissue cysts from a suitable intermediate host—that is, the ability of oocysts to initiate gametogenesis in the definitive host has been lost; and (3) these species can be successfully propagated asexually by mechanical transmission from intermediate host to intermediate host by blood-sucking arthropods. Other details of what little we know about the life cycle of various *Besnoitia* species have been summarized by Leighton and Gajadhar (2001) and Duszynski and Couch (2013).

SPECIES DESCRIPTION

ORDER DIDELPHIMORPHIA GILL, 1872

FAMILY DIDELPHIDAE GRAY, 1821 (17 GENERA, 87 SPECIES)

GENUS *DIDELPHIS* L., 1758 (6 SPECIES)

BESNOITIA DARLINGI (BRUMPT, 1913) MANDOUR, 1965

Synonyms: Sarcocystis sp. Darling, 1910; *Sarcocystis darlingi* Brumpt, 1913; *Besnoitia panamensis* Schneider, 1965; *Besnoitia sauriana* Garnham, 1966; *Fibrocystis darlingi* (Brumpt, 1913) Babudieri, 1932.
Definitive type host: Unknown.
Type locality: SOUTH AMERICA: Panama.

FIGURES 8.1, 8.2 **8.1.** Photomicrograph of a sporulated oocyst of *Besnoitia darlingi* from the feces of an experimentally infected cat. **8.2.** Photomicrograph of a section through an intact cyst of *B. darlingi* in the lamina propria of an experimentally infected mouse. Both figures in Smith and Frenkel, 1977, with permission from the Editor of the *Journal of Parasitology*.

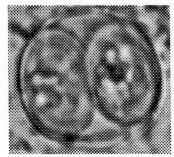 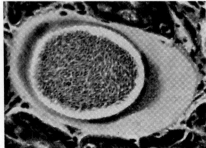

Other definitive hosts: *Felis catus* L., 1758, Domestic Cat (see Smith and Frenkel, 1977).

Intermediate type host: *Didelphis marsupialis* L., 1758, Common Opossum.

Other intermediate hosts: **Marsupials**: *Caluromys derbianus* (Waterhouse, 1841), Brown-eared Woolly Opossum (experimental); *Didelphis aurita* (Wied-Neuwied, 1826), Big-eared Opossum; *Didelphis virginiana* Kerr, 1792, Virginia Opossum; *Philander opossum* (L., 1758), Gray Four-eyed Opossum (experimental); **Other mammals**: *Carollia perspicillata* (L., 1758), Seba's Short-tailed Bat (experimental); *Mesocricetus auratus* (Waterhouse, 1839), Golden Hamster (experimental); *Mus musculus* L., 1758, House Mouse (experimental); *Saguinus geoffroyi* (Pucheran, 1845), Geoffroy's Tamarin (experimental); *Sciurus granatensis* Humboldt, 1811, Red-tailed Squirrel (experimental); *Sciurus* (*Sciurus*) *variegatoides* Ogilby, 1839, Variegated Squirrel (experimental); **Lizards**: *Ameiva ameiva* L., 1758, Giant Ameiva; *Ameiva praesignis* (Baird and Girtard, 1852), Amazon Racerunner; *Basiliscus basiliscus* L., 1758, Common Basilisk; *Basiliscus vittatus* Wiegmann, 1828, Brown Basilisk; *Holcosus leptophrys* (Cope, 1893) (syn. *Ameiva leptophrys* Dunn, 1940), Delicate Ameiva.

Geographic distribution: CENTRAL AMERICA: Belize (formerly British Honduras); Panama; NORTH AMERICA: USA: Illinois, Kansas, Kentucky, Missouri; SOUTH AMERICA: Brazil.

Description of sporulated oocyst: Oocyst shape: subspheroidal; number of walls: 1; wall characteristics: thin, smooth; L×W: 12.0×10.3 (11–13×10–12); L/W ratio: 1.2 (Smith and Frenkel, 1977) or L×W: 12×12; L/W ratio: 1.0 (Smith and Frenkel, 1984); M, OR, PG: all absent. Distinctive features of oocyst: small spheroidal to subspheroidal oocyst similar to those of *Toxoplasma gondii*.

Description of sporocyst and sporozoites: Sporocyst shape: ellipsoidal; L×W: 7.9×5.4 (6–9×5–6); L/W ratio: 1.5; SB, SSB, PSB: all absent; SR: present, granular; SZ: ~5×2 (Smith and Frenkel, 1977). Distinctive features of sporocyst: None.

Prevalence: Myocardial cysts were found in 2/2 (100%) *D. marsupialis* in Panama (Schneider, 1967a); Conti-Diaz et al. (1970) found a *Besnoitia* sp. consistent with both *B. darlingi* and *B. jellisoni* in the lungs, and to a lesser extent in the liver of 1/5 (20%) *D. marsupialis*, in Kentucky; Flatt et al. (1971) found it in many tissues of 8/13 (61.5%) *D. virginiana*, in Missouri and Illinois; Smith and Frenkel (1977) found it in 2/5 (40%) road-killed *D. virginiana* in Kansas. Naiff and Arias (1983) found what presumably was *B. darlingi* in 15/224 (7%) *D. marsupialis* collected in Amazônica, Brazil. (Note: There is a question regarding the identity of the opossums some of these investigators examined. According to Walker et al. (1975), *D. marsupialis* occurs from Mexico southward to northern Argentina, while *D. virginiana* occurs from southern Canada, southward into Central America. However, the form in the United States has been called *D. marsupialis* until recently, and it is uncertain to me which species Darling (1910), Schneider (1965, 1967a,b,c), and Garnham (1964, 1965, 1966) were dealing with.) Stabler and Welch (1961) found what was probably this species in an opossum in Texas. Houk et al. (2010) examined blood of *D. virginiana* for antibodies to six protozoan parasites including *B. darlingi*; they found that 14/30 (47%) demonstrated antibodies against *B. darlingi* using an indirect immunofluorescent antibody test (IFAT) against *in vitro*-produced antigens.

Sporulation: Oocysts sporulated in 2–3 days in 2% sulfuric acid at room temperature (Smith and Frenkel, 1977).

Prepatent and patent periods: The prepatent period was 13 (11–14) days, and the patent period lasted 6 (5–10) days (Smith and Frenkel, 1977).

Site of infection, definitive host: Unknown.

Site of infection, intermediate host: Found in numerous locations, dependent upon the host: (1) Found in the lungs, kidney, heart, spleen, brain, muscle, fibrous tissue, and peritoneal fluid of experimentally infected laboratory mice and a tamarin; (2) Tachyzoites are found in the lungs and lymph nodes of experimental mice (Schneider, 1967a; Smith and Frenkel, 1977); (3) Found in the tongue, ears, mesenteries, gastrointestinal tract, adrenal glands, kidneys, abdominal muscles, and uterus of opossums (Smith and Frenkel, 1977). Smith and Frenkel (1977) also noted that the concentration of cysts was greatest in the adrenals; they postulated that since opossums (and other mammals) predominately secrete cortisol, the higher concentration of this steroid in the adrenal cortex may delay the development of immunity locally, permitting *B. darlingi* to proliferate longer than in other tissues and, thus, develop a greater number of cysts in that organ.

Endogenous stages, definitive host: Unknown, but likely intestinal epithelial cells.

Endogenous stages, intermediate host: Meronts (in lizards) are ovoidal or spheroidal, often appearing lobed, with a three-layered wall: outer is 2.5–3 thick, middle contains a large N, and the inner consists of a thin membrane; the combined walls are ~12 thick (Garnham, 1966). Meronts were 62–156 × 66–300, each with thousands of merozoites, also in lizards (Schneider, 1965) or 693 (438–827) wide in opossums (Smith and Frenkel, 1977). Merozoites in peritoneal fluid are crescent-shaped, spindle-shaped, piriform, or ovoidal, 7–11 × 1–2, while merozoites in meronts from lizards are crescentic to banana-shaped, 7–8 × 1–2 (Schneider, 1965). Trophozoites isolated from noncompartmentalized tissue cysts in *D. marsupialis* were 6.1 × 2.1 (6–9 × 1.7–4). Conti-Diaz et al. (1970) found cysts in *D. marsupialis* "visible to the naked eye,…as white spherical bodies not exceeding 1 mm in diameter," while the crescent-shaped cyst organisms were 7.6 × 1.7 (4–9 × 1–2).

Cross-transmission: Darling (1910) infected a guinea pig with an opossum strain by intramuscular injection of merozoites. Schneider (1965) infected white mice, golden hamsters, and a marmoset (tamarin, *S. geoffroyi*) by intraperitoneal injection of merozoites from a basilisk lizard, *B. basiliscus*, and/or the giant ameiva, *A. ameiva*; the mice and tamarin died, but the hamsters remained healthy until they were killed. Schneider (1965) was not able to infect the guinea pig, laboratory rabbit, a rhesus monkey, a white-faced monkey (*Cebus capucinus imitator*), or pigeons, with merozoites of this species from *B. basiliscus*. Later (1967a), Schneider produced fatal infections in laboratory mice, with a strain from the opossum and transmitted it from these mice to other white mice, the golden hamster, the tamarin, two species of squirrels, *S. granatensis*, and *S. (S.) variegatoides*, and to a woolly opossum (*C. derbianus*) and one four-eyed opossum (*P. opossum*), causing acute, fatal infections in both of them. He was not able to transmit it to the guinea pig, laboratory rat, night monkey (*Aotus trivirgatus*), rhesus monkey (*Macaca mulatta*), an iguana (*Iguana iguana*), or a baby caiman (*Caiman sclerops*). Schneider (1966) infected six of 11 short-tailed bats, *Carollia panamensis*, by intraperitoneal injection with merozoites of lizard origin, which he had adapted to white mice; the bats remained healthy. Schneider (1967c) found that the marmoset, *S. geoffroyi*, could be infected either by intraperitoneal (**IP**) injection or orally (**per os**) with lizard and opossum strains causing a fatal infection. Garnham (1966) was able to infect white mice with his strain of "*B. sauriana*" from the basilisk lizard. Smith and Frenkel (1977) could not infect the dog with their strain from the opossum, but one cat fed infected tissues began shedding unsporulated oocysts in its feces on the 11th day PI, and continued shedding oocysts for 10 days. Once sporulated, these oocysts were inoculated per os into three mice, all of which died 11–14 days after infection. To complete Koch's postulates, Smith and Frenkel (1977) inoculated three new cats with carcasses of *Besnoitia*-infected mice, and all three began shedding oocysts with a prepatent periods of 11–14 days and patency that lasted 5–8 days. Conti-Diaz et al. (1970) found that their strain from the opossum, from Kentucky, was highly pathogenic for the golden hamster, but had little or no pathogenicity for white Swiss mice; it could not be transmitted to adult guinea pigs by IP inoculation.

Pathology: Highly variable, as noted in cross-transmission studies (above). Smith and Frenkel (1977) found that 6/7 (86%) mice and 7/8 (88%) hamsters inoculated with tissue cysts from infected opossums, died 10–14 and 9–10 days PI, respectively. Brown (1988) found 19/27 (70%) *D. virginiana*, from near Baton Rouge, Louisiana, USA, had endogenous lipid pneumonia, and in 5/19 (26%) she found tissue stages she identified as *B. darlingi*. Endogenous lipid pneumonia is characterized by hyperplasia of Type II pneumocytes, overproduction of surfactant, and consequent accumulation of lipid-laden macrophages, but she was cautious to mention that most of the foci, in the *D. virginiana* she examined, were subpleural, and not usually in the vicinity of the parasite-induced granulomas.

Materials deposited: None.

Remarks: This species was first found in Panama, in the opossum *D. marsupialis*, by Darling (1910). Barretto (1940) reported it from *D. aurita* in Brazil. Schneider (1965) found it in the basilisk lizard *B. basiliscus*, and in the "borriguero" lizard, *A. a. praesignis*, and named it *B. panamensis*. Later, Schneider (1967a) rediscovered it in *D. marsupialis* in Panama, was able to establish the strain in mice, and then transferred it from them into hamsters, marmosets, squirrels, a woolly opossum, a four-eyed opossum, wild-caught *D. marsupialis*, and a lizard, *Ameiva ameiva*; this raised the question about the validity of other named species reported from the Western Hemisphere, especially those found in Central American lizards. Garnham (1964, 1965, 1966) found what was presumably the same species in the basilisk lizards, *B. basiliscus* and *B. vittatus*, in British Honduras (Belize) and named it *B. sauriana*, because it differed in morphology in several ways from the one described by Schneider (1965) in Belize. Once Schneider (1967b) established

evidence that there was strong cross-immunity between his *B. panamensis* and *B. darlingi*, Schneider (1967c) synonymized the lizard forms (*B. panamensis*, *B. sauriana*) from Central America, with *B. darlingi*. Smith and Frenkel (1977) speculated how *B. darlingi* might be transmitted to this and other intermediate hosts in nature. They noted that cat/opossum interactions are probably few and far between, but that as common road kills, it is likely cats occasionally feed on opossum carcasses, and eventually produce oocysts. Opossums are not known to be coprophagous, so it is unlikely they get oocysts from cat feces; they are, however, insectivorous, and ingest many beetles, which might bridge the food web between infected cat feces as a source of infection. Opossums also are well-known carrion feeders, and can be cannibalistic, both habits that easily can transmit bradyzoites to these intermediate hosts.

Finally, Yamada et al. (1981) reported "only a host case of the kangaroo has been reported on the *Besnoitia jellisoni* (Frenkel, 1953)," suggesting that *B. jellisoni* also infects marsupials. However, there likely was an error in translation because Frenkel (1953) reported *B. jellisoni* from kangaroo rats (*Dipodomys*).

TOXOPLASMATINAE: TOXOPLASMA IN MARSUPIALS

Toxoplasma gondii may be the most ubiquitous parasite on Earth; it certainly is the most common parasite of all warm-blooded vertebrates, and it is not uncommon in poikilotherms (except snakes). The history of its discovery, general biology, and life cycle stages have been reviewed many times (Dubey and Beattie, 1988; Weiss and Kim, 2007) and were detailed briefly by Duszynski and Upton (2010), so I will not repeat them here. My comments below are generally restricted to what we now know about *T. gondii* in marsupials.

SPECIES DESCRIPTION

TOXOPLASMA GONDII (NICOLLE AND MANCEAUX, 1908) NICOLLE AND MANCEAUX, 1909

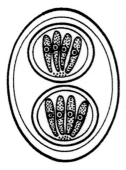 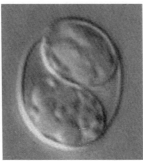

FIGURES 8.3, 8.4 **8.3.** Line drawing of a sporulated oocyst of *Toxoplasma gondii* from Dubey and Odening, 2001 (their Figure 17.11), with permission of the senior author and from John Wiley & Sons, owner of the Iowa State University Press. 8.4. Photomicrograph of a sporulated oocyst of T. gondii (original, courtesy of S.J. Upton).

Synonyms: Numerous (see Levine, 1977).

Definitive type host: *Felis catus* L., 1758, Domestic Cat.

Type locality: Worldwide.

Other definitive hosts: Most, perhaps all, other cats in the Felidae.

Intermediate type host: *Ctenodactylus gundi* (Rothmann, 1776), Common Gundi.

Other intermediate hosts: Most/all warm-blooded and many cold-blooded vertebrates can become intermediate hosts. Among the marsupials, the following have documented infections with T. gondii: **Order Dasyuromorphia**: *Antechinomys laniger* (Gould, 1856) (syn. *Antechinomys spenceri* Thomas, 1906), Kultarr (Attwood et al., 1975); *Antechinus minimus* (É. Geoffroy, 1803), Swamp Antechinus (O'Donoghue and Adlard, 2000); *Antechinus swainsonii* (Waterhouse, 1840), Dusky Antechinus (O'Donoghue and Adlard, 2000); *Dasycercus cristicauda* (Krefft, 1867), Mulgara (Attwood et al., 1975); *Dasyuroides byrnei* Spencer, 1896, Kowari (Attwood et al., 1975);

Dasyurus viverrinus (Shaw, 1800), Eastern Quoll (O'Donoghue and Adlard, 2000); *Dasyurus* sp. (O'Donoghue and Adlard, 2000); *Myrmecobius fasciatus* Waterhouse, 1836, Numbat (Canfield et al., 1990); *Parantechinus apicalis* (Gray, 1842) (syn. *Antechinus apicalis*), Southern Dibbler (Attwood et al., 1975); *Phascogale tapoatafa* (Meyer, 1793), Brush-tailed Phascogale (O'Donoghue and Adlard, 2000); *Pseudantechinus macdonnellensis* (Spencer, 1896) (syn. *Antechinus macdonnellensis*), Fat-tailed False Antechinus (Attwood et al., 1975); *Sminthopsis crassicaudata* (Gould, 1844), Fat-tailed Dunnart (Attwood et al., 1975); *Sminthopsis macroura* (Gould, 1845) (syn. *Sminthopsis larapinta* Spencer, 1896), Striped-faced Dunnart (Attwood et al., 1975); *Sminthopsis leucopus* (Gray, 1842), White-footed Dunnart (Attwood et al., 1975); **Order Didelphimorphia**: *Didelphis albiventris* Lund, 1840, White-eared Opossum (Siqueira et al., 2013); *Didelphis aurita* (Wied-Neuwied, 1826), Big-eared Opossum (Siqueira et al., 2013); *Didelphis marsupialis* L., 1758, Common Opossum (Burridge et al., 1979); *Micoureus demerarae* (Thomas, 1905), Woolly Opossum (Siqueira et al., 2013); *Marmosa murina* (L., 1758), Linnaeus's Mouse Opossum (Siqueira et al., 2013); *Monodelphis domestica* (Wagner, 1842), Gray Short-tailed Opossum (Siqueira et al., 2013); *Metachirus nudicaudatus* (E. Geoffroy, 1803), Brown Four-eyed Opossum (Siqueira et al., 2013); **Order Diprotodontia**: *Dendrolagus lumholtzi* Collett, 1884, Lumholtz's Tree-kangaroo (O'Donoghue and Adlard, 2000); *Lasiorhinus latifrons* (Owen, 1845), Southern Hairy-nosed Wombat (Munday, 1970; Doube, 1981); *Macropus agilis* (Gould, 1842), Agile Wallaby (O'Donoghue and Adlard, 2000); *Macropus eugenii* (Desmarest, 1817), Tammar Wallaby (syn. *Thylogale* (*Wallabia*) *eugenii*, Derby Kangaroo) (Dobos-Kovacs et al., 1974a,b; Lynch et al., 1993; Dubey and Crutchley, 2008); *Macropus fuliginosus* (Desmarest, 1817), Western Grey Kangaroo (Dubey et al., 1988); *Macropus giganteus* Shaw, 1790, Eastern Grey Kangaroo (O'Donoghue and Adlard, 2000); *Macropus parma* Waterhouse, 1846, Parma Wallaby

(O'Donoghue and Adlard, 2000); *Macropus robustus* Gould, 1841, Wallaroo (Riemann et al., 1974; Boorman et al., 1977); *Macropus rufogriseus* (Desmarest, 1817), Red-necked Wallaby (syn. *Macropus bennetti* Waterhouse, 1838, Bennett's Wallaby) (Ratcliffe and Worth, 1951; Grünberg, 1959; Mandelli et al., 1966; Johnson et al., 1988; Adkesson et al., 2007; Basso et al., 2007; Dubey and Crutchley, 2008); *Macropus rufus* (Desmarest, 1822), Red Kangaroo (Hackel et al., 1953; Barker et al., 1963); *Petrogale xanthopus* Gray, 1855, Yellow-footed Rock-wallaby (O'Donoghue and Adlard, 2000); *Phascolarctos cinereus* Blainville, 1816, Koala (Canfield et al., 1990; Hartley et al., 1990); *Setonix brachyurus* (Quoy and Gaimard, 1830), Quokka (Gibb et al., 1966); *Thylogale billardierii* (Desmarest, 1822), Tasmanian Pademelon (Obendorf and Munday, 1983; Johnson et al., 1988; Dubey et al., 1991); *Trichosurus vulpecula*, (Kerr, 1792), Common Brushtail (Cook and Pope, 1959; Presidente, 1984; Canfield et al., 1990; Viggers and Spratt, 1995; Eymann et al., 2006); *Vombatus ursinus* (Shaw, 1800), Common Wombat (Coutelen, 1932; Munday, 1970; Presidente, 1982; Skerratt et al., 1997; Skerratt, 1998; Hartley and English, 2005; Canfield et al., 1990); *Wallabia bicolor* (Desmarest, 1804), Swamp Wallaby (O'Donoghue and Adlard, 2000); **Order Peramelemorphia**: *Isoodon obesulus* (Shaw, 1797), Southern Brown Bandicoot (Pope et al., 1957); *Macrotis lagotis* (Reid, 1837), Greater Bilby (Canfield et al., 1990); *Perameles gunnii* Gray, 1838, Eastern Barred Bandicoot (Obendorf et al., 1996); *Perameles nasuta* E. Geoffroy, 1804, Long-nosed Bandicoot (Pope et al., 1957).

Geographic distribution: Worldwide.

Description of sporulated oocyst: Oocyst shape: spheroidal to slightly ellipsoidal; number of walls: 2; wall characteristics: both layers colorless; L×W: 13×11; L/W ratio: 1.2; M, OR, PG: all absent. Distinctive features of oocyst: very small size with two transparent wall layers.

Description of sporocyst and sporozoites: Sporocyst shape: ellipsoidal; L×W: 8×6; L/W ratio: 1.3; SB, SSB, PSB: all absent; SR: present; SR characteristics: composed of disbursed granules; SZ: sausage-shaped, with a subterminal to central N, but no visible RBs. Distinctive features of sporocyst: very small size, ellipsoidal shape, only a few, scattered SR granules, and lack of SB, SSB, and PSB.

Prevalence: Found in about 30% or more of warm-blooded mammals worldwide (Weiss and Kim, 2007). Mandelli et al. (1966) isolated *T. gondii* in mice inoculated with tissues from 3/3 (100%) *M. rufogriseus* (syn. *M. bennetti*) that died in a zoo in Italy. In Budapest, Hungary, Dobos-Kovács et al. (1974a,b) fed tissues of 2/2 (100%) *M. eugenii* (syn. *T. eugenii*) that eventually died in a zoo, to a cat that subsequently shed oocysts of *T. gondii*. Attwood et al. (1975) did a histopathological survey of dasyurid marsupials in Australia; the animals examined were wild-caught and either killed or maintained in the laboratory, laboratory-reared, or found dead in the field. Of the 240 marsupials examined, 122/240 (51%) were identified as positive for *T. gondii* by various methods (serology, mouse passage, tissue cysts). Eight of nine species examined were positive including: 9/12 (75%) *A. laniger* (syn. *A. spenceri*); 5/9 (56%) *P. apicalis* (syn. *A. apicalis*); 9/14 (64%) *P. macdonnellensis* (syn. *A. macdonnellensis*); 34/51 (67%) *D. cristicauda*; 52/107 (49%) *D. byrnei*; 4/7 (57%) *S. crassicaudata*; 1/2 (50%) *S. macroura* (syn. *S. larapinta*); 8/17 (47%) *S. leucopus*, but all 21 *Antechinus stuartii* Macleay, 1841, the brown antechinus, examined were negative for *T. gondii*. Boorman et al. (1977) chronicled an outbreak of toxoplasmosis in *Macropus robustus* Gould, 1841, Wallaroo, from a zoo in central California, USA. In a colony of 22 animals, four died within a three-week period, and histopathological findings of brain, lung, and heart tissues confirmed that all died of *T. gondii*. Within four months of the last death, serum was drawn from nine of the remaining 18 wallaroos and tested for antibodies against *T. gondii* using the indirect hemagglutination test; all nine had positive titers ranging from 1:64 to 1:131,072.

Burridge et al. (1979) collected serum samples from 27 mammal species in Florida, USA, and tested them for antibodies to *T. gondii* using the indirect hemagglutination test; they found that opossums, *D. marsupialis*, were among the four mammal species with the highest prevalence (11%) of antibody titers to *T. gondii*. Obendorf and Munday (1983) were among the first to document *T. gondii* in 2/2 (100%) wild Tasmanian pademelons, *Ty. billardierii*, when a carcass of each sex was brought to their laboratory. O'Callaghan and Moore (1986) found no hemagglutinating antibody in 30 brushtail possums (*T. vulpecula*) from Kangaroo Island, South Australia. Johnson et al. (1988) isolated *T. gondii* by mouse inoculation from the brains of 6/17 (35%) *M. rufogriseus* and 4/17 (23.5%) *Ty. billardierii* from Tasmania, Australia. Johnson et al. (1988) used an enzyme-linked immunosorbent assay to detect antibody against *T. gondii* in serum from 236 macropods collected from 21 locations in Tasmania and Flinders Island; *T. gondii* antibody was detected in 20/236 (8%) animals including 15 *Ty. billardierii* and five *M. rufogriseus*. Hartley et al. (1990) found *Toxoplasma*-like organisms in the heart, kidney, liver, lung, lymph node, spleen, small intestine, and stomach of two koalas (*P. cinereus*) that died suddenly in a faunal park in Sydney, Australia; they confirmed their identification of *T. gondii* by immunohistochemical staining. Obendorf and Munday (1990) studied a toxoplasmosis outbreak in Eastern barred bandicoots (*P. gunnii*) at two locations in southern Tasmania, and examined the tissues of three bandicoots that had died; 3/3 (100%) had *T. gondii* cysts in the brain and lungs. On the other hand, Oakwood and Pritchard (1999) collected tissues from 28 road-killed northern quolls, *D. hallucatus* Gould, 1842, and examined histologically their brains, liver, lungs, cardiac, and skeletal muscles, and found no *T. gondii* cysts; additionally, they examined 22 of the serum samples for antibodies, via the latex agglutination test, and also found no evidence of infection with

this parasite. Dubey et al. (1991) did a case report on a female koala that died at the San Francisco Zoo, and found that it had numerous tissues infected with *T. gondii*. Obendorf et al. (1996) did a histopathological examination of eight dead Eastern Barred Bandicoots, and confirmed toxoplasmosis in seven (87.5%); in each positive case, both the direct (DAT) and modified agglutination tests (MAT), using formalin-treated tachyzoites as the antigen, gave titers >64. They then examined sera from 150 *P. gunnii*, using the same DAT and MAT and found that 10/150 (7%) diagnosed as positive in both. Bettiol et al. (2000a) infected two wild-caught, and seronegative, *P. gunnii* with 100 sporulated oocysts of a highly virulent strain of *T. gondii* to chart the progression of pathology; both bandicoots became infected and died on days 12 and 17 PI. Hartley and English (2005) examined the sera of 23 common wombats (*V. ursinus*) from the Southern Tablelands of New South Wales. Their sera were examined for antibodies to *T. gondii* using three serological tests, and 6/23 (26%) were found to be positive. Eymann et al. (2006) also did a serological survey of 142 common brushtail possums (*T. vulpecula*), and found that 9/142 (6%) had positive titers for antibodies to *T. gondii* using the MAT. Houk et al. (2010) examined blood serum of *D. virginiana* for antibodies to six protozoan parasites including *T. gondii*; they found that 8/30 (27%) demonstrated antibodies against *T. gondii* using an indirect immunofluorescent antibody test (IFAT) against *in vitro*-produced antigens. Using the same serum samples, a modified DAT revealed that 9/30 (30%) had antibodies to *T. gondii*. Siqueira et al. (2013) looked for seroprevalence of *T. gondii* in wild marsupials from Pernambuco State, Brazil; using the MAT, they found that 15/223 (7%) individuals in the Didelphidae they sampled had positive titers of >25 or higher including: 9/77 (12%) *D. albiventris*; 1/26 (4%) *D. aurita*; 1/43 (2%) *M. demerarae*; 1/43 (2%) *M. murina*; 1/10 (10%) *M. domestica*; and 2/21 (10%) *M. nudicaudatus*.

Sporulation: Occurs in 1–5 days, depending upon aeration and temperature (Dubey and Odening, 2001).

Prepatent and patent periods: Prepatency is 3–10 days after cats ingest tissue cysts (with **bradyzoites**), 18 or more days after they ingest oocysts, and 13 or more days after ingesting **tachyzoites**. Less than 50% of cats shed oocysts after ingesting tachyzoites or oocysts, but almost all cats shed oocysts after ingesting tissue cysts.

Site of infection, definitive host: Intestinal epithelium of the felid.

Site of infection, intermediate host: Cells in virtually any tissue in the body.

Endogenous stages, definitive host: Five morphologically distinct merogonous stages (types A–E) develop in the intestinal epithelial cells before gamogony (Dubey and Odening, 2001).

Endogenous stages, intermediate host: After entering host cells by active penetration, tachyzoites become surrounded by a parasitophorous vacuole, and then rapidly multiply asexually via repeated endodyogeny until the host cell is filled. These cysts remain intracellular as their bradyzoites divide by endodyogeny. Young cysts may be as small as 5 wide, or grow up to 60–100 wide (Dubey and Odening, 2001).

Cross-transmission: Too numerous to list.

Pathology: Clearly, *T. gondii* can and does cause fatal infections in many marsupial species, and Australian marsupials, especially, seem to be highly susceptible to infection and to death. Thompson and Reed (1957), using histological techniques, looked at toxoplasmosis in the swamp wallaby, *W. bicolor*. Hilgenfeld (1965) was among the first to describe and document an enzootic outbreak in a flock of kangaroos observed for six years in which 20 animals died. He observed macroscopic changes in the lungs, intestinal tract, central nervous system, myocardium, muscles, adrenal glands, genital organs, urinary bladder, and eyes of dead kangaroos. Dobos-Kovacs et al. (1974) described an outbreak in which three derby kangaroos, *M. eugenii* (syn. *T. eugenii*), died in the Budapest Zoo that was caused by eating fodder contaminated with cat feces. Boorman et al. (1977) described an outbreak in *M. robustus* in a central California zoo in which 4/22 (18%) animals died within three weeks. Wilhelmsen and Montali (1980) described the histological stages of toxoplasmosis in the parma wallaby, *M. parma*. Doube (1981) noted that captive wombats (both *L. latifrons* and *V. ursinus*) appear to be quite susceptible to infection with *T. gondii*, and death with associated pneumonia and encephalitis is common. Presidente (1982) reported that toxoplasmosis was a major cause of death in hand-reared young *V. ursinus*, within which it manifests in interstitial pneumonia and focal encephalitis. Obendorf (1983) said that many species of small dasyurid marsupials (e.g., antechinuses, dunnarts, others) are affected by a variety of abnormalities including altered behavior, blindness, incoordination, and paralysis suggestive of central nervous system dysfunction; he also said that these animals are sometimes found dead without prior obvious symptoms. In Australia, one instance was cited where deaths due to toxoplasmosis rose steadily over a five-year period in a captive colony of small dasyurids that had been fed fresh mutton, but that no cases of toxoplasmosis were reported after their diet was changed to pre-frozen mutton and beef (Attwood and Woolley, 1973a,b; Attwood et al., 1975; Obendorf, 1983). Dickens (1978), also in Australia, reported the presence of *Toxoplasma*-like organisms in tissue sections of the liver, heart, kidney, pancreas, and brain of an unspecified number of koalas that died suddenly. Obendorf and Munday (1983), who documented *T. gondii* in two wild *Ty. billardierii*, reported from their accompanying history that several wallabies had been found dead, and many were found blind and/or uncoordinated; apparently, up to 50 wallabies consisting of pademelons and Bennett's wallabies (*M. r. rufogriseus*), exhibited these disease symptoms on a farm at Lucaston, in southern Tasmania. Obendorf and Munday's (1983) examination of the dead pademelons revealed myocarditis, encephalitis, hepatic necrosis, and congested and edematous lungs, with numerous *T. gondii* cysts in and around these lesions. Phillips (1986) studied the pathology of *T. gondii* in tissue sections of *P. xanthopus*, the yellow-footed rock-wallaby, and Patton et al. (1986) studied the epizoology of toxoplasmosis in *P. tridactylus*, and other marsupials in the Knoxville Zoo in Tennessee, USA. Obendorf and Munday (1990) reported that infected bandicoots (*P. gunnii*) showed signs of incoordination, blindness, erratic staggering movements, and unnatural daytime activity. Upon necropsy and histological examination, three infected bandicoots had numerous focal areas of nonsuppurative meningo-encephalitis in their brains characterized by necrotic infiltration of lymphocytes and cysts typical of *T. gondii*, and the lungs were congested and edematous with infiltration of lymphocytes into the alveolar wall around *T. gondii* cysts. Canfield et al. (1990) summarized the clinical signs, necropsy findings, and histopathological lesions for 43 macropods (*Macropus* spp.), two common wombats (*V. ursinus*), six possums (species unknown), 15 dasyurids (species unknown), two numbats (*My. fasciatus*), eight bandicoots (species unknown), and one bilby (*M. lagotis*) that either died suddenly or exhibited serious respiratory, neurological, or enteric disease. All lesions were consistent with toxoplasmosis. Hartley et al. (1990) examined two koalas that died of toxoplasmosis in Sydney, Australia, and found a few to many small multifocal areas of inflammatory necrosis, often associated with free or small aggregates of tachyzoites in their hearts, livers, stomachs, and small intestinal musculature. In the lungs of the koalas there was mild to moderate alveolar edema with alveolar histiocytosis, and there were free zoites present in septal capillaries. Dubey et al. (1991b) found *T. gondii* in the heart, brain, liver, spleen, lymph nodes, urinary bladder, kidney, and adrenal glands of a captive adult female koala (*P. cinereus*) that died suddenly at the San Francisco Zoo. Predominant lesions were encephalitis, myocarditis, and

necrosis of the pancreas and adrenal glands. Reddacliff et al. (1993) experimentally dosed 13 Tammar wallabies (*M. eugenii*) orally with 500, 1000, or 10,000 sporulated oocysts of *T. gondii*; 11 wallabies died of acute toxoplasmosis 9–15 days PI, although all 13 were infected. The remaining two wallabies had chronic infections with small, focal, noninflammatory lesions in the brain, heart, and skeletal muscles four months PI. Skerratt et al. (1997) euthanized an eight-year-old female wombat (*V. ursinus*) from Victoria, Australia, after an illness of 36 days manifested by lethargy, inappetence, and terminal coma with respiratory failure. Skerratt et al. (1997) histological diagnosis showed granulomatous encephalitis, focal myocarditis, interstitial pneumonia, and severe adrenal cortical necrosis, and the presence of large numbers of *T. gondii* tachyzoites within focal necrotic lesions of the brain, myocardium, and adrenal cortices. An incidental finding of Skerratt et al. (1997) was calcification in the media of the ascending aorta and proximal parts of the major arteries that likely contributed to the pulmonary edema observed. Focal calcified deposits also occurred in the renal cortical tubules. Bettiol et al. (2000a) charted the pathology of two bandicoots (*P. gunnii*) they experimentally infected with 100 oocysts of a pathogenic strain of *T. gondii*. The bandicoots died 12 and 17 days PI; notable postmortem findings included congestion, edema, and patchy consolidation of the lungs, excess and slightly blood-tinged abdominal fluid, petechial hemorrhage in the gastric and small intestinal serosa, edematous mesentery and enlargement of the mesenteric lymph nodes, distinctly enlarged spleen and liver with multifocal areas of necrosis, extensive interstitial pneumonia of the lungs and cellular infiltrates into alveolar tissues along with focal fibrinous necrosis, focal areas of nonsupportive interstitial inflammation, and myonecrosis in the heart. Numerous tachyzoites and tissue cysts were found in association with all of these lesions. These numerous pathogenic manifestations suggested to Bettiol et al. (2000a) that bandicoots are highly susceptible to infection with *T. gondii* and that in nature they likely die within weeks of infection. Dubey and Crutchley (2008) examined the pathology due to *T. gondii* in five infected wallabies; two male *M. rufogriseus* (raised in the USA; Nos. 4, 5), two female *M. rufogriseus* (wild-caught, South Island, New Zealand; Nos. 2, 3), and one female *M. eugenii* (wild-caught, North Island, New Zealand; No. 1). Wallaby No. 1 was in poor health upon arrival in Philadelphia, Pennsylvania, and was treated with various drugs (ivermectin, amprolium, sulfadimethoxine, pyrimethamine) for 3 months after arrival at which time it died.

Wallabies 2 and 3 were in good condition upon arrival in Philadelphia, but three months later, they became lethargic and also received treatment (pyrimethamine, sulfadimethoxine, leucovorin, vitamin E). After the first week of this treatment, the two wallabies became lethargic, progressively lost weight, developed incoordination while hopping, began listing to the right while standing, and had progressive loss of vision. At this time, administration of pyrimethamine, sulfadimethoxine, and leucovorin was stopped and changed to atovaquone (100 mg/kg, oral, every 24 h, along with peanut oil). Ophthalmic examination of the two wallabies showed raised spots of yellow exudate, bilateral retinal damage, splotchy pigment changes with areas of atrophy, papilledema with blurring of the optic disc margin, and behavior that indicated complete blindness. Interestingly, five days after atovaquone treatment began, the papilledema resolved, and eyesight steadily improved and their sight began to return. At eight weeks after beginning atovaquone, retinal changes were stable and their coordination improved quickly. Due to other complications, wallabies No. 2 and 3 were killed 2.5 and three years, respectively, from the time toxoplasmosis was diagnosed. Wallabies No. 4 and 5 had bouts with various symptoms of toxoplasmosis and treatments with atovaquone; they were killed at five and four years of age, respectively.

Microscopic lesions were found in their brains and were characterized by mild gliosis and perivascular infiltrations with mononuclear cells in the cerebrum. *Toxoplasma gondii* was isolated from the tissues of four of the five wallabies (Nos. 1, 3, 4, 5) while the fifth wallaby (No. 2) had an antibody titer of >3200 in the MAT.

Materials deposited: None, to my knowledge.

Remarks: See Weiss and Kim (2007) for the most comprehensive exposition on *T. gondii*, or any introductory parasitology text (e.g., Roberts and Janovy, 2009), for general information and an overview of pathology caused by this species in vertebrates. Siqueira et al. (2013) felt that finding *T. gondii* in wild marsupials (and rodents) in Brazil was important because the animals they studied are prey for felids, which can then shed oocysts into the environment. These prey also can be, and are, consumed by humans, who also can encounter oocysts from water and plant materials contaminated with oocysts shed by felines.

Toxoplasma gondii causes serious disease and death in Australian marsupials, both in the wild (Attwood et al., 1975; Obendorf and Munday, 1983; Johnson et al., 1989; Canfield et al., 1990) and in zoos, there and abroad (Boorman et al., 1977; Jensen et al., 1985; Patton et al., 1986; Dubey et al., 1988; Miller et al., 1992; Adkesson et al., 2007). From the few studies that have documented pathology, it seems that Australasian marsupials, especially wallabies in which it causes clinical disease and death, demonstrate a vulnerability to toxoplasmosis that is not apparent in larger kangaroos (Dubey and Crutchley, 2008). It is also clear that other Australian marsupials, especially free-ranging Tasmanian marsupials such as the Eastern barred bandicoot (*P. gunnii*), are highly susceptible to disease and death due to acute toxoplasmosis.

Obendorf and Munday (1990) suggested that although the source of *T. gondii* infection for the bandicoots they studied was unknown, "it is highly likely that mechanical transport hosts such as earthworms, arthropods and other soil and pasture invertebrates were involved." Later, Bettoil et al. (2000b) confirmed their hypothesis when they infected two bandicoots (*P. gunnii*) with artificially cultured earthworms that were maintained in autoclaved nutrient-enriched soil contaminated with *T. gondii* oocysts. Both bandicoots died on the 11th and 14th day PI and necropsy findings were consistent with acute toxoplasmosis similar to that seen in their earlier study (Bettoil et al., 2000a). Two bandicoots fed earthworms maintained on sterilized uncontaminated soil, and two bandicoots fed earthworms initially from soil contaminated with *T. gondii* oocysts, but later transferred through three changes of sterile soil, all remained uninfected and healthy.

Many marsupials have become reasonably well-adapted to increasing urbanization, resulting in them having greater interactions with humans and their domestic animals, both livestock and pets. For example, opossums (*Didelphis* spp.) in North and South American cities, and brushtail possums (*Trichosurus* spp.) in Australian cities, have become quite common and wild bandicoots (Obendorf et al., 1996) and quokkas (Gibb et al., 1966) also become acclimated quite easily to human habitations (see Eymann et al., 2006). This puts them at a higher risk of exposure to zoonotic pathogens, and they may become infected by parasites hosted by cats (*T. gondii*) and dogs (*Neospora caninum*) (Eymann et al., 2006). In Australia, marsupials evolved in the absence of *T. gondii* and have only recently been exposed to it as there were no cats before European settlements arrived. This likely makes Australian marsupials highly susceptible for toxoplasmosis, and infections are now known to be debilitating and fatal in both captive and free-ranging populations.

Domestic cats, especially when present in such large numbers that many become feral around human habitats, can seed their environments with oocysts for years. A seroprevalence study on domestic cats in Melbourne, showed that ~40/103 (39%) cats were positive for *T. gondii* (Summer and Ackland, 1999), and in Sydney, 20/80 (25%) domestic cats were seropositive (Watson et al., 1982). Cats may be infective for only a short time before acquiring immunity, but millions of oocysts may be released in the feces in a single day. Although only a few cats may be shedding *T. gondii* oocysts at any given time, the enormous numbers produced, and their resistance to destruction, ensure widespread contamination (Dubey, 2004).

DISCUSSION AND SUMMARY

I mentioned in the previous chapter that the Sarcocystidae, as a family, is likely the most successful protist clade in nature because its family members are capable of taking up residence in the cells of virtually all vertebrate species, using them either as intermediate or definitive hosts, or as both. This ability to infect most cells in most vertebrates, to be the supreme generalist as an agent of infection, is certainly true for *T. gondii*, likely the most ubiquitous protist parasite on Earth. In this chapter, I point out two "givens" about *T. gondii*. The first is that, in time, it truly may become almost ubiquitous in marsupials; it is now found in about 41 species, in four orders (Tables 11.1 and 11.2); those are either just the species in which it has been looked for or the animals were sick and dying, and it was found to be the etiological agent of that distress. The second obvious point to reiterate is that in marsupials, at least in Australian marsupials, *T. gondii* can be, and is, highly pathogenic and often fatal. The likely reason for this susceptibility is that Australian marsupials evolved without *T. gondii* on their continent, until Europeans brought their domestic cats to seed the continent with infective oocysts.

Cryptosporidiidae: *Cryptosporidium* in Marsupials

CRYPTOSPORIDIIDAE: CRYPTOSPORIDIUM IN MARSUPIALS

INTRODUCTION

As noted earlier (Duszynski and Couch, 2013), the genus *Cryptosporidium* represents a distantly related lineage of the Apicomplexa, that possess features of both the coccidia and the gregarines. Zhu et al. (2000) argued that this group emerged very early at the base of the Apicomplexa lineage, and asked a question that still has gone unanswered, "Are we ready to move the *Cryptosporidium* group out of the coccidia-proper to form a new group (Class?), perhaps on an equal status with the Haematozoa and the Gregarina?" I'm still curious why coccidian and cryptosporidian systematists haven't yet taken time to work together and take the lead to make this change.

Cryptosporidium species are transmitted directly via the fecal–oral route with their oocysts contaminating food and water, and they constitute an important enteric parasite of most vertebrates: native, feral, domesticated, and humans. Their oocysts are environmentally stable, are resistant to commonly used drinking water disinfectants, and are able to survive routine wastewater treatment (Fayer et al., 2000; Ryan and Power, 2012). At least 24

Cryptosporidium species have been identified and named to date (Ryan and Power, 2012), of which seven are known to infect humans; additionally, there are about 40 cryptic species, called genotypes, that have been identified across a wide range of taxa (Fayer, 2010; Power, 2010). About 19 species of marsupials (Table 11.2) are known to host 16 forms, "species," or genotypes (Table 11.1) of *Cryptosporidium*. Because some species (e.g., *Cryptosporidium parvum*) show little host specificity, zoonotic transmission from and between domestic, native, and feral animals and humans, especially vis-a-vis their ability to contaminate water supplies, can have serious public health implications (see Power, 2010 for review). In Australia, marsupials are a dominant component of the landscape, with densities in some areas of >500 per square km, but little is known about their contribution of human pathogenic strains of *Cryptosporidium* oocysts to recreational and drinking water catchments. Ryan and Power (2012) focused on the available genotyping data of *Cryptosporidium* species in wildlife and domestic animals, and tried to quantify the impact they had on contaminating drinking water catchments in Australia; information from studies like theirs is vital to improve our understanding of the public health implications involved. Similar studies, to my knowledge, have not been attempted with any American marsupials.

One of the great difficulties in studying this genus in wild animals is that the oocysts are very small and they exhibit limited morphological variation; and because of their small size, they are difficult to find and study in fecal smears, and via the standard concentration techniques (saturated sugar or salt solutions) usually used to collect and study coccidian oocysts. Thus, molecular analyses (genotyping data) have become the key to initial detecting, identifying, classifying, and even "source tracking" *Cryptosporidium* species (Power et al., 2009; Power, 2010).

CRYPTOSPORIDIUM IN MARSUPIALS

To date, *Cryptosporidium* species have been identified in two American and in 17 Australian marsupial species (Ryan and Power, 2012; Tables 11.1 and 11.2) as detailed below and in Chapter 10 (*Species Inquirendae*); comments below address what is known and pertains to the *Cryptosproidium* species in each marsupial host genus. The three marsupial orders with named, described species are listed alphabetically.

SPECIES DESCRIPTIONS

ORDER DIDELPHIMORPHIA GILL, 1872

FAMILY DIDELPHIDAE GRAY, 1821 (17 GENERA, 87 SPECIES)

GENUS *DIDELPHIS* L., 1758 (6 SPECIES)

CRYPTOSPORIDIUM PARVUM TYZZER, 1912

Type host: *Mus musculus* (L., 1758), House Mouse.

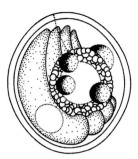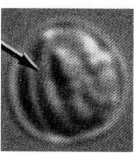

FIGURES 9.1, 9.2 **9.1.** Line drawing of the sporulated oocyst of *Cryptosporidium parvum*. **9.2.** Photomicrograph of a sporulated oocyst of *C. parvum*. Both figures from Upton and Current, 1985 (their Figures 8, 5), with permission from the senior author and from the Editor of the *Journal of Parasitology*.

Type locality: NORTH AMERICA: USA: Massachusetts, Cambridge.

Other hosts: >150 known mammalian species (Robinson and Chalmers, 2009) including: *Homo sapiens* L., 1758, Humans; ruminants including Cattle, Sheep/Lambs, Pigs, and Goats; Lagomorphs (i.e., rabbits); reptiles including Snakes and Turtles; laboratory Rodents; **Marsupials**: *Didelphis virginiana* Kerr, 1792, Virginia Opossum (experimentally; Lindsay et al., 1988 infected five nursing joeys with *C. parvum* oocysts of calf origin), pregnant female collected in the wild from Lee County, Alabama, USA (32° 36′ N, 85° 36′ W); *Macropus giganteus* Shaw, 1790, Eastern Grey Kangaroo (Ng et al., 2011; Ryan and Power, 2012); *Isoodon obesulus* (Shaw, 1797), Southern Brown Bandicoot (?); *Trichosurus vulpecula* (Kerr, 1792), Common Brushtail (?); *Wallabia* sp. (?) (Ryan and Power, 2012).

Geographic distribution: Cosmopolitan.

Description of sporulated oocyst: Oocyst shape: spheroidal; number of walls: 1; wall characteristics: ~0.4 thick, smooth, with a suture along one side; L×W: 5.2×4.6 (5–6×4–5); L/W ratio: 1.1–1.2 (Duszynski and Upton, 2001) or, L×W: 5.0×4.5 (4.5–5×4–5); L/W ratio: 1.1–1.2 (Upton and Current, 1985); M: absent; OR: present; OR characteristics: spheroidal, 2.4×2.5 (2–4×2–4), composed of numerous small granules, and a spheroidal, membrane-bound globule, 1.5×1.6

(1–2×1–2); PG: absent. Distinctive features of oocyst: small size and a faint, subterminal suture present at one pole that extends diagonally across oocyst to about half of its width (Upton and Current, 1985).

Description of sporozoites: Four SZ occur within each oocyst; L×W: 4.9×1.2 (4.5–6×1.0–1.4), they lie parallel along one side of oocyst, tightly enclosing the OR (Upton and Current, 1985).

Prevalence: Highly variable; cryptosporidiosis may occur sporadically or as outbreaks following zoonotic transmission from farm animals, person-to-person spread, or the contamination of water supplies (Casemore, 1991). Lindsay et al. (1988) used a nursing adult female *D. virginiana*, and infected five of her eight joeys (~75 days old) with $5×10^6$ *C. parvum* oocysts of calf origin. All inoculated joeys, and two of their three noninoculated pouch mates, acquired infection based on examination of their feces and tissue sections.

Sporulation: Endogenous. Sporulated oocysts are discharged in the feces.

Prepatent and patent periods: Prepatent period is generally four days and patency generally lasts 7–10 days in immune-competent hosts, but it is not known if these times apply to infected opossums.

Site of infection: The preferred site of infection is the ileum, although other sites also are colonized in heavy infections (Duszynski and Upton, 2001). In the young *D. virginiana*, developmental stages of *C. parvum* were found in the ileum, cecum, and colon of five animals, but only in the cecum and colon of the other two (Lindsay et al., 1988).

Endogenous stages: More is known about the endogenous development of this species than any other member of the genus, and the details on merogony and gamogony have been published elsewhere (Duszynski and Upton, 2001; Duszynski and Couch, 2013). To summarize, in mice, meronts are spheroidal, ~5 wide at their maximum, but many segmenting forms are much smaller; merozoites vary in size from 5–7×2.5–5 (Tyzzer, 1912). These meronts are termed Type I meronts and they produce eight merozoites that rupture from the host cell, enter other cells, and undergo merogony again; the second meront is termed Type II, and it produces only four merozoites. The second generation merozoites eventually produce micro- and macrogametes (see Duszynski and Upton, 2001, for details). Unfortunately, nothing is known about the sizes of any of these stages in opossums.

Cross-transmission: Numerous examples exist in the literature (see Duszynski and Upton, 2001) that *C. parvum* lacks host specificity, and can infect species in multiple genera, families, and even orders; however, these are all eutherian (placental) mammals. In the only known cross-transmission to a metatherian (marsupial) mammal, the American opossum, Lindsay et al. (1988) transmitted oocysts of *C. parvum* from cattle to juvenile *D. virginiana*. Most of our solid information about host specificity (or lack thereof) on *Cryptosporidium* species is based on such cross-transmission work. Thus, *C. parvum* seems to be able to infect vertebrate hosts, even in different evolutionary lineages (placental vs marsupial). However, as Power (2010) cautioned, "Given that the opossums were infected with a high dose of *C. parvum*, that juvenile marsupials are highly immune naïve, and that naturally occurring *C. parvum* infections have not been identified in marsupials, it appears likely that marsupials are not susceptible to natural infection by *C. parvum*."

Pathology: None of the juvenile opossums died as a result of infection with *C. parvum*, and the only clinical sign was that they all had semiformed, dark brown fecal material in their colons and rectums. When tissue sections were examined, two of the seven infected joeys had mild villous atrophy in their ilea on days 6 and 7 postinoculation (PI). Neither developmental stages of *C. parvum*, nor microscopic lesions, were seen in other tissues that were examined (lung, liver, kidney, spleen, pancreas, stomach, duodenum, jejunum). Thus, *C. parvum* seems to be only mildly pathogenic for opossums.

Material deposited: None.

Remarks: Because so many mammalian species can be infected with *C. parvum*, a large potential zoonotic reservoir exists in wild, domestic, and companion animals. Numerous studies have demonstrated or correlated transmission of this parasite from various other animals to humans, especially to children, and such cases usually involve direct exposure to infected animals or their feces, or exposure to contaminated raw milk, food, or water (Duszynski and Upton, 2001).

The reports and identifications of *C. parvum* in kangaroos (*M. giganteus*), a wallaby (no species identification), the brushtail possum (*T. vulpecula*), and bandicoots (*I. obesulus*) were based on direct DNA extraction from feces and subsequent PCR screening, but in all cases, *Cryptosporidium* could be amplified only at the multicopy 18S rDNA locus (Ryan and Power, 2012, and others). In these studies, the marsupials sampled were living in areas associated with humans, so it is not clear whether these marsupials were actually infected with *C. parvum* or whether they were simply passively transmitting oocysts they had ingested by feeding on fecal-contaminated vegetation (Hill et al., 2008; Ng et al., 2011; Ryan and Power, 2012).

Infection with *C. parvum* is of concern for humans and other animals because the ingestion of even small numbers of oocysts can cause severe diarrhea in people (Angus, 1987). The oocysts survive well outside the host and are resistant to chlorination levels used for disinfection of tap water. Many wild mammals have been identified as reservoirs of *C. parvum*, and the infection in most of these mammals appears to be asymptomatic, but oocysts shed in their feces may pose a threat to human health in urban and rural environments, particularly for individuals who may have frequent contact with animal feces, such as field and farm workers or veterinarians.

ORDER DIPROTODONTIA OWEN, 1866

SUBORDER MACROPODIFORMES AMEGHINO, 1889 (3 FAMILIES, 16 GENERA, 76 SPECIES)

FAMILY MACROPODIDAE GRAY, 1821 (11 GENERA, 65 SPECIES)

SUBFAMILY MACROPODINAE GRAY, 1821 (10 GENERA, 64 SPECIES)

GENUS MACROPUS SHAW, 1790 (14 SPECIES)

CRYPTOSPORIDIUM FAYERI RYAN, POWER, AND XIAO, 2008

Type host: *Macropus rufus* (Desmarest, 1822), Red Kangaroo.

Type locality: AUSTRALIA: Western Australia, Perth.

Other hosts: *Macropus fuliginosus* (Desmarest, 1817), Western Grey Kangaroo; *Macropus giganteus* Shaw, 1790, Eastern Grey Kangaroo; *Phascolarctos cinereus* (Goldfuss, 1817), Koala; *Petrogale xanthopus* Gray, 1855, Yellow-footed Rock Wallaby; *Perameles bougainville* Quoy and Gaimard, 1824, Western Barred Bandicoot; *Wallabia bicolor* (Desmarest, 1804), Swamp Wallaby.

Geographic distribution: AUSTRALIA.

Description of sporulated oocyst: Oocyst shape: ellipsoidal to slightly ovoidal; number of walls: 1; wall characteristics: thin, smooth; $L \times W$ (n = 50): 5×4.3 (5×4–5); L/W ratio: 1.1 (1.0–1.2); M, PG: both absent; OR: present. Distinctive features of oocyst: typical cryptosporidid oocyst, very small size, and lack of sporocysts.

Description of sporozoites: Four SZ occur within each oocyst, but they were not measured.

Prevalence: Not known for the type host (Ryan et al., 2008), but *Cryptosporidium* species oocysts were found in 239/3557 (7%) *M. giganteus*; of the positive samples that were genotyped, 61% proved to be *Cryptosporidium fayeri*, while the remaining 39% were *Cryptosporidium macropodum*, (Power et al., 2005).

Sporulation: Endogenous, oocysts were passed fully sporulated in the feces.

Prepatent and patent periods: Unknown.

Site of infection: Intestine.

Endogenous stages: Microvillus border of intestinal epithelial cells.

Cross-transmission: Sporulated oocysts of *C. fayeri* (kangaroo origin) were inoculated into one-day-old Swiss mice, but the mice showed no signs of infection, and when the gastrointestinal tract, gut contents, and feces were screened by PCR, the parasite could not be demonstrated (Ryan et al., 2008).

Pathology: Several authors have noted a distinct absence of clinical signs in infected marsupial hosts, despite excretion of high oocyst numbers (Power et al., 2005; Thompson, 2007; Power and Ryan, 2008; Ryan et al., 2008). However, *C. fayeri* was more recently reported in a 29-year-old immunocompetent female, who suffered prolonged gastrointestinal disease in Sydney, in 2009 (Waldron et al., 2010).

Material deposited: A phototype of sporulated oocysts and GenBank accession numbers for eight gene loci (see Table 2, Ryan et al., 2008) were sent to the Australian Registry of Wildlife Health, Taronga Zoo, Mosman, New South Wales, Australia, ARWH Reference No. 5924/1.

Etymology: This species was named in honor of Dr. Ronald Fayer for his contribution to *Cryptosporidium* research.

Remarks: Oocysts of this species are morphologically indistinguishable from *C. macropodum* (Power and Ryan, 2008), and from *C. parvum*, a pathogen readily transmissible to humans from a variety of wild and domestic mammals. Prior to their convincing arguments to name this species in honor of Dr. Fayer, Ryan et al. (2008) summarized

the brief history of what was known about *Cryptosporidium* infections in Australian marsupials, and the specific hosts in which they had been recorded; their review is worth reiterating here.

Ryan et al. (2008) reported *Cryptosporidium* infections in Australian marsupials to include at least 12 host species in 10 genera in 3 orders: **Dasyuromorphia**: brown antechinus (*Antechinus stuartii*, Barker et al., 1978); **Diprotodontia**: Eastern grey kangaroo (*M. giganteus*, Power et al., 2004, 2005); Western grey kangaroo (*M. fuliginosus*); red kangaroo (*M. rufus*, O'Donoghue, unpub. observ.); tammar wallaby (*Macropus eugenii*, Power et al., 2003); Tasmanian pademelon (*Thylogale billardierii*, Obendorf, unpub. observ.); yellow-footed rock wallaby (*P. xanthopus*, Power et al., 2003); brushtail possum (*T. vulpecula*, Power et al., 2003); koala (*P. cinereus*, Phillips et al., unpub. observ.; Morgan et al., 1997, 1999a); swamp wallaby (*W. bicolor*, Ryan et al., unpub. observ.; Ryan and Power, 2012); **Peramelemorphia**: greater bilby (*Macrotis lagotis*, Warren et al., 2003); Southern brown bandicoot (*Isoodon obseulus*, O'Donoghue, unpub. observ.); Western barred bandicoot (*P. bougainville*, Wielinga et al., unpub. observ.). Since 2008, those numbers for Australian marsupials have increased to 19 marsupial species (Table 11.2).

Initially, many of these infections were attributed to *Cryptosporidium* sp. because all *Cryptosporidium* oocysts are nearly identical, with only slight differences in size. However, Morgan et al. (1997) were the first to analyze and sequence a gene locus (18S rRNA) in an isolate from a koala (*P. cinereus*), and they determined it to be genetically distinct from *C. parvum*. Since then, many authors have used multiple other gene loci (actin, internal transcribed spacers 1, 2 (ITS1, 2), *Cryptosporidium* oocyst wall protein (COWP), heat shock protein 70 (HSP70), dihydrofolate reductase thymidylate synthase) to help them confirm genetic distinctness between *Cryptosporidium* species, with similar-looking oocysts, from multiple host species (Morgan et al., 1999a,b; Power et al., 2004, 2005; Sulaiman et al., 2000; Warren et al., 2003; Xiao et al., 1999a,b, 2002).

In addition, because of the many problems associated with determining the identification and taxonomy of *Cryptosporidium* species, four basic guidelines have evolved over time, and are now established by those who work with them: (1) the oocyst and sporozoites should be measured in detail, photographed, and photomicrographs deposited in an accredited, well-recognized museum (e.g., National Museum of Natural History, Washington, DC; see Chapter 11, under The Value of Archiving Types, for detailed instructions.); (2) each isolate must be characterized genetically; (3) there should be a demonstration of natural and, if possible, experimental cross-transmission work to establish host specificity (or not); and (4) naming a new species must comply with the International Code of Zoological Nomenclature (Xiao et al., 2004; Ryan et al., 2008).

Working with different genotypes to satisfy the conditions noted above, Morgan et al. (1977, 1999a,b), Power et al. (2004, 2005), Warren et al. (2003), Xiao et al. (1999a,b, 2000, 2002), and Sulaiman et al. (2000) identified marsupial genotypes I and II, opossum genotypes I and II, and a *Cryptosporidium muris* genotype in the greater bilby. Based on careful analysis of loci examined and neighbor-joining analysis of several of the gene sequences identified, Ryan et al. (2008) firmly established that marsupial genotype I is a distinct species that they named *C. fayeri*. Finally, Power et al. (2009) analyzed the diversity within the GP60 locus of 25 isolates from *M. giganteus* (grey kangaroo, 21 isolates), *P. xanthopus* (yellow-footed rock wallaby, one isolate), *P. cinereus* (koala, two isolates), and *P. bougainville* (Western barred bandicoot, one isolate), and concluded that *C. fayeri* isolates could be assigned to six subtypes that were associated with host species and locality. This intraspecific diversity that Power et al. (2009) saw in *C. fayeri* suggested to them that it was host adapted, but it was still less than the diversity for human pathogenic species; it also led them to believe that the GP60 locus in marsupials is under less selective pressure in them than in more host-adapted species.

Finding *C. fayeri* to cause gastrointestinal illness in a resident of Sydney (Waldron et al., 2010) is of concern for water catchment authorities in the city region, because its main water supply, the Warragamba Dam, is surrounded by national forest inhabited by a diverse and abundant array of marsupial species (Ryan and Power, 2012).

CRYPTOSPORIDIUM HOMINIS MORGAN-RYAN, FALL, WARD, HIJJAWI, SULAIMAN, FAYER, THOMPSON, AND OLSON, 2002

Type host: *Homo sapiens* L., 1758, Humans.

Type locality: AUSTRALIA: Western Australia: Perth.

Other hosts: *Capra hircus* L., 1758, Goat (natural, Giles et al., 2009); *Dugong dugon* (Müller, 1776), Dugong (natural, Morgan et al., 2000); *Sus scrofa domesticus* L., 1758, Domestic Pig (experimental in gnotobiotic pigs, Widmer et al., 2000); *Ovis aries* L., 1758, Domestic Sheep (experimental and natural, Giles et al., 2001, 2002); *Macropus giganteus* Shaw, 1790, Eastern Grey Kangaroo (Ng et al., 2011; Ryan and Power, 2012).

Geographic distribution: Worldwide; likely to be found wherever humans are found.

Description of sporulated oocyst: Oocyst shape: spheroidal to slightly subspheroidal; number of walls: one; wall characteristics: thin, smooth; L × W: 5.2 × 4.9 (4–6 × 4–5); L/W ratio: 1.1 (1.0–1.1); M, PG: both absent; OR: present. Distinctive features of oocyst: a typical cryptosporidid oocyst, small in size, lacking sporocysts, and containing four SZ.

Description of sporozoites: Four SZ occur within each oocyst, but they were not measured.

Prevalence: Unknown.

Sporulation: Endogenous. Oocysts are passed fully sporulated.

Prepatent and patent periods: Unknown.

Site of infection: Microvillus border of the intestinal epithelial cells in the ileum and colon of inoculated pigs (Morgan-Ryan et al., 2002).

Endogenous stages: Unknown.

Cross-transmission: Morgan-Ryan et al. (2002) inoculated oocysts into mice (*Mus musculus* L., 1758), nude mice, rats (*Rattus norvegicus* Berkenhout (1769)), cats (*Felis catus* L., 1758), and dogs (*Canis lupus familiaris* L., 1758), but all remained uninfected.

Pathology: Only mild lymphoid hyperplasia was observed in the ileum and colon of infected pigs. There was mild or no mucosal attenuation, which was restricted to the ileum and colon (Morgan-Ryan et al., 2002).

Material deposited: A phototype of sporulated oocysts and GenBank accession numbers (Morgan-Ryan et al., 2002, their Table 2) are deposited in the United States National Parasite Collection, Beltsville, Maryland, USA, USNPC No. 092045.

Etymology: This species was named to reflect its type host (Morgan-Ryan et al., 2002).

Remarks: *Cryptosporidium hominis* is commonly found to infect humans (Casemore et al., 1997), and it seems to be widespread in the environment (Arrowood, 1997). Since the oocysts of *C. hominis* overlap in size with those of *C. parvum* (bovine genotype) to make them morphologically identical, the correct distinction between them (and other *Cryptosporidium* species) in clinical and epidemiological studies has important public health implications. However, the two species can be distinguished on the basis of genetic differences at multiple loci (see Table 2, Morgan-Ryan et al., 2002), and by the fact that *C. hominis* is not transmissible to mice, nude mice, rats, cats, or dogs, unlike *C. parvum*.

McLauchlin et al. (2000) examined 1705 human fecal samples in the UK and found distinct geographic and temporal variations in the distribution of two species; *C. parvum* was more common during spring, while *C. hominis* was significantly more common in patients infected during late summer–autumn, especially in those with a history of foreign travel (McLauchlin et al., 2000). Other European studies have reported that *C. parvum* is more common in humans than *C. hominis* (Alves et al., 2001; Guyot et al., 2001; McLauchlin et al., 1999; Pedraza-Diaz et al., 2001),

whereas in Australia, the US, and South America, reports show *C. hominis* to be the most common *Cryptosporidium* species infecting humans (Morgan et al., 1998; Sulaiman et al., 1998; Widmer et al., 2000; Xiao et al., 1999b, 2001d).

The only reports of *C. hominis* infecting marsupials are those found in *M. giganteus* (Ng et al., 2011; Ryan and Power, 2012).

CRYPTOSPORIDIUM MACROPODUM POWER AND RYAN, 2008

Type host: *Macropus giganteus* Shaw, 1790, Eastern Grey Kangaroo.

Type locality: AUSTRALIA: New South Wales: Sydney, watershed of Lake Burragorang.

Other hosts: *Macropus fuliginosus* (Desmarest, 1817), Western Grey Kangaroo; *Macropus rufus* (Desmarest, 1822), Red Kangaroo; *Perameles bougainville* Quoy and Gaimard, 1824, Western Barred Bandicoot; *Petrogale xanthopus* Gray, 1855, Yellow-footed Rock Wallaby; *Phascolarctos cinereus* (Goldfuss, 1817), Koala; *Wallabia bicolor* (Desmarest, 1804), Swamp Wallaby.

Geographic distribution: AUSTRALIA.

Description of sporulated oocyst: Oocyst shape: ellipsoidal to slightly ovoidal; number of walls: 1; wall characteristics: thin, smooth; L × W: 5.4 × 4.9 (5–6 × 4.5–6); L/W ratio: 1.1–1.2; M, PG: both absent; OR: present. Distinctive features of oocyst: a typical cryptosporidid oocyst of small size, lacking sporocysts, and containing four SZ.

Description of sporozoites: Four SZ occur within the oocysts, but they have not been measured.

Prevalence: *Cryptosporidium* species oocysts were found in 239/3557 (7%) *M. giganteus*; of the positive samples that were genotyped, 39% proved to be *C. macropodum*, while the remaining 61% were *C. fayeri* (Power et al., 2005). Thompson (2007) identified 6/10 (60%) *M. fuliginosus* and 3/30 (10%) *M. rufus* to be infected with *C. macropodum*.

Sporulation: Endogenous. Sporulated oocysts are discharged in the feces.

Prepatent and patent periods: Unknown.

Site of infection: Intestine.

Endogenous stages: Unknown.

Cross-transmission: None to date.

Pathology: Several authors have noted a distinct absence of clinical signs in infected marsupial hosts despite excretion of high oocyst numbers (Power et al., 2005; Thompson, 2007; Power and Ryan, 2008).

Material deposited: A photomicrograph of sporulated oocysts has been deposited at the Australian Registry of Wildlife Health, Taronga Zoo, Mosman, New South Wales, Australia, ARWH Reference 5966.1.

Etymology: This species was named after the Macropodidae, the family of hosts in which it is found.

Remarks: Oocysts of this species are morphologically indistinguishable from *C. fayeri* (Ryan et al., 2008), and from other previously described species including *C. hominis*, *C. parvum*, *C. canis*, and *C. suis*, all of which are found in places inhabited by marsupials in Australia (Power and Ryan, 2008). However, genetic characterization at four loci, 18S rRNA, ITS1, COWP, and HSP70, confirmed its genetic distinctness. In addition, phylogenetic analyses of the 18S rRNA, actin, and HSP70 loci demonstrated that this species is genetically distinct from all previously described *Cryptosporidium* species, including others found in marsupials (e.g., *C. fayeri*).

In two of the surveys mentioned above, some interesting shedding patterns of oocysts were noticed. In *M. giganteus*, oocyst shedding of *C. macropodum* dominated during the cooler months, while *C. fayeri* oocyst shedding dominated during periods when kangaroo populations contained high numbers of juveniles (Power et al., 2005). In contrast, Thompson (2007) noted that *C. macropodum* was the only species found in captive *M. fuliginosus* and *M. rufus* during the summer.

Finally, although *C. macropodum* and *C. fayeri* are found in the same marsupial species and are closely related genetically, the data presented by Power and Ryan (2008) seem to confirm that they are two distinct species.

CRYPTOSPORIDIUM XIAOI FAYER AND SMITH, 2009

Type host: *Ovis aries* L., 1758, Sheep.

Type locality: NORTH AMERICA: USA: Maryland, Beltsville.

Other hosts: *Bos grunniens* L., 1766, Yak (Karanis et al., 2007); *Capra aegagrus hircus* (L., 1758), Goat (Feng et al., 2007); *Macropus fuliginosus* (Desmarest, 1817), Western Grey Kangaroo (Yang et al., 2011).

Geographic distribution: AFRICA: Tunisia; ASIA: China; AUSTRALIA: Western Australia; EUROPE: Spain; United Kingdom; NORTH AMERICA: USA: Maryland.

Description of sporulated oocyst: Oocyst shape: subspheroidal to spheroidal; number of walls: 1; wall characteristics: thin, smooth; L×W (n=25): 3.9×3.4 (3–4×3–4); L/W ratio: 1.1; M, PG: both absent; OR: present. Distinctive features of oocyst: a typical cryptosporidid oocyst, very small size, lacking sporocysts, but containing four SZ.

Description of sporozoites: Four SZ occur within the oocysts, but they were not measured.

Prevalence: Unknown.

Sporulation: Endogenous, sporulated oocysts are shed in the feces.

Prepatent and patent periods: Prepatent period is 7–8 days, and the patent period is 13–15 days (Fayer and Smith, 2009).

Site of infection: Unknown.

Endogenous stages: Unknown.

Cross-transmission: Oocysts from sheep were not infectious for BALB/c mice (*M. musculus*), *Bos taurus* calves, or *C. a. hircus* kids.

Pathology: Unknown.

Material deposited: A phototype and description of oocysts are deposited in the United States National Parasite Collection, Beltsville, Maryland, USA, as USNPC No. 101171.

Etymology: This species was named for Dr. Lihua Xiao, who has contributed greatly to taxonomy and molecular epidemiology of *Cryptosporidium* species.

Remarks: This species is commonly found in sheep, but it was found in other native mammals in irrigation catchments in the southwest of Australia (McCarthy et al., 2008). It also was identified in six wild Western grey kangaroos, *M. fuliginosus*, in Western Australia by Yang et al. (2011). Their identification in the kangaroo suggested to Ryan and Power (2012) that the kangaroos picked up the infection from grazing on sheep pastures. However, it is not certain whether the kangaroos were actually infected or simply passing oocysts they had ingested. Fayer and Smith (2009) also produced gene sequence data for HSP70, actin, and SSU rDNA genes.

GENUS *PETROGALE* GRAY, 1837 (16 SPECIES)

CRYPTOSPORIDIUM FAYERI RYAN, POWER, AND XIAO, 2008

Type host: *Macropus rufus* (Desmarest, 1822), Red Kangaroo.
Remarks: Power et al. (2009) found this species in *P. xanthopus* (Ryan and Power, 2012).

GENUS *WALLABIA* TROUESSART, 1905 (MONOTYPIC)

CRYPTOSPORIDIUM MACROPODUM POWER AND RYAN, 2008

Type host: *Macropus giganteus* Shaw, 1790, Eastern Grey Kangaroo.
Remarks: Ryan and Power (2012) reported this species in *W. bicolor* (as part of their unpublished work).

CRYPTOSPORIDIUM PARVUM TYZZER, 1912

Type host: *Mus musculus* (L., 1758), House Mouse.
Remarks: Ng et al. (2011) found this species in a *Wallabia* sp. (no species identified) according to Ryan and Power (2012).

SUBORDER VOMBATIFORMES BURNETT, 1830 (2 FAMILIES, 3 GENERA, 4 SPECIES)

FAMILY PHASCOLARCTIDAE OWEN, 1839 (1 GENUS, 1 SPECIES)

GENUS *PHASCOLARCTOS* DE BLAINVILLE, 1816 (MONOTYPIC)

CRYPTOSPORIDIUM FAYERI RYAN, POWER, AND XIAO, 2008

Type host: *Macropus rufus* (Desmarest, 1822), Red Kangaroo (see type host for complete description).
Remarks: Morgan et al. (1997) reported *C. fayeri* in the koala, *P. cinereus*, in New South Wales, Australia (Ryan and Power, 2012).

ORDER PERAMELEMORPHIA AMEGHINO, 1889

FAMILY THYLACOMYIDAE BENSLEY, 1903 (1 GENUS, 2 SPECIES)

GENUS *MACROTIS* REID, 1837 (2 SPECIES)

CRYPTOSPORIDIUM MURIS (TYZZER, 1907) TYZZER, 1910

Type host: *Mus musculus* L., 1758, House Mouse.

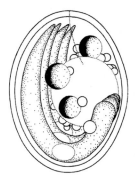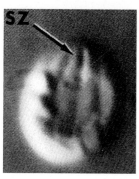

FIGURES 9.3, 9.4 **9.3.** Line drawing of the sporulated oocyst of *Cryptosporidium muris*. **9.4.** Photomicrograph of a sporulated oocyst of *C. muris*. Both figures from Upton and Current, 1985 (their Figures 7, 2), with permission from the senior author and from the Editor of the *Journal of Parasitology*.

Other hosts: *Bos taurus* L., 1758, Domestic Cow (Anderson, 1988; Esteban and Anderson, 1995); *Camelus bactrianus* L., 1758, Bactrian Camel (Anderson, 1991; Fayer et al., 1991); *Canis lupus familiaris* L., 1758, Domestic Dog (Iseki et al., 1989; Aydin, 1991); *Cavia porcellus* L., 1758, Domestic Guinea Pig (Iseki et al., 1989; Aydin, 1991); *Felis catus* L., 1758, Domestic Cat (Iseki et al., 1989; Aydin, 1991); *Macrotis lagotis* (Reid, 1837), Greater Bilby (Warren et al., 2003); *Mesocricetus auratus* (Waterhouse, 1839), Golden Hamster (Rhee et al., 1999); *Oryctolagus cuniculus* L., 1758, European (Domestic) Rabbit (Iseki et al., 1989; Aydin, 1991); *Phodopus roborovskii* (Satunin, 1903), Rovorovski's Desert Hamster (Pavlásek and Lavička, 1995); *Rattus norvegicus* (Berkenhout, 1769), Brown Rat (Iseki, 1979, 1986).

Geographic distribution: Cosmopolitan, probably worldwide.

Description of sporulated oocyst: Oocyst shape: subspheroidal; number of walls: 1; wall characteristics: thin, smooth, colorless, ~0.5 thick, with a faint, longitudinal suture that extends from one pole of oocyst down each side to about ½ of the oocyst length; L×W: 8.4×6.3 (7.5–10×5.5–7); L/W ratio: 1.4 (Duszynski and Upton, 2001) or, L×W: 7.4×5.6 (7–8×5–6.5); L/W ratio: 1.3 (1.1–1.5) (Upton and Current, 1985); M, PG: both absent; OR: present, a spheroidal or ovoidal, membrane-bound globule, 3.4×3.3 (3–5×3–4),

and usually surrounded by 2–40 smaller granules. Distinctive features of oocyst: a typical cryptosporidid oocyst, small size, no sporocysts, containing four SZ, larger oocysts than those of *C. parvum*, and with a faint, longitudinal suture that extends from one pole of oocyst down each side to about half of the oocyst length.

Description of sporozoites: Four vermiform SZ occur within each oocyst; L×W: 11.1×1.0 (10–12.5×1), and lying parallel to each other along one side of oocyst, tightly enclosing the OR (Upton and Current, 1985).

Prevalence: This species has been documented in 3/64 (5%) *Rattus* species in Osaka, Japan (Iseki, 1979, 1986); in 15/58 (26%) mice (*M. musculus*) on a farm in Moreton Morrell, in the UK (Chalmers et al., 1994); possibly in one Bactrian Camel (*Camelus bactrianus*) from the National Zoological Park, Virginia, USA, because cross-transmission showed that mice could be infected with these oocysts suggesting it was truly *C. muris* (Anderson, 1991); *C. muris* was found in 11/28 (39%) bilbies that were housed at a captive breeding colony in Western Australia (Warren et al., 2003).

Sporulation: Endogenous, oocysts were passed fully sporulated in the feces.

Prepatent and patent periods: Prepatency is about six days (Rhee et al., 1991b) and patency exceeds two months (Rhee et al., 1995).

Site of infection: In the microvillar surface of gastric glands of the stomach of rodents.

Endogenous stages: Tyzzer (1907, 1910) reported only a single autoinfective merogonous generation from the gastric mucosa, and no one, as yet, has reported additional types. However, Duszynski and Upton (2001) speculated that there may be more than one type of asexual stage in this life cycle.

Cross-transmission: Iseki et al. (1989) and Aydin (1991) demonstrated that dogs, guinea pigs, rabbits, and especially cats can be successfully infected, and some think that *Cryptosporidium* species reported from camels may represent *C. muris*, as their oocysts are similar in size, and are transmissible to rodents (Anderson, 1991; Fayer et al., 1991; Esteban and Anderson, 1995; Duszynski and Upton, 2001).

Pathology: Infections tend to be chronic and subclinical. Neither Iseki (1986) nor Iseki et al. (1989) noted clinical signs in animals infected with *C. muris*; however, histological examination of infected rodents showed enlargement of the lumens of the gastric glands, flattening and atrophy of epithelial cells, and reduction in the number of microvilli (Aydin, 1991; Yoshikawa and Iseki, 1992; Özkul and Aydin, 1994).

Material deposited: None, to my knowledge.

Remarks: There is an interesting history in the discovery and naming of *C. muris*. Clarke (1895) found a dead white laboratory mouse "in a place previously occupied by rabbits." He examined the gut for coccidia and found an "abnormal feature" in the cardiac opening of the stomach. He then placed the intestinal contents on damp blotting paper in a Petri dish kept at room temperature and, over the next eight days, observed what we now know to be the sporulation process in oocysts that may have been *Eimeria falciformis* (Eimer, 1870) Schneider, 1875. After 22 days exposure to the air, he fed a young mouse "with bread-sop containing some of the material taken from the Petri dish." On day 6 after exposure, the mouse's coat became rough, the abdomen was distended, and the thighs drawn up toward the body; on day 7 PI, he noticed blood discharged in the feces and that "the animal was distinctly ill and suffering, so it was killed." Upon histological examination, he observed minute bodies on the epithelial cells of the gastric glands in the cardiac end of the stomach that he believed to be the "swarm-spore" stage of *E. falciformis*.

Ernest Edward Tyzzer, MD (1875–1965), the George Fabyan Professor of Comparative Pathology in the Harvard Medical School (1916–1942), was a world-renowned physician and scientist, not only in parasitology/protistology, but also in oncology, pathology, virology, and bacteriology (R.B. Williams, pers. comm.). A dozen years after Clarke's work, Tyzzer (1907) first named this genus, and the type species, in a brief preliminary description, but in reality it was a *species inquirenda*, since he did not provide a separate description as "gen. nov." and "sp. nov.," nor did he provide a drawing or photomicrograph to accompany this description. However, Tyzzer (1910) redescribed *C. muris* in detail and included the notations, "gen. nov." and "sp. nov." and his expanded description was accompanied by line drawings and photomicrographs of asexual and sexual stages, and of oocysts in tissue sections. Thus, the type species name and/or the genus name are sometimes dated as 1907, because of the confusion involving these two publications.

This species is commonly found in rodents, but Warren et al. (2003) identified it in bilbies (*M. lagotis*) in Australia. Their identification combined oocyst morphology with molecular analyses to confirm its identity as *C. muris*. Prior to their identifying *C. muris* in the bilbies, a mouse had been trapped in the breeding enclosures, and was determined to be positive for *C. muris*. They considered it likely that the bilbies got infected from mice in the colony via fecal contamination of their food and water (Warren et al., 2003; Ryan and Power, 2012). The identification of *C. muris* in bilbies represents the only reported case of a natural cryptosporidium infection in marsupials by a species other than *C. fayeri*, or *C. macropodum*, opossum genotype II, and the brushtail possum genotype I, which are all thought to be marsupial specific and host adapted (Power, 2010).

FAMILY PERAMELIDAE GRAY, 1825 (6 GENERA, 18 SPECIES)

SUBFAMILY PERAMELINAE GRAY, 1825 (2 GENERA, 7 SPECIES)

GENUS *PERAMELES* E. GEOFFROY, 1804 (4 SPECIES)

CRYPTOSPORIDIUM FAYERI RYAN, POWER, AND XIAO, 2008

Type host: *Macropus rufus* (Desmarest, 1822), Red Kangaroo.

Remarks: Ryan and Power (2012) reported that their colleagues, P.R. Wielinga, A. de Vries, T.H. van der Goot, T. Mank, M.H. Mars, L.M. Kortbeek, and J.W. van der Giessen, had unpublished observations of *C. fayeri* in *P. bougainville* Quoy and Gaimard, 1824, the Western barred bandicoot.

DISCUSSION AND SUMMARY

Here I present the information known through 2014, on the *Cryptosporidium* species reported, described, and named from marsupials. It quickly becomes clear that there is not a great deal of information known about the general biology, endogenous development, host specificity, pathogenicity, geographic distribution, or epidemiology of *Cryptosporidium* in marsupials. One of the great difficulties in studying this parasite genus in wild animals is that its oocysts are very small, and they exhibit limited morphological variation; thus, molecular analyses (genotyping data) have become the key to initial detecting, identifying, classifying, and even "source tracking" *Cryptosporidium* species (Power et al., 2009; Power, 2010).

The first two *Cryptosporidium* species to be genetically characterized were called marsupial genotype I (from a koala, Morgan et al., 1997) and marsupial genotype II (from the Eastern grey kangaroo, Power et al., 2004); later analyses at multiple gene loci confirmed that the two forms were genetically distinct from each other and they were named *C. fayeri* (Ryan et al., 2008) and *C. macropodum* (Power and Ryan, 2008), respectively. To date, 24 *Cryptosporidium* species have been identified and named (Ryan and Power, 2012), of which seven are known to infect humans; additionally, there are about 40 cryptic species (genotypes) that have been identified across a wide range of taxa (Fayer, 2010; Power, 2010).

About 16, probably more, distinct species, and/or forms, and/or genotypes of *Cryptosporidium* are now known to infect 19 marsupial species in four orders, eight families, and 11 genera (Tables 11.1 and 11.2), with only two species from the Americas, and the other 17 from Australia. Focusing only on Australia, this indicates a broad host distribution across their marsupial taxa. In addition, *Cryptosporidium* species are geographically widespread across Australia, having been reported from four states (New South Wales, South Australia, Victoria, Western Australia) and in New Zealand (Chilvers et al., 1998) in brushtail possums, *T. vulpecula*, which were introduced from Australia in 1837 (Power, 2010) to establish the fur trade.

In Australia, of course, marsupials comprise a major component of the natural landscape, with densities in some areas of >500 animals/km^2. We know that *Cryptosporidium* oocysts are stable in the environment, resistant to commonly used drinking water disinfectants, and are able to survive routine wastewater treatment (Fayer et al., 2000; Ryan and Power, 2012). Because some species (e.g., *C. parvum*) show little host specificity, zoonotic transmission from and between domestic, native, feral, and zoo animals, and humans, especially *vis-a-vis* their ability to contaminate water supplies, can have serious public health implications (see Power, 2010 for review). Given that many infected marsupials, especially kangaroos, can shed millions of oocysts into the environment, there is concern that *Cryptosporidium* oocysts can contaminate recreational and drinking water catchments and watersheds used by cities. What effect might these ubiquitous oocysts have on humans and wildlife, and what threat might they pose to human health and/or biodiversity of other species in these environments?

Ryan and Power (2012) were among the first to focus on the available genotyping data of *Cryptosporidium* species in wildlife and domestic animals so that an attempt could be made to quantify the impact they had on contaminating drinking water catchments in Australia. From the limited data available to them, they drew several general conclusions: (1) *Cryptosporidium* species have evolved in close association with marsupials and, thus, are host adapted; (2) confirmation (via gene sequence data) of human-infectious species from marsupials is rare;

(3) There is a need to confirm whether detection of zoonotic *Cryptosporidium* species, via molecular methods (i.e., DNA extraction), is associated with actual infections; and (4) the detection of one or more atypical *Cryptosporidium* species in a few marsupial host animals does not indicate that the parasite will be successful in any other or all marsupials. Information from studies like theirs is vital to improve our understanding of the public health implications involved, if any. Similar studies, to my knowledge, have not been attempted with any American marsupials.

Marsupial and placental mammals diverged about 180 MYA, long before the radiation of extant eutherian mammals (~100 MYA). The marsupial lineage radiated from North America, even though only one extant species is now found there (*D. virginiana*), while all other species are found in South America (~93 species; opossums, shrew opossums, Monito del Monte) and Australia (~242 species; possums, kangaroos, koalas, many small insectivores, carnivores) (Mikkelsen et al., 2007; Wilson and Reeder, 2005; Baker et al., 2015). Given that marsupial evolution predates that of placentals, Power (2010) expected the marsupial *Cryptosporidium* species to have diverged before those from placental mammals, assuming that this host–parasite system was, indeed, coevolving. However, after making some preliminary phylogenetic inferences

from the limited sequence data available (see her Figure 1), she (Power, 2010) concluded that at this stage in the development of our knowledge, congruence between *Cryptosporidium* and their vertebrate hosts cannot be reliably inferred using current coevolutionary analytical methods.

Although there is a sufficient and growing amount of genetic data from placental mammals (domestic and humans), there is not very much from diverse wildlife hosts from different geographic regions to confidently infer the evolutionary history of *Cryptosporidium*. To help resolve this shortage of the right kind of genetic information, Power (2010) suggested we need genetic analyses of all newly characterized isolates to include at least three commonly used loci to help strengthen phylogenetic inferences. For example, because of their similarities, *C. fayeri* isolates from Australian and American marsupials could suggest that this species was present in marsupial stock prior to the separation of the continents, or at least until greater than 40 MYA, when the land bridge via Antarctica began to unzip, permanently splitting the continents. The presence of *C. fayeri* in both American and Australian marsupials, however, also could be due to human influence and relocation of marsupial species, particularly to the United States. For the present, the origin of marsupial *Cryptosporidium* species remains unclear.

Species *Inquirendae* in Marsupials

INTRODUCTION

Before listing the apicomplexan organisms that have been found in a wide variety of marsupials in Australia and the Americas, but have not been well described, or described at all, I want to make some comments on a few key papers in the older literature, to try to clear up some of the confusion these may have caused, and so that authors who follow don't have to redo this effort. After attempting to explain the

seven points I want to make, I list all the "species" from marsupials that I am aware of that either have not been named, or that have been improperly named, or about which there is just not enough known and which I think best belong in this group called the *species inquirendae*.

Earlier workers named a number of organisms that they saw in sections of the intestine, and these organisms have been a source of nomenclatural and taxonomic confusion ever since. Many (but not all) likely were, as Pellérdy

(1974) said, "very probably developmental stages of known or as yet unknown *Eimeria* species." Since one of the reasons for confusion is the fact that various authors have lumped some or all of them together, they will be discussed separately below. There are seven of these "forms/issues" that need clarification.

One. In 1884, Raphael Blanchard autopsied a female Rock Wallaby, *Petrogale penicillata* (Gray, 1827), at the Paris Garden of Acclimatâtion. It had been dead for 4–5 days. He found meronts in the submucosa of the large intestine that were 700–1200 × 600–900. They contained a "prodigieux" number of reniform merozoites, 10–12 × 4–5.5. He published his observations (1885a,b) calling the organism *Balbiania mucosa*. Minchin (1903) assigned it to the genus *Sarcocystis*, and Nöller (1920) to *Globidium*, calling it *G. mucosum*. Wenyon (1926) accepted Nöller's designation, as did Triffitt (1926), and Babudieri (1932). Coutelen (1933) restudied Blanchard's material, finding it in poor condition, and concluded that the organism belonged to the genus *Sarcocystis*. Mackerras (1958) called it *Globidium mucosae* (Blanchard, 1885a,b) Wenyon, 1926, but she was apparently not aware of Coutelen's work. Recalling that the name *Globidium* is now recognized to be a synonym of *Eimeria*, Levine (1979) believed that the form seen by Blanchard (1885a,b) and others was a giant meront of an *Eimeria* species, or similar coccidium, and called it *Eimeria* (?) *mucosa* (Blanchard, 1885a,b) Levine, 1979. However, O'Donoghue et al. (1987) solved this mystery. They redescribed *Sarcocystis mucosa* in rock wallabies (*Petrogale assimilis*) and Bennett's wallabies (*Macropus rufogriseus*), noting that the parasite's sarcocysts were found in the submucosa of the gastrointestinal walls of the forestomach, small intestine, and colon. Their observations matched those of the previous authors.

Two. Gilruth and Bull (1912) found meronts of an organism they called *Sarcocystis macropodis* in the submucosa of the entire small intestine of three recently captured wallabies, identified only as *Petrogale* sp., in the Melbourne Zoo, Australia. The mature meronts were roughly spheroidal, 360–700 wide. They had a wall composed of an outer radiate, fringelike layer that was uniformly ~20 thick in early stages, but extremely irregular in thickness as the meront aged; the inner layer was described only as "deeply staining." They contained 60–80 (in median section), mostly spheroidal, "blastophores" which had many N that gradually developed into mature merozoites. Mature meronts ("cysts") were 334–750 in size, and the mature merozoites were ovoidal or falciform, 7–12 × 3–5 in alcohol-fixed smears, with a large, poorly staining "nucleus" nearer the narrow end than the center. Henry and Masson (1932) assigned it to *Gastrocystis* (a synonym of *Globidium*, which is a synonym of *Eimeria*). Pellérdy (1974) thought that it was very probably the developmental stage of an *Eimeria* species, and Levine (1979) agreed with him. Once again, O'Donoghue et al. (1987) came to the rescue to solve this mystery, when they examined *M. rufogriseus*, and noted that their parasite was found in the submucosa of the gastrointestinal walls of the forestomach, small intestine, and colon. Thus, they were able to synonymize *S. macropodis* with *S. mucosa*.

Three. Gilruth and Bull (1912) found some large cysts, sometimes singly, but generally in clusters of three to eight that they called *Ileocystis macropodis* in the submucosa and, less frequently, in the epithelium of the small intestine of a kangaroo, *Macropus* sp., in Australia. Multinuclear and mature forms were present only in the submucosa. Meronts were present in circular groups, 70–334 wide. Each meront had a "fringelike external coat," ~8 thick, with striations much finer and more regular than those of the *Petrogale* meronts described above. In the early stages, the meronts were 13–15 wide and crowded with N, each ~1.7 wide. As the meronts grew, these nuclei multiplied greatly, and at times were arranged mulberry-fashioned around a central mass. They gradually became surrounded by a spindle-shaped mass of cytoplasm with blunt ends, which attained dimensions of 4–5 × 2. In none of the sections did these cells appear to be mature. Gilruth and Bull

(1912) called these meronts "large cysts." Chatton (1912) assigned this organism to the genus *Gastrocystis* (a synonym of *Globidium*, which is a synonym of *Eimeria*). Alexeieff (1913) thought that it was the same as *Lymphocystis macropodis* (see **Four**, below). Nöller (1920) called it *Globidium mucosa*, and Triffitt (1926) agreed. Wenyon and Scott (1925) thought that it might belong to the genus *Globidium* (*Gastrocystis*) or be *Eimeria macropodis*. Mackerras (1958) called it *Globidium macropodis* (Gilruth and Bull, 1912) Wenyon, 1926. Pellérdy (1965, 1974) considered it a coccidium of uncertain taxonomic position. These organisms are now thought to represent different developmental stages of one or more *Eimeria* species (Pellérdy, 1974; O'Donoghue et al., 1987).

Four. Gilruth and Bull (1912) found a form in the small intestine of the same kangaroo in which they found *I. macropodis* and called it *L. macropodis*; they said it had small meronts and, "All the villi in our sections…are greatly swollen, and almost all are denuded of epithelium. The majority are crowded especially toward the base with large cells 8.4 in diameter, containing parasites, which have pushed the nucleus to one side…In these parasites nearly all the stages of schizogony, from that of division into four nuclei, can be observed." They saw meronts with four to many nuclei, and said that the host cell became enlarged to three or four times its original diameter. Eventually, spindle-shaped merozoites, 4–5.5 × 2–2.5 developed and escaped into the intestinal lumen. They believed that the host cells were not epithelial cells because they were always found in the basement membrane of the villi; thus, they considered them to be mononuclear leukocytes. Alexeieff (1913) thought that this was the same species as *I. macropodis*. Nöller (1920) assigned it to the genus *Globidium* without giving it a specific name, and Triffitt (1926) agreed. She said the specific name (*macropodis*) fell as a homonym because the species was placed in the genus *Globidium*, but she did not give it a new name. Wenyon and Scott (1925) thought that it might be a stage of *E. macropodis*

or possibly *Globidium* (*Gastrocystis*). Mackerras (1958) called it *Globidium* sp. Wenyon, 1926. Pellérdy (1965, 1974) considered it a coccidium of uncertain taxonomic position. Under the circumstances, I believe that this is its best position for the present. Many species of *Eimeria* have been named from kangaroos and wallabies (Chapter 4), but the only one whose meronts have been described is *E. macropodis* (see **Three**, above), and its meronts are in the epithelial cells of the small intestinal villi, so *L. macropodis* cannot be this species.

Five. Gilruth and Bull (1912) found a form which they called *Ileocystis wombati* in the small intestine of the Southern Hairy-nosed Wombat, *Lasiorhinus latifrons* (Owen, 1845) (syn. *Phascolomys latifrons* Owen, 1845) that had died 24 h previously in the Melbourne Zoo, Australia. The small intestinal villi were greatly hypertrophied by meronts generally attached to their surface, but also crowding and distending the glands of Lieberkühn. These meronts were spheroidal or ellipsoidal, 93–113 in greatest diameter, with a thin wall, and contained many small nuclei. Chatton (1912) assigned this species to *Gastrocystis*. Wenyon (1926) assigned it to *Globidium*, and Mackerras (1958) did the same. Pellérdy (1965, 1974) considered it a coccidium of uncertain taxonomic position. This is now *Eimeria wombati* (Gilruth and Bull, 1911) Barker, Munday and Presidente, 1979.

Six. Wenyon and Scott (1925) and Triffitt (1926) found what they considered to be *I. macropodis* in a Red-necked Wallaby, *M. rufogriseus*, in the London Zoo. They found no oocysts that could be attributed to this species, and based their identification solely on the endogenous stages. Oocysts of *E. macropodis*, Wenyon and Scott, 1925, were reported from the same host, but Triffitt (1926) said that its meronts were in the epithelial cells of the small intestinal villi, so it cannot be this species. The actual identity of this form remains to be determined by future cross-transmission experiments and/or molecular analysis.

Seven. Wenyon and Scott (1925) and Triffitt (1926) found what they considered to be *L. macropodis* in a Red-necked Wallaby, *M. rufogriseus*, in the London Zoo. They found no oocysts that could be attributed to this species, and based their identification solely on the endogenous stages. Oocysts of *E. macropodis* Wenyon and Scott, 1925 were reported from the same host, but Triffitt (1926) said that its meronts were in the epithelial cells of the small intestinal villi, so it cannot be this species. Whether this form is actually *L. macropodis* remains to be determined by future cross-transmission experiments and molecular characterization.

SPECIES INQUIRENDAE (68+)

BESNOITIA SP. OF CONTI-DIAZ ET AL., 1970

Original host: *Didelphis virginiana* Kerr, 1792, Virginia Opossum.
Remarks: Conti-Diaz et al. (1970) found a *Besnoitia* sp. which they considered consistent with both *Besnoitia darlingi* and *Besnoitia jellisoni*, in the lungs, and to a lesser extent in the liver, of 1/5 (20%) *D. virginiana* in Kentucky, USA, but it is not certain which species, if either, they found.

BESNOITIA SP. OF STABLER AND WELCH, 1961

Original host: *Didelphis marsupialis* L., 1758, Common Opossum.
Remarks: Stabler and Welch (1961) found what they called *B. jellisoni* in an opossum in Texas, USA, but it may have been *B. darlingi*.

COCCIDIUM SP. OF JOHNSTON, 1910a

Original host: *Macropus eugenii* (Desmarest, 1817) (syn. *Halmaturus* (*Thylogale*) *eugenii* Gray, 1837 (syn. *Halmaturus thetis* Lesson, 1828)), Tammar Wallaby.

Remarks: It was reported in the Proceedings of the Linnaean Society of New South Wales that "Mr T.H. Johnston (1910a) exhibited a series of Entozoa comprising the following...(3) *Coccidium* sp., from the intestinal walls of *M. thetidis* (N.S.W.), not previously known from this host, but apparently the same as that recently found by him in a similar situation in *Macropus parryi* Benn., from near Brisbane."

COCCIDIUM SP. OF JOHNSTON, 1910b

Original host: *Macropus giganteus* Shaw, 1790, Eastern Grey Kangaroo.
Remarks: It was reported in the Proceedings of the Linnaean Society of New South Wales that "Mr T.H. Johnston (1910b) exhibited...(2) portion of the small intestine of a Kangaroo, *Macropus giganteus* Zimm., showing the presence of *Coccidium* sp., (collected by Mr O.S. Lesouëf at Coonamble, N.S. Wales). Neither of the above parasites had been previously recorded from these hosts in Australia."

CRYPTOSPORIDIUM: BRUSHTAIL POSSUM GENOTYPE I OF RYAN AND POWER, 2012

Original host: *Trichosurus vulpecula* (Kerr, 1792), Common Brushtail Possum.
Remarks: Chilvers et al. (1998), in New Zealand, detected *Cryptosporidium* in 5/39 (13%) *T. vulpecula* using only sugar and salt flotation and centrifugation. Later, Hill et al. (2008), in Australia, using immunomagnetic separation coupled to PCR, reported *Cryptosporidium* prevalence in *T. vulpecula* to be 11.3% in urban environments versus 5.6% of those captured in woodland environments. This genotype, so far, has been found only in the Brushtail Possum, which has a range of habitats throughout Australia (Ryan and Power, 2012). It seems

to be genetically distinct at two gene loci (18S rDNA, actin), one of the major criteria now used to delimit species of *Cryptosporidium* (Hill et al., 2008; Ryan and Power, 2012). This genotype has not yet been reported from people, so its potential zoonotic importance, if any, is unknown. This seems to be a host-adapted strain of *Cryptosporidium* (Ryan and Power, 2012).

CRYPTOSPORIDIUM PARVUM/HOMINIS-LIKE OF RYAN AND POWER, 2012

Original hosts: *Macropus giganteus* Shaw, 1790, Eastern Grey Kangaroo; *Isoodon obesulus* (Shaw, 1797), Southern Brown Bandicoot; *Perameles nasuta* É. Geoffroy, 1804, Long-nosed Bandicoot; *Trichosurus vulpecula* (Kerr, 1792), Common Brushtail.

Remarks: The reports and identifications of *Cryptosporidium parvum* in kangaroos (*M. giganteus*), a wallaby (no species identification), the brushtail possum (*T. vulpecula*), and bandicoots (*I. obesulus, P. nasuta*) were based on direct DNA extraction from feces, and subsequent PCR screening, but in all cases, *Cryptosporidium* could be amplified only at the multicopy 18S rDNA locus (Ryan and Power, 2012). In these studies, the marsupials sampled were living in areas associated with humans, so it is not clear whether these marsupials were actually infected with *C. parvum* and/or *Cryptosporidium hominis* or whether they were simply passively transmitting oocysts they had ingested by feeding on fecal-contaminated vegetation (Hill et al., 2008; Ng et al., 2011; Ryan and Power, 2012).

CRYPTOSPORIDIUM SP.: KANGAROO GENOTYPE I OF YANG ET AL., 2011

Original host: *Macropus fuliginosus* (Desmarest, 1817), Western Grey Kangaroo.

Remarks: This genotype, so far, has been found only in the Western grey kangaroo (Yang et al., 2011; Ryan and Power, 2012). Like the genotype found in the brushtail possum (above) it also seems to be genetically distinct at two gene loci (18S rDNA, actin), one of the major criteria now used to delimit species of *Cryptosporidium* (Ryan and Power, 2012). Similarly, this genotype has not yet been reported from people, so its potential zoonotic importance, if any, is unknown. This seems to be a host-adapted strain of *Cryptosporidium* (Ryan and Power, 2012).

CRYPTOSPORIDIUM SP. OF BARKER ET AL., 1978

Original host: *Antechinus stuartii* Macleay, 1841, Brown Antechinus.

Remarks: Barker et al. (1978) mentioned finding a *Cryptosporidium* sp. in *A. stuartii*, the marsupial mouse, but no other data were presented. Based on the number of *Cryptosporidium* species now known to infect Australian marsupials, it is impossible to even guess the identity of this one.

CRYPTOSPORIDIUM SP. OF OBENDORF, UNPUB. OBSERV. (IN RYAN ET AL., 2008)

Original host: *Thylogale billardierii* (Desmarest, 1822), Tasmanian Pademelon.

Remarks: Ryan et al. (2008) listed in her Table 1 that Obendorf had some unpublished data that *Cryptosporidium* was found in this marsupial species.

CRYPTOSPORIDIUM SP. OF O'DONOGHUE, 1985

Original host: *Antechinus* sp.

Remarks: O'Donoghue (1985) mentioned finding a *Cryptosporidium* sp. in "the marsupial mouse," but no other data were presented. Based on the number of *Cryptosporidium* species now known to infect Australian marsupials, it is impossible to guess the identity of this one.

CRYPTOSPORIDIUM SP. OF O'DONOGHUE, UNPUB. OBSERV. (IN RYAN ET AL., 2008)

Original host: *Macropus rufus* (Desmarest, 1822), Red Kangaroo.

Remarks: Ryan et al. (2008) listed in her Table 1 that O'Donoghue had some unpublished data that *Cryptosporidium* was found in this marsupial species.

CRYPTOSPORIDIUM SP. OF PHILLIPS ET AL., UNPUB. OBSERV. (IN RYAN ET AL., 2008)

Original host: *Phascolarctos cinereus* (Goldfuss, 1817), Koala.

Remarks: Ryan et al. (2008) listed in her Table 1 that Phillips et al., had some unpublished data that *Cryptosporidium* was found in this marsupial species.

CRYPTOSPORIDIUM SP. OF POWER ET AL., 2003

Original host: *Macropus eugenii* (Desmarest, 1817), Tammar Wallaby.

Remarks: Power et al. (2003) mentioned finding oocysts of *Cryptosporidium* in this host marsupial, while examining a flow cytometry technique.

CRYPTOSPORIDIUM SP. OF ZANETTE ET AL., 2008

Original host: *Didelphis albiventris* Lund, 1840, White-eared Opossum.

Remarks: Zanette et al. (2008) reported finding *Cryptosporidium* oocysts in the feces of 3/6 (50%) *D. albiventris* from southern Brazil, using zinc flotation methods, but did not attempt to name the organism.

EIMERIA KOGONI OF MYKYTOWYCZ, 1964

Original host: *Macropus giganteus* Shaw, 1790 (syn. *Macropus canguru* aka Mykytowycz, 1964), Eastern Grey Kangaroo.

Remarks: Mykytowycz (1964) reported this species in 16/149 (11%) *M. giganteus* in New South Wales and Queensland. His description was insufficient to consider this species valid. Oocysts were described as elongate-ovoidal, pointed at one end with a conspicuous M; they measured 36.6 × 21.2 (33–42 × 20–23). Sporocysts were ovoidal, 13.3 × 10.0 (12–15 × 9–11), with a large SR. No other structural information was given. Barker et al. (1989) examined hundreds of fecal samples from grey kangaroos from the type locality (Mount Hope, N.S.W.) and elsewhere in Australia, but were unable to find oocysts corresponding with those described as *Eimeria kogoni*. The oocysts of this species look very much like those of *Eimeria wilcanniensis* from *M. rufus* (see Chapter 4) and this "species" may well be a synonym. For the present, however, it is best to consider it a *species inquirenda*.

EIMERIA RUFUSI OF PRASAD, 1960

Original host: *Macropus rufus* (Desmarest, 1822), Red Kangaroo.

Remarks: Prasad (1960) described this form from two red kangaroos in the London Zoo. He said the oocysts were subspheroidal to spheroidal, with three wall layers, and measured, L × W: 24.7 × 21.5 (22.5–27 × 20–23), and were without M, OR, and PG. The sporocysts were spheroidal to subspheroidal, L × W: 6.2 × 5.5 (6–6.5 × 5–6), without SB, SSB, or PSB, but an SR was present

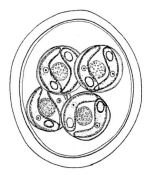

FIGURE 10.1   Line drawing of the sporulated oocyst of *Eimeria rufusi* from Prasad, 1960 (his Figure 4), with permission from Springer-Verlag publishers of *Parasitology Research* (formerly *Zeistchrift für Parasitenkunde*).

as a mass of tiny granules (line drawing). Mykytowycz (1964) examined 523 wild and captive *M. rufus* from four sites in Queensland and New South Wales, Australia, and never found this species. Barker et al. (1989) examined 97 wild and captive *M. rufus* from three locations in New South Wales and South Australia, and did not find this species. Between them, they examined >600 individuals of 11 other *Macropus* species throughout Australia, and reported no oocysts from them that resembled *Eimeria rufusi* (Mykytowycz, 1964; Barker et al., 1989). This evidence led Barker et al. (1989) to regard *E. rufusi* as a *species inquirenda*, a decision with which I can agree. Prasad (1960) published a reasonable line drawing that I feel obligated to include here.

EIMERIA SP. OF BARKER ET AL., 1963

Original host: *Macropus giganteus* Shaw, 1790 (syn. *Macropus canguru* aka. Mykytowycz, 1964), Eastern Grey Kangaroo.

Remarks: Barker et al. (1963) reported an outbreak of coccidiosis in young kangaroos in their laboratory, with lesions similar to those described by Winter (1959) in *M. rufus*, and said that five kangaroos died from the disease. They also did not identify the species.

EIMERIA SP. OF BARKER ET AL., 1988B

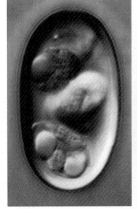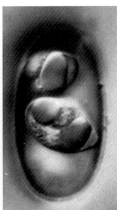

FIGURES 10.2, 10.3   **10.2.** Photomicrograph of a sporulated oocysts of *Eimeria* sp., from Barker et al. (1988b, Figure 12), with permission of all three authors, and kind permission from Elsevier, publishers of *The International Journal for Parasitology*. **10.3.** Photomicrograph of a sporulated oocysts of *Eimeria* sp., original (from M. O'Callaghan).

Original host: *Lagorchestes conspicillatus* Gould, 1842, Spectacled Hare-wallaby.

Remarks. Barker et al. (1988b) surveyed wallabies and kangaroos in five genera of Macropodidae and, in addition to describing 11 new eimerian species, they found a single oocyst of an *Eimeria* sp. The oocyst was a blunt ellipsoid, L×W: 33.6×19.2, L/W 1.75, with a thick (~1.6) two-layered smooth wall; M, OR: both absent; PG: present. Ovoidal sporocysts were, L×W: 14.4×8.8, L/W 1.6, with an inconspicuous SB, and an SR of a few scattered granules. SZ had finely granular cytoplasm and each had a large RB, 8.0×6.0 wide. Oocysts with this configuration of features have not been further described since its initial discovery.

EIMERIA SP. OF BARKER ET AL., 1988C

Original host: *Petrogale penicillata* (Gray, 1827), Brush-tailed Rock Wallaby.

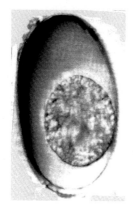

FIGURE 10.4 Photomicrograph of an unsporulated oocyst of *Eimeria* sp. from Barker et al. (1988c, their Figure 21), with permission from all four authors, and from Elsevier, publishers of *The International Journal for Parasitology*.

Remarks: Barker et al. (1988c) found large numbers of unsporulated oocysts in only one *P. penicillata* from "Kilmorey," Injune, Queensland, Australia. The ovoidal to ellipsoidal oocysts had a two-layered, smooth outer wall that was ~1.6 thick, and a colorless inner wall, ~0.4 thick; L × W (n = 20): 43.6 × 27.4 (41–47 × 25–29); L/W ratio: 1.6; M: absent. The authors felt like these large oocysts represented an *Eimeria* species, because they never found oocysts of any other genera of coccidia in the feces of >30 species of macropod marsupials.

EIMERIA SP. OF MACKERRAS, 1958

Original host: *Isoodon macrourus* (Gould, 1842), Northern Brown Bandicoot.

Remarks: Mackerras (1958) and Mackerras and Mackerras (1960) reported finding oocysts in the feces of the Northern brown bandicoot in Australia, but did not describe them. This also was mentioned by Bennett and Hobbs (2011), who said that no measurements or description of sporulated oocysts was given for this unknown eimerian.

EIMERIA SP. OF OBENDORF AND MUNDAY, 1990

Original host: *Perameles gunnii* Gray, 1838, Western Barred Bandicoot.

Remarks: Obendorf and Munday (1990) mentioned an eimerian species from the Western barred bandicoot. This was reiterated by Bennett and Hobbs (2011), who said that no measurements or description of sporulated oocysts were given for this unknown eimerian.

EIMERIA SP. OF O'CALLAGHAN AND MOORE, 1986

Original host: *Trichosurus vulpecula* (Kerr, 1792), Common Brushtail.

Remarks: O'Callaghan and Moore (1986) mentioned finding eimerian oocysts of an undescribed species in the fecal samples 11/40 (27.5%, eight male, three female) *T. vulpecula* collected on Kangaroo Island, South Australia. To my knowledge, there was never a formal description of this species.

EIMERIA SP. OF O'DONOGHUE, 1997

Original host: *Pseudocheirus peregrinus* (Boddaert, 1785), Common Ringtail Possum.

Remarks: O'Donoghue (1997) reported finding oocysts of what might be an eimerian in the feces of the common ringtail.

EIMERIA SP. OF O'DONOGHUE, 1997

Original host: *Macropus rufus* (Desmarest, 1822), Red Kangaroo.

Remarks: O'Donoghue (1997) reported finding oocysts of what might be an eimerian in the feces of the red kangaroo. O'Donoghue and Adlard (2000) also listed an unidentified *Eimeria* in the feces of this host.

EIMERIA SP. OF O'DONOGHUE AND ADLARD, 2000

Original host: *Macropus agilis* (Gould, 1842), Agile Kangaroo.

Remarks: O'Donoghue and Adlard (2000), referring to a previous paper by O'Donoghue (1997) reported finding oocysts of what might be an eimerian in the feces of the agile kangaroo.

EIMERIA SP. OF O'DONOGHUE AND ADLARD, 2000

Original host: *Macropus parryi* Bennett, 1835, Pretty-faced Wallaby.

Remarks: O'Donoghue and Adlard (2000), referring to references by four other authors reported finding oocysts of what might be an eimerian in the feces of *M. parryi*.

EIMERIA SP. OF SPEARE ET AL., 1984

Original host: *Hemibelideus lemuroides* (Collett, 1884), Lemuroid Ringtail Possum.

Remarks: O'Donoghue and Adlard (2000), referring to a previous paper by Speare et al. (1984) reported finding oocysts of what might be an eimerian in the intestines of *H. lemuroides*.

EIMERIA SP. OF SPEARE ET AL., 1984

Original host: *Pseudochirops* (syn. *Pseudocheirus*) *archeri* (Collett, 1884), Green Ringtail Possum.

Remarks: O'Donoghue and Adlard (2000), referring to a previous paper by Speare et al. (1984) reported finding oocysts of what might be an eimerian in the intestines of *P. archeri*.

EIMERIA SP. OF SPEARE ET AL., 1989

Original host: *Macropus dorsalis* (Gray, 1837), Black-striped Wallaby.

Remarks: O'Donoghue and Adlard (2000), referring to a previous paper by Speare et al. (1989) reported finding oocysts of what might be an eimerian in the intestines of *M. dorsalis*.

EIMERIA SP. OF WINTER, 1959

Original host: *Macropus giganteus* Shaw, 1790, (syn. *Macropus canguru* aka. Mykytowycz, 1964), Eastern Grey Kangaroo.

Remarks: Winter (1959) looked at an outbreak of coccidiosis in pet kangaroos in Queensland, Australia, but focused his attention on the pathology of the disease. At autopsy he reported an increase in serous fluid in the abdominal, thoracic, and pericardial cavities, the lungs were hyperemic and edematous; the most significant changes were seen in the small intestine and included hemorrhage and edema of the mucous membrane. He did not describe or identify the species of *Eimeria* that purportedly caused the outbreak, but he did state that it differed from all known species at that time. He also said that two animals recovered after the incorporation of sulfadimidine in their rations.

EIMERIA SPP. 1 AND 2 OF BENNETT AND HOBBS, 2011

Original host: *Isoodon obesulus* (Shaw, 1797), Southern Brown Bandicoot.

Remarks: Bennett and Hobbs described *Eimeria quenda* from this host (2011) and concluded their paper by saying, "there are two other morphologically distinct sporulated oocyst types recovered from *Isoodon obesulus* feces (both in 1999), recorded in the archives of the Parasitology Department, Murdoch University School of Veterinary and Biomedical Sciences." Thus, there are clearly other coccidians of bandicoots in Western Australia (and in most vertebrates worldwide) awaiting description. This would be a great Masters' thesis.

EIMERIA SPP. OF SPEARE ET AL., 1984

Original host: *Pseudochirulus* (syn. *Pseudocheirus*) *herbertensis* (Collett, 1884), Herbert River Ringtail.

Remarks: Speare et al. (1984) reported on diseases of this ringtail and on other rain forest possums, and mentioned that intestinal coccidia were common in them, and appeared to be nonpathogenic. There are no eimerian coccidia yet described from the four genera/species in this family (Pseudocheiridae); nonetheless, I took the liberty to assume that the "common intestinal coccidian" oocysts seen by Speare et al. (1984) belong to the genus *Eimeria*. Here is another host that needs to be reexamined to determine what species of intestinal coccidia parasitize it.

"EIMERIINA" SP. OF YAMADA ET AL., 1981

Original host: *Macropus fuliginosis* (Desmarest, 1817), Grey Kangaroo; likely the Western Grey Kangaroo, since it had been imported to the Tokushima Zoo, Japan, from the Zoological Gardens, south Perth, Australia.

Remarks: A pair of grey kangaroos imported by Japan, died one month after arrival due to severe bleeding of the intestinal mucosa. Necropsy and histological examination, determined that the intestinal epithelium had been

destroyed, and replaced with necrotic degeneration from the stomach to the jejunum. The authors found a peculiar cyst-forming apicomplexan in the intestinal epithelium, but not in the peritoneum, that allowed them to conclude it was not a *Besnoitia* species. They studied the histopathological changes and showed that the intestinal epithelium was replaced by hemorrhagic necrosis and composed of "highly swollen cells which looked like giant cells." This led them to suggest that the host cell enlarged to form giant cells within which they found spindle-shaped tachyzoites. The giant cells measured up to 1 mm in diameter and were surrounded by a thick wall. Yamada et al. (1981) acknowledged that the exceptional thickening of the cyst walls resembled somewhat the host cell reaction of *Besnoitia* in mice and cats, but that it differed from known *Besnoitia* species by parasitizing the glandular epithelium from the stomach through the small intestine, but did not form cysts in the muscularis mucosa. To date, *B. darlingi* is the only species in the genus known to infect marsupials, but only in opossums from the Americas (Leighton and Gajadhar, 2001; see Chapter 8).

ISOSPORA SP. OF ERNST ET AL., 1969

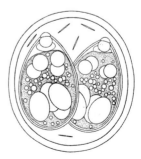

FIGURE 10.5 Line drawing of the sporulated oocyst of *Isospora* sp. from Ernst et al., 1969 (their Figure 2), with permission from the Managing Editor, *Journal of Wildlife Diseases* (formerly, *Bulletin of the Wildlife Disease Association*).

Original host: *Didelphis virginiana* Kerr, 1792, Virginia Opossum.

Remarks: Ernst et al. (1969) recovered oocysts in the feces of an opossum from Alabama, USA. The oocysts they described were subspheroidal, spheroidal, or ellipsoidal with a thin, one-layered wall, ~1 thick, light brown, tending to be slightly darker on the inner surface; oocyst: L × W: 21.6 × 20.5 (18–26 × 18–24); L/W: 1.1 (1.0–1.3); OR, M: both absent; PG: consisted of 5–15 splinterlike fragments, often scattered throughout oocyst. SP: distinctly ovoidal with one end pointed and the other rounded; L × W: 15.1 × 9.8 (13–17 × 8–11); L/W, 1.6; SB: present at pointed end of SP; SSB: present, ~2 times larger than SB (line drawing), and had a "satellite body" (?) partially surrounding it; PSB: absent; SR: present, composed of discrete coarse granules; SZ: were nondistinct, but each had a large, clear RB at one end and a smaller one at the other. Ernst et al. (1969) were not sure whether this was a true parasite of the opossum or a parasite of some bird that the opossum had eaten.

ISOSPORA SP. OF JOSEPH, 1974

Original host: *Didelphis virginiana* Kerr, 1792, Virginia Opossum.

Remarks: Joseph (1974) recovered oocysts in the feces of an opossum from Indiana, USA. The oocysts he measured were spheroidal to subspheroidal, with a smooth, one-layered wall, ~1 thick, and measured, L × W: 21 × 20 (18–24 × 15–23). Sporocysts were ovoidal, with conspicuous SB and SSB. Each SZ had two clear RB, one ~3 wide, and the other ~1.5 wide. Joseph (1974) said that the only difference between this form, and that described by Ernst et al. (1969), was that his form lacked a satellite body (?) of the SSB. He too, like Ernst et al. (1969), thought that it might be the parasite of some bird the opossum had eaten.

ISOSPORA SP. OF LAINSON AND SHAW, 1989

Original host: *Philander opossum opossum* (L., 1758), Gray Four-eyed Opossum.

Remarks: Lainson and Shaw (1989) described an isosporan from *P. o. opossum* in Brazil that they thought might be *Isospora boughtoni* Volk, 1948. We now know that the thin-walled oocysts they saw, along with the small ellipsoidal sporocysts without SB and SSB, are best identified as *Sarcocystis* species. I think that the sporocysts they observed were either those of *Sarcocystis falcatula* or *Sarcocystis lindsayi*, both of which are known to parasitize opossums as definitive hosts in South America.

KLOSSIELLA SP. OF BARKER ET AL., 1975

Original host: *Potorous tridactylus* (Kerr, 1792), (syn. *Potorous apicalis* (Gould, 1851)), Long-nosed or Southern Potoroo.

Remarks: Barker et al. (1975) found this form in 2/3 (67%) *P. tridactylus* from Winkleigh, Tasmania. They did not see oocysts, but they said they saw a few bodies, L × W: up to 30 × 12 that contained merozoites ~3 × 1. Their interpretation was that these were meronts "of a *Klossiella* sp. which lack sufficient distinction to merit a name at present." The stages seen were in the glomeruli and epithelial cells of proximal convoluted tubules of the kidneys.

KLOSSIELLA SP. OF MACKERRAS, 1958

Original host: *Perameles nasuta* É. Geoffroy, 1804, Long-nosed Bandicoot.

Remarks: Mackerras (1958) said he found this form in the kidneys of the long-nosed bandicoot in Australia, but he did not describe it.

KLOSSIELLA SP. OF SPEARE ET AL., 1984

Original host: *Pseudochirops* (*Pseudocheirus*) *archeri* (Collett, 1884), Green Ringtail Possum.

Remarks: Speare et al. (1984) reported on diseases of rain forest possums and mentioned that *Klossiella* was commonly found in *P. archeri* in the epithelial cells of the kidney. This form was mentioned again by O'Dounghue and Adlard (2000) in their catalog of protozoan parasites recorded in Australia.

KLOSSIELLA SP. OF SPEARE ET AL., 1984

Original host: *Pseudochirulus* (syn. *Pseudocheirus*) *herbertensis* (Collett, 1884), Herbert River Ringtail.

Remarks: Speare et al. (1984) reported on diseases of rain forest possums and mentioned that *Klossiella* was commonly found in *P. herbertensis* in the epithelial cells of the renal cortex. They said that the parasitized cells were enlarged, and probably destroyed by the parasites, but that the damage was minimal and there was no inflammatory response by the host.

"SARCOCYSTIDAE" SP. OF MERINO ET AL., 2008

Original host: *Thylamys elegans* (Waterhouse, 1839), Elegant Fat-tailed Mouse Opossum.

Remarks: Merino et al. (2008) surveyed the blood of 16 adult *T. elegans* near Santiago, Chile, for parasites and found 15 (94%) to be infected. Initially, based on the morphology of the intraerythrocytic forms found, the parasite was identified as *Hepatozoon didelphydis* (d'Utra e. Silva and Arantes, 1916) Wenyon, 1926 (see Smith, 1996). However, after amplification (PCR), a DNA fragment of 18S rDNA was sequenced and then analyzed phylogenetically. To their surprise, their analyses indicated that the parasite was not a *Hepatozoon* species, but clearly belonged instead within the cyst-forming Sarcocystidae. In the past, *Hepatozoon* species have been identified based solely on the morphology of their blood stages, and these have been reported from a number of marsupials including *Didelphis marsupialis*, *Philander opossum*, and *Metachirus nudicaudatus* (Ayala et al., 1973; Deane and Deane, 1961; de Thoisy et al., 2000; d'Utra e. Silva and Arantes, 1916; Garnham and Lewis, 1958; Regendanz and Kikuth, 1928). Clearly, molecular analyses will be required in future studies to help determine where within the Apicomplexa these parasites really belong. Thus, the parasite found infecting the red blood cells of *T. elegans* appeared to the authors to require assignment to the family Sarcocystidae and likely incorporated into a new, and as yet unnamed, genus.

"SARCOCYSTIDAE" SP. OF MERINO ET AL., 2009

Original host: *Dromiciops gliroides* Thomas, 1894, Monito del Monte.

Remarks: Merino et al. (2009) collected blood and DNA samples from individuals of *D. gliroides*; 35/73 (48%) blood smears were found to be infected with an intraerythrocytic banana-shaped parasite that was morphologically identified as a *Hepatozoon* species. However, as in their previous work (Merino et al., 2008, above), and that of Zhu et al. (2009, below), their phylogenetic analysis based on a sequence of DNA fragments (small subunit (SSU) rRNA gene) found that the *Hepatozoon* lineages, found in *D. gliroides* and in an Australian bandicoot, were not closely related to each other, or to the *Hepatozoon* lineage found in other Australian marsupials, or to the lineages in other American vertebrates (anurans, marsupials, rodents, reptiles, carnivores). This indicates that the parasite in *D. gliroides* may correspond to an intraerythrocytic sarcocystidian.

"SARCOCYSTIDAE" SP. OF ZHU ET AL., 2009

Original host: *Petaurus australis* Shaw, 1791, Yellow-bellied Glider.

Remarks: Zhu et al. (2009) examined the blood of two yellow-bellied gliders from Australia and found them to be infected with an intraerythrocytic parasite that usually would have been identified as a hemogregarine/*Hepatozoon* species. However, after using molecular techniques that targeted the parasite's SSU- and large subunit (LSU) rDNA, they found that their blood parasite was most closely related to the cyst-forming coccidia (Sarcocystidae) including *Besnoitia*, *Cystoisospora*, *Hammondia*, *Hyaloklossia*, *Neospora*, *Sarcocystis*, and *Toxoplasma* species.

A year later, Merino et al. (2010) found that the intraerythrocytic parasites of both the South American mouse opossum, *T. elegans* (above), and the yellow-bellied glider, *P. australis* from Australia, were monophyletic using their SSU- and LSU rDNA sequences. Merino et al.'s (2010) phylogenetic reconstruction unambiguously placed both species within the Apicomplexan family Sarcocystidae, indicated that they shared a common ancestor, and suggested that they share similar parasites in spite of the time since separation of both continents. The life cycle(s) of these intraerythrocytic parasites of marsupials remain(s) unknown, and the authors suggested they represent an, as yet, unnamed genus, which they predicted will show typical isosporan oocysts with two sporocysts, each having four sporozoites. Sequences of both the South American and Australian parasites have been placed in GenBank and deserve further attention and analyses.

SARCOCYSTIS BETTONGIAE BOURNE, 1934

Original host: *Bettongia lesueur grayii* Gould, 1841, Boodie or Short-nosed "Rat" Kangaroo.

Remarks: Bourne (1934) described small sarcocysts, up to 1000 long with sickle-shaped merozoites (bradyzoites), in muscles of the Boodie. Mandour (1965) called this a *nomen nudum* because the name "was proposed solely on the basis of the host." Some authors in the older literature often gave new names to forms of organisms they saw, but with no other information. These names become "nude names," or *nomen nuda* (pl.) according to the *International Code of Zoological Nomenclature* (Ride et al., 2000). The *Code* also defines a *species inquirenda* as one of doubtful identity that needs further investigation. Implicit in that definition is that the taxonomic species has been named in some published document, but without the existence of a type specimen of any kind, and without sufficient quantitative and qualitative data to distinguish it from other closely related species. Although there was mention of the size of a sarcocyst, there was little other information given, but the paper *was* published. Thus, I think it is best to regard this species as a *species inquirenda*, especially because no other *Sarcocystis* forms/species have been described from this host genus since the initial mention by Bourne (1934). The name can be resurrected at a later time if a systematic survey of *Bettongia* species in Australia finds and documents similar forms in the muscles.

SARCOCYSTIS SP. OF CARINI, 1939

Synonym: *Isospora lutreolina* Carini, 1939.

Original host: *Lutreolina crassicaudata* (Desmarest, 1804), Lutrine Opossum.

Remarks: Carini (1939) found sporulated oocysts in the subepithelial tissues of the anterior small intestinal villi in a lutrine opossum from Brazil, South America. He described these endogenous oocysts as dumbbell-shaped, with a thin wall that sinks between the sporocysts; these oocysts were, L × W: 22–20 × 17–19, and the ellipsoidal sporocysts were, L × W: 12–14 × 9–10, without an SB, but with an SR, all features typical of a *Sarcocystis* species. The oocysts were scarce in the feces, but abundant in intestinal scrapings and sections. I am confident that this species is actually a form of *Sarcocystis*, since its oocysts are already sporulated in the tissues. Carini (1939) was unable to infect two opossums, *Didelphis aurita*, with sporulated oocysts of this species, further suggesting that he was dealing with a *Sarcocystis* species in which the opossum was the definitive host.

SARCOCYSTIS SP. OF DUBEY ET AL., 2001b

Original host: *Merops nubicus* Gmelin, 1788, Northern Carmine Bee-eater.

Remarks: Dubey et al. (2001b) found a male *M. nubicus* in a zoo in Florida, that was infected with a species of *Sarcocystis*, which their data suggested may be different from *S. falcatula*-like parasites described from other avian hosts. They suspected, as did Box and Smith (1982), that *S. falcatula* is a mixture of more than one species, based on the broad range of intermediate hosts reported to harbor it. I include this form here because parasites in both the lungs and muscles of the bee-eater reacted with varying intensity with polyclonal rabbit antisera to both *Sarcocystis neurona* and *S. falcatula* which, of course, share the opossum (*D. virginiana*) as a definitive host.

SARCOCYSTIS SP. OF DUSZYNSKI AND BOX, 1978

Original definitive host: *Didelphis virginiana* Kerr, 1792, Virginia Opossum.

Original intermediate host: *Anas acuta* L., 1758, Northern Pintail Duck.

Remarks: Duszynski and Box (1978) found a hunter-killed pintail duck from Galveston County, Texas, to have sarcocysts in its breast muscle that were round and measured, L × W: 5.0 × 1.0 mm. They fed this sarcocyst-infected muscle to an opossum, which began to discharge sporocysts of *Sarcocystis* in its feces 13–18 days after ingestion. Giemsa-stained zoites in dried, ethanol-fixed smears measured 10.9 × 3.2. They chose not to name the species.

SARCOCYSTIS SP. OF MACKERRAS, 1958

Original host: *Dasyurus* (syn. Satanellus) *hallucatus* Gould, 1842, Northern Quoll.

Remarks: Mackerras (1958) did not describe this form.

SARCOCYSTIS SP. OF MACKERRAS ET AL., 1953

Original host: *Isoodon obesulus* (Shaw, 1797), Southern Brown Bandicoot.

Remarks: Mackerras et al. (1953) found sarcocysts in the muscles of the body wall of the bandicoot in Australia, but did not describe it further.

SARCOCYSTIS SP. OF MUNDAY ET AL., 1978

Original host: *Petrogale penicillata* (Gray, 1825), Brush-tailed Rock Wallaby.

Remarks: O'Donoghue and Adlard (2000) listed that Munday et al. (1978) had found a sarcocyst in the muscles of *P. penicillata*.

SARCOCYSTIS SP. 1 OF MUNDAY ET AL., 1978

Original host(s): *Antechinus stuartii* Macleay, 1841, Brown Antechinus; *Antechinus swainsonii* (Waterhouse, 1840), Dusky Antechinus.

Remarks: Munday et al. (1978) found sarcocysts of this form in the skeletal muscles of 4/44 (9%) *A. stuartii* and in 1/12 (8%) *A. swainsonii* (Dasyuridae) in Australia. They considered the forms in both host species to be the same *Sarcocystis* species (Type B). These sarcocysts were thin walled and contained small merozoites. Sarcocysts were up to 800 × 45, and their walls were simple, with undulations and many invaginations. No other structural information was given.

SARCOCYSTIS SP. 2 OF MUNDAY ET AL., 1978

Original host: *Dasyurus maculatus* (Kerr, 1792), Tiger Quoll or Tiger Cat.

Remarks: Munday et al. (1978) found sporocysts of this form in the feces of 1/11 (9%) *D. maculatus* (Dasyuridae) in Australia. The sporocysts were similar to those from the Tasmanian devil, but larger, L × W: 11.5 × 8. No other structural information was given. They said it was not possible to be sure that these sporocysts had originated in the intestinal mucosa and, therefore, they could have been pseudoparasites derived from a prey species. Since *Sarcocystis* sporocysts have not been found in any prey animal, this possibility seems unlikely.

SARCOCYSTIS SP. 3 OF MUNDAY ET AL., 1978

Original host: *Isoodon macrourus* (Gould, 1842), Northern Brown Bandicoot.

Remarks: Munday et al. (1978) found sarcocysts of this form in the muscles of 1/1 *I. macrourus* (Peramelidae) in Australia. The sarcocysts were

thin walled (Type B) and contained well-defined merozoites; the largest sarcocysts were. L × W: 200 × 50. They gave no further information.

SARCOCYSTIS SPP.(?) 4 A AND B OF MUNDAY ET AL., 1978

Original host: *Macropus rufus* (Desmarest, 1822), Red Kangaroo.

Remarks: Munday et al. (1978) found sarcocysts in the skeletal muscles, but not the heart, of 7/47 (15%) *M. rufus* in Australia, including Type A and B sarcocysts. Type A sarcocysts in one animal were, L × W: 2500 × 175, had a thin wall, and were compartmentalized, but with relatively few merozoites. "Other Kangaroos in the same area had a steatitis associated with schizonts in the fat cells. Some organisms were round to oval and others were triangular due to compression by fat globules. The schizonts were up to 90 in length and 45 in width and contained zoites measuring 7 × 1.2. Possibly these were *Sarcocystis* meronts because O'Donoghue (pers. comm.) has found schizonts of *Sarcocystis ovicanis* in adipose tissue of lambs." Six of the seven (86%) infected *M. rufus* had Type B sarcocysts, but they did not mention these. No further information was given.

SARCOCYSTIS SP. (SPP.?) 5 OF MUNDAY ET AL., 1978

Original hosts: *Macropus agilis* (Gould, 1842), Agile Wallaby; *Macropus giganteus* (Shaw, 1790), Eastern Grey Kangaroo; *Macropus rufogriseus* (Desmarest, 1817), Red-necked Wallaby; *Wallabia bicolor* (Desmarest, 1804), Swamp Wallaby; *Thylogale billardierii* (Desmarest, 1822), Tasmanian Pademelon.

Remarks: Munday et al. (1978) found sarcocysts of this form(s) in the muscles, tongue, and diaphragm, but not the heart in 2/18 (11%) *M. giganteus*, 1/3 (33%) *M. agilis*, 14/105 (13%) *M. rufogriseus*, 1/2 (50%) *W. bicolor*, and 2/123

(2%) *T. billardierii* in Australia. All of the cysts were Type B sarcocysts. The sarcocysts were all thin walled, with no detectable trabeculae, and all had small merozoites. The sarcocysts varied considerably in size, with the longest one being L×W: 500×200. They gave no further information except to say that they detected no sarcocysts in macropods collected from islands where dasyurid marsupials were unknown.

SARCOCYSTIS SP. 6 OF MUNDAY ET AL., 1978

Original hosts: *Petrogale* (syn. *Peradorcas*) *concinna* Gould, 1842, Nabarlek or Little-rock Wallaby; *Petrogale brachyotis* (Gould, 1841), Short-eared Rock Wallaby (syn. *Petrogale venustula* (Thomas, 1926)).

Remarks: Munday et al. (1978) found sarcocysts of this form in the skeletal muscles and tongue, but not the heart, of 2/3 (67%) *P.* (syn. *Peradorcas*) *concinna* and 3/4 (75%) *P. brachyotis* (syn. *P. venustula*) in Australia. Sarcocysts in both species were Type A, which were variable in size. Those in the tongue had a wall 2–4 thick with striations, no detectable trabeculae, and small merozoites. Those in the limb muscles had walls 1–2 thick containing protrusions or villi, 1–2×1, but these had no detectable trabeculae, and also had small merozoites. The longest sarcocyst they measured was, L×W: 410×40 in *P. brachyotis*, while the largest sarcocysts in *P. cocinna* were, L×W: 140×75. They gave no further information, and they did not suggest that these may be different species.

SARCOCYSTIS SP. 7 OF MUNDAY ET AL., 1978

Original hosts: *Perameles gunnii* Gray, 1838, Eastern Barred Bandicoot; *Perameles nasuta* É. Geoffroy, 1804, Long-nosed Bandicoot.

Remarks: Munday et al. (1978) found sarcocysts of this form in the muscles of 3/31 (10%) *P. gunnii*, and in 1/2 (50%) *P. nasuta* in

Australia; they considered both as Type B sporocysts, with thin walls, and containing small merozoites. They gave no further information, but they did write, "On the basis of morphology these latter organisms were tentatively identified as *Toxoplasma* which was supported in one instance by the fact that cysts were present in adrenal gland as well as muscle."

SARCOCYSTIS SP. 8 OF MUNDAY ET AL., 1978

Original host: *Pseudochirops* (syn. Pseudocheirus) *archeri* (Collett, 1884), Green Ringtail.

Remarks: Munday et al. (1978) found sarcocysts of this form in the muscles of 1/1 *P. archeri* in Australia. According to them, these sarcocysts were Type A, thick walled, up to 5 thick, with a wall containing fingerlike cytophaneres, 4–5×1; the longest sarcocyst found was, L×W: 1200×145. No other information was given.

SARCOCYSTIS SP. 9 OF MUNDAY ET AL., 1978

Original host: *Sarcophilus harrisii* (Boltard, 1841), Tasmanian Devil.

Remarks: Munday et al. (1978) found sporocysts of this form in the feces of 1/50 (2%) *S. harrisii* in Australia. Sporocysts were, L×W: 10×7.2, and occurred in pairs wrapped within a "fine" oocyst wall. No further information was given.

SARCOCYSTIS SP. 10 OF MUNDAY ET AL., 1978

Original host: *Sarcophilus harrisii* (Boltard, 1841), Tasmanian Devil.

Remarks: Munday et al. (1978) also found Type B sarcocysts in the skeletal muscles and diaphragm, but not in the heart, of 1/29 (3%) *S. harrisii* in Australia. The sarcocysts were thin walled, L×W: up to 2000×52, and contained small merozoites. They gave no further information.

SARCOCYSTIS SP (SPP.?) 11 OF MUNDAY ET AL., 1978

Original hosts: *Trichosurus vulpecula* (Kerr, 1792), Common Brushtail; *Trichosurus caninus* (Ogilby, 1836), Short-eared Possum.

Remarks: Munday et al. (1978) found this (these?) species in 1/155 (0.6%) *T. vulpecula* and 2/44 (4.5%) *T. caninus*; they said that the sarcocysts in both were Type B, thin walled, and contained small merozoites. They found only one sarcocyst in *T. vulpecula* in a distorted extrinsic muscles of the eye, that measured, L×W: 330×180. In *T. caninus* they found relatively numerous sarcocysts, L×W: 220×72, in the tongues of both infected possums.

SARCOCYSTIS SP. OF SENEVIRATNA ET AL., 1975

Original host: *Didelphis virginiana* Kerr, 1792, Virginia Opossum.

Remarks: Seneviratna et al. (1975) found sarcocysts in the muscles of the 3/19 (16%) opossums collected from the Detroit metropolitan area, Michigan, USA. They did not describe this form further.

SARCOCYSTIS SP. OF SCHOLTYSECK ET AL., 1982

Original host: *Didelphis virginiana* Kerr, 1792, Virginia Opossum.

Remarks: Scholtyseck et al. (1982) examined one naturally-infected opossum in southwestern Michigan, USA, and found both sarcocysts in the skeletal and tongue muscles, and sporulated oocysts and sporocysts in intestinal scraping and in the feces. They examined the spindle-shaped

tissue cysts by both light and electron microscopy (TEM). Grossly, the sarcocysts in muscles measured, L×W: 140×70, and they provided measurements of the cyst wall, metrocytes and merozoites when viewed by TEM, but they did not measure oocysts or sporocysts. In 1982, there were only two valid species of *Sarcocystis* in the opossum, *Sarcosystis didelphidis* (Venezuela) and *Sarcosystis garnhami* (Belize), both described from *D. marsupialis*. Scholtyseck et al. (1982) felt that the species they examined was different enough from both, and since it came from a different host species (although a congener), that "it is likely that a new species of *Sarcocystis* is represented in our study," but they did not name it. Opossums are known to be able to serve as both intermediate and definitive hosts to different *Sarcocystis* species, but it is unlikely, in my opinion, that the intestinal stages they saw (but did not describe) were the same species as the sarcocysts in the muscles that they did study.

SARCOCYSTIS SP. OF SPEARE ET AL., 1989

Original host: *Dendrolagus lumholtzi* Collett, 1884, Lumholtz's Tree Kangaroo.

Remarks: O'Donoghue and Adlard (2000) listed that Speare et al. (1989) had found a sarcocyst in the muscles of *D. lumholtzi*.

SARCOCYSTIS SP. OF TRIFFITT, 1927

Original host: *Macropus rufogriseus* (Desmarest, 1817), Red-necked Wallaby (syn. *Macropus bennetti* Waterhouse, 1838, Bennett's Wallaby).

Remarks: Triffitt (1927) reported finding sarcocysts in the mucosal and serosal wall of the small and large intestine of a wallaby that died in the Zoological Gardens in London. Smaller forms were spheroidal, ~0.5mm wide, while larger forms were more ovoidal, 1.75×1.0mm.

When parts of the intestinal wall were fixed, embedded, and sectioned, she found these cysts in the muscle layers of the gut where they caused, "considerable distension but no definite lesion" and no tissue reaction. The cysts in the longitudinal muscle layer caused projections on the serous surface of the intestine, and those within the circular muscle layer caused distortion of the mucosa. Zoites within the cysts were sickle-shaped, 17–19 × 4.5–5. She found it curious that no other tissues throughout the body showed infection with cysts, although she did not have access to skeletal muscle to examine for sectioning. Triffitt (1927) attempted to transmit this parasite to a "mouse" (species unknown) by feeding it "a great number of spores." Two months PI, the mouse was killed and examined; while the intestinal walls showed no cysts, there were sarcocysts present in the skeletal muscles, but "these were probably due to a natural infection of *S. muris*" (Triffitt, 1927).

TOXOPLASMA SP. OF MUNDAY ET AL., 1978

Original host(s): *Perameles gunnii* Gray, 1838, Eastern Barred Bandicoot; *Perameles nasuta* E. Geoffroy, 1804, Long-nosed Bandicoot.

Remarks: Munday et al. (1978) found what they considered to be Type B sporocysts in both *Perameles* species; they had thin walls, and contained small merozoites. They gave no further information, but they wrote, "On the basis of morphology these latter organisms were tentatively identified as *Toxoplasma* which was supported in one instance by the fact that cysts were present in adrenal gland as well as muscle."

TOXOPLASMA SPP. OF O'DONOGHUE AND ADLARD, 2000

Original host(s): *Antechinus minimus* (Geoffroy, 1803), Swamp Antechinus; *Antechinus swainsonii* (Waterhouse, 1840), Dusky Antechinus; *Dasyurus viverrinus* (Shaw, 1800), Eastern Quoll; *Phascogale tapoatafa* (Meyer, 1793), Brush-tailed Phascogale.

Remarks: O'Donoghue and Adlard (2000), in their catalog of protozoan parasites recorded in Australia, cited the work of five other papers stating that they had found *Toxoplasma* sp. in these hosts.

TYZZERIA SP. OF BARKER ET AL., 1988C

Original host: *Thylogale thetis* (Lesson, 1828), Red-necked Pademelon.

Remarks: Barker et al. (1988c) did a survey of five genera of wallabies and kangaroos (Macropodidae) for coccidia and mentioned that they found oocysts in the feces of the red-necked pademelon that contained eight SZ. They interpreted these to be either a species of *Tyzzeria* (perhaps) or *Pfeifferinella* (unlikely, found only in invertebrates) and said, "since their status as parasites of *T. thetis* is not certain they are not described."

DISCUSSION AND SUMMARY

Pick one of the 68+ *species inquirendae* above, and there is a research project awaiting your attention.

Discussion, Summary, and Conclusions

Within the Apicomplexan order Eucoccidiorida, four families of parasitic protists have been found to parasitize marsupials. A general overview of what we now know—and more importantly do not know—about the parasites in each of these families is summarized below. Following those summaries, I have included sections on type specimens, the value of archiving types, molecular tools, revisionary trends, and the future of taxonomy of the Apicomplexa since they seem germane to the topics presented.

ADELIIDAE

Only one genus in this family has members known to parasitize marsupials and, to date, 11 *Klossiella* species have been found in three marsupial orders, Didelphimorphia, Diprotodontia, and

Peramelemorphia (Tables 11.1 and 11.2); 10 of these named forms occur in Australian marsupials. As in the Eimeriidae species (below), we know virtually nothing about the biology of the named species other than one or two tissue stages that have been observed in histological sections of kidneys. For example, a sporulated oocyst with sporocysts and its sporozoites is known for only 1/11 (9%) named species. In seven other species, immature sporocysts (sporoblasts) were measured, but only in tissue sections, and not their sporozoites. We know nothing about the prepatent or patent periods of any species. All species seem to undergo endogenous development in host kidney cells, but only one or two of the endogenous stages are known for 6/11 (55%) of the named species. No complete life cycle is known and no cross-transmission studies have been attempted. Five of the 11 species were said to be nonpathogenic, one seems to be mildly pathogenic, and nothing is known about the pathology of the remaining five named species. Type materials have been deposited in accredited museums for only 2/11 (18%) named species. Our knowledge of these apicomplexan parasites in marsupials is minimal, even though they seem to be regular inhabitants of marsupial kidneys once we look for them. The fault seems to be that our old habits and traditions are difficult to change. As parasitologists working in the field, we need to incorporate collecting urine into our field protocols so we can gain some sense of what oocysts and sporocysts of *Klossiella* really look like, what variation exists among and between the various species, and what a reasonable incidence of infection may be in any host population sampled. Collecting kidney and related tissue samples for squash preparations/smears to be stained on slides, and blocks of tissue to be fixed, embedded, sectioned, and prepared for histological examination, is crucial in future surveys. What a nice discovery it would be for someone to infect a marsupial species with oocysts/sporocysts, and be able to trace the development of a complete life cycle. And, most importantly in all future studies, it is imperative that DNA be collected and sequenced so that we

gain an exact sense of the nature and affinity of these very interesting parasites—about which we know so little—to other species groups within the Eucoccidiorida. There are almost uncountable potential research projects waiting for eager young (and old) minds to explore and solve.

CRYPTOSPORIDIIDAE

To date, *Cryptosporidium* species have been identified in two American and in 17 Australian marsupial species (Table 11.2); these include 16 forms, "species," or genotypes (Table 11.1) in four orders, eight families, and 11 genera. Because some species (e.g., *C. parvum*) show little host specificity, zoonotic transmission from and between domestic, native, and feral animals and humans, especially focusing on their ability to contaminate water supplies, might have serious public health implications, especially in Australia, where marsupials are a dominant component of most landscapes. Unfortunately, we know very little about their contribution of human pathogenic strains of *Cryptosporidium* oocysts to recreational and drinking water catchments.

The major difficulty in studying this genus in wild animals is that the oocysts are very small and exhibit virtually no morphological variation. Because of their small size, they are difficult to find, let alone study in fecal smears, even when concentration and/or specialized staining techniques are used. Thus, molecular analyses are truly the key to detecting, identifying, naming, and classifying *Cryptosporidium* species.

EIMERIIDAE

Coccidia within the Eimeriidae (*Eimeria*, *Isospora* species) have been found in three Marsupial orders: Didelphimorphia, Diprotodontia, and Peramelemorphia. Only 7/14 (50%) extant families, 23/60 (38%) extant genera, and 46/249 (18%) extant marsupial species in these orders have been examined for, and found to be infected with, intestinal coccidia. From this very modest sample, 56 *Eimeria* and one *Isospora* species have been identified, and at least the majority seems to be valid species. With the exception of genera in the Macropodidiae and Hypsiprymnodontidae (Diprotodontia), most of the species examined for intestinal coccidia in the eight other families (Didelphidae, Peramelidae, Phalangeridae, Phascolarctidae, Potoridae, Pseudocheiridae, Thylacomyidae, and Vombatidae) in these three orders had only very small numbers of individuals, from limited geographic areas, sampled for coccidia. I am convinced that these factors contributed to the fact that so few eimeriid coccidians (mostly one, sometimes two, see Table 11.2) were described from these other species.

We know almost nothing about the biology of these intestinal coccidians from the three marsupial orders that harbor so many species. The amount of time it takes for oocysts to sporulate once they leave the confines of their host's intestinal tract has been determined, to some degree, for 12/57 (21%) of the known *Eimeria* and *Isospora* species. We know the prepatent and/or patent periods for only 3/57 (5%) of these eimeriid species. We know the site of infection, where endogenous development takes place, in only 6/57 (10.5%) eimeriid species. We know only partial details of one or two endogenous tissue stages in 4/56 (7%) of these species, but we *do* know the complete life cycle, and all of the endogenous stages, for 1/57 (<2%) species, *E. marmosopos*. This later work (Chinchilla et al., 2015) marks a milestone of sorts because it is the only complete endogenous life cycle known for any marsupial intestinal coccidian. Only 2/57 (3.5%) species, *E. haberfeldi* and *Isospora arctopitheci*, have been cross-transmitted to other host species. We know that at least 5/57 (9%) species including *E. marmosopos* (mild) (Didelphimorphia), *E. wombati* (mild), *E. arundeli* (severe), *E. macropodis* (severe) (Diprotodontia), and *E. kanyana* (mild) (Peramelemorphia) can be pathogenic in the three orders of marsupials sampled.

SARCOCYSTIDAE

Only one genus within the Sarcocystinae, *Sarcocystis*, has at least 10 recognized species known to parasitize marsupials either as intermediate hosts (*S. didelphidis, S. garnhami, S. greineri, S. inghami, S. marmosae, S. mucosa*), in which sarcocysts are found in the muscles, or as definitive hosts (*S. falcatula, S. lindsayi, S. neurona, S. speeri*), in which sporocysts are discharged in the feces. Of these 10, only *S. mucosa* has been recorded from four Australian marsupial species, while the others have been studied and defined in six species of American opossums; thus, 10 *Sarcocystis* species in 10 marsupial species in seven genera. However, there are more than 20 *Sarcocystis*-like organisms, identified mostly from muscle sarcocysts that have been reported from an additional 18 marsupial species in 12 more genera. All told, we now know that *Sarcocystis* species have been reported in four marsupial orders representing eight families, at least 19 genera, and about 30 or more host species (Chapter 10, Tables 11.1 and 11.2). With <10% of all marsupial species worldwide having been examined for these parasites, it portends that there is still a gold mine of new *Sarcocystis* species yet to be discovered.

In spite of the rewards of such new discoveries, future researchers must proceed with caution. Sarcocysts in tissues look very similar and young sarcocysts look different than older ones of the same species. Sporocysts found in feces all look identical and their differences in sizes are trivial and not definitive. Some *Sarcocystis* species may (or may not) be specific for their definitive hosts, but less specificity should be expected in their intermediate hosts; thus, a new host species in which one stage or the other is found is no indicator of having found a new *Sarcocystis* species.

Tissues with sarcocysts must be collected and properly preserved for LM and TEM studies and, when possible, for cross-transmission to potential definitive hosts. Sporocysts should be collected and preserved in both 2% aqueous (w/v) potassium dichromate solution ($K_2Cr_2O_7$)

to collect mensural date for morphological study, and in 70–100% ethanol for DNA extraction. Bioassay and molecular methods were developed at a rapid pace in the last decade and have begun to help distinguish the sporocysts of different *Sarcocystis* species in fecal samples, and these should be used at every opportunity. One of the more reliable bioassays to help distinguish between sporocysts in feces of some *Sarcocystis* species is the use of knockout mice and budgerigars in cross-transmission studies because some are not infective to one or the other or both. In addition, molecular methods and/or markers are now in place to distinguish many species, one from the other, including 18S rRNA markers, phylogenetic resolution using the ITS-1 locus within the 18S rRNA gene array to look distinct nucleotide differences, panels of random amplified polymorphic DNA (RAPD) markers, and others.

Within the Toxoplasmatinae, two genera, *Besnoitia* and *Toxoplasma*, are known to infect marsupials. *Besnoitia darlingi* is the only species known to infect marsupials, and it is found in about four American opossum species; no *Besnoitia* species are yet reported from Australian marsupials. Pathology of *B. darlingi* in opossums seems to be variable in time and space and dependent upon the host it infects. To the untrained eye, tissue cysts of *Besnoitia* species can be mistaken for those of *Sarcocystis* species (except they are not found in striated muscles) and the oocysts, shed in the feces unsporulated, are very small and often missed or overlooked as are those of *Toxoplasma*. These two features of the life history likely contribute to *Besnoitia* species either being misidentified or being underrepresented during survey work.

Toxoplasma is quite common, and pathogenic, in dozens of marsupial hosts, especially those in Australia. In Australia, marsupials evolved in the absence of *T. gondii* as there were no Felidae there before Europeans arrived. We now know that Australian marsupials are highly susceptible to *T. gondii* and infections are debilitating and fatal in both captive and free-ranging populations. This parasite is known in at least 35 species, in four

marsupial orders (Tables 11.1 and 11.2); I believe these are just the species in which it has been looked for, or the animals were sick and dying, and it was found to be the etiological agent of that distress.

SPECIES INQUIRENDAE

Earlier workers named a number of organisms that they saw in sections of the intestine, or in host feces and these organisms have become a source of nomenclatural and taxonomic confusion ever since. Other authors simply took shortcuts and did not produce species descriptions that were complete enough, or they made very simple observations of stages seen in the tissues or in the feces, and gave their identifications only at the genus level. After reviewing all the marsupial "species" that either were not named, were improperly/incorrectly named, or about which there is just not enough known, I found at least 68 apicomplexan forms, in nine genera, that must be relegated to a group that can only be called *species inquirendae*, because their validity must remain in question. These include two *Besnoitia*, two *Coccidium*, 10 *Cryptosporidium*, 19+ *Eimeria*, three *Isospora*, four *Klossiella*, 25 *Sarcocystis*, two+ *Toxoplasma*, and one *Tyzzeria* "species." They provide interesting insights into work that can be followed up and completed to verify their true identities.

TYPE SPECIMENS

After researchers find what they believe may be new species of intestinal eimeriids, they usually observe, study, measure, preserve (in some way), describe, and then name them. This naming reflects the use of the *International Code of Zoological Nomenclature* but, in fact, our work as parasitologists has not been consistent with the intent of the Code, which recommends the designation of *type specimens* for each new species. This "name-bearing type of a nominal taxon provides the objective standard of reference for the application of the name it bears" and "no matter how the boundaries of the taxon may vary…the valid name of such a taxon is determined from the name-bearing type" (Articles 61.1 and 61.1.1, p. 63, Ride et al., 2000). The Code says that the type *is* the specimen, with the implication that the type: (1) is intended to be unchanging and objective, whereas the limits of a nominal species are recognized to be subjective and transient; (2) serves as an anchor for the name (to some extent it is the name); and (3) will be available for future study. Unfortunately, this "type" tradition has been lacking among taxonomists working with the Eimeriidae. It has only been in the last 15 years, or so, that we have begun to archive actual specimens (e.g., phototypes/photosyntypes, symbiotype hosts, tissue sections with endogenous stages, DNA). In this regard, we have archived parasite stages, symbiotype host specimens, and/or gene sequences into accredited museums or GenBank for only 21/86 (24%) of the named apicomplexan species in the four families covered in this book: phototypes/photosyntypes of oocysts or sporocysts have been archived for: *Cryptosporidium fayeri, C. hominis, C. macropodum, C. xiaoi, Eimeria auritanensis, E. caluromydis, E. cochabambensis, E. kanyana, E. marmosopos, E. micouri, E. philanderi, E. quenda, E. trichosuri, Isospora arctopitheci,* and *Sarcocystis lindsayi*; tissue sections of kidney, intestine, or muscle tissues on slides have been archived for *E. arundeli, Klossiella tejerai, K. quimrensis, S. greineri, S. inghami, S. lindsayi, S. marmosae, S. neurona,* and *S. speeri*; preserved sporocysts in formalin have been archived only for *K. tejerai*; accession numbers for gene loci have been archived in GenBank for *C. fayeri, E. macropodis,* and *E. trichosuri*; and the **symbiotype** host has been archived for *E. caluromydis, E. cochabambensis, E. marmosopos,* and *E. micouri*. These numbers show that we are light years behind our vertebrate and botanical colleagues in appreciating, knowing, and having access and reference to their specimens of interest.

THE VALUE OF ARCHIVING TYPES

Regarding the value of archiving specimens in established, accredited museums, this concept seems to fall on deaf ears among most parasitologists. It is exceptionally important for us to adopt the habit of archiving at least the symbiotype host from which new species are discovered and described, **and** to archive oocysts in 70–100% ethanol; in both instances access to such specimens will help future workers to collect and analyze DNA to better comprehend species identities and relationships to similar forms, to find and identify cryptic species, and to more accurately define biodiversity on Earth. Natural history and research museums should be considered our most important libraries of life; they do not hold books, but they do maintain, in perpetuity, plant and animal specimens that have been carefully collected and curated over centuries by explorers, naturalists, and scientists. These specimens, including our parasites and their type hosts, serve as the foundation of our system of taxonomy, and they are integral to our understanding of the origins, interrelationships, and even the threats to biodiversity (Lujan and Page, 2015). These collections of former life forms are critical to modern biologists because, like the literature of books and maps, each and every specimen allows reinterpretation by every person who examines it. A parasitologist looking to confirm whether or not the type host, or the parasite were properly identified, or one who is looking for genetic differences between host and/or a coccidian species, will find the same specimens of each one valuable, but for different reasons. And, advancements in molecular biology (e.g., high-throughput DNA sequencing) can allow parasitologists to make new discoveries and draw conclusions from decades- (or even centuries-)old specimens. If only we had centuries-old specimens of symbiotype hosts and the oocysts they produced; we, as parasitologists, can no longer afford to deny the value of such archived specimens. By doing so, we only accept embracing ignorance of many of the prerequisites needed to understand the evolution, ecology, and extent of biodiversity of our organisms.

So where should our parasite specimens be archived in perpetuity? The United States National Parasite Collection (USNPC) has been the cornerstone of North American and global parasitology for over 120 years. Initially it was maintained in Washington, D.C., but for the last 70+ years the collection has been curated in the Beltsville Area Research Center in Maryland. The current holdings include over 100,000 cataloged specimen lots (potentially thousands of individuals per lot) of animal parasites; included are about 3000 holotypes and 7000 type series. Historically, this has been the most active parasite collection in the world with a growth rate of about 1000–1500 specimen lots added annually. In 2013, an agreement was reached between the USNPC and the Smithsonian Institution to transfer the entire collection to the National Museum of Natural History (NMNH) in Washington, D.C. The current collections staff, including senior curator Dr. Eric P. Hoberg and support scientists and managers, will accompany the transfer that was scheduled to occur on or about June 2, 2014; the conditions of this agreement should provide continuity and assistance for curation, and accessibility during and after the relocation. New curatorial controls will be established under NMNH guidance by Dr. Anna J. Phillips. Smithsonian protocols will be adopted and stakeholders and users of the collection are asked to refer directly to the NMNH. Information about procedures for donation of specimens, policies for loans, and so on, can be found on the Web site for the NMNH Department of Invertebrate Zoology (http://invertebrates.si.edu/collections.htm). During the transition, the final version of the USNPC database (as of May 30, 2014) is available as a single downloadable Excel file from the above Web site. Migration of this database into the Electronic Museum management system (EMu) platform of the NMNH is anticipated to take about two years. New specimens or other parasitological materials should be sent with advance notice to: William Moser, Department of Invertebrate Zoology, Smithsonian Museum Support Center, 4210 Silver Hill Road, Suitland, MD 20746, USA (Hoberg and Phillips, 2014a) (you also can call or email for more information (301-238-1761; moserw@si.edu). In addition to your donation of new specimens, you will need to submit a Deed of Gift Form; this can be downloaded from http://invertebrates.si.edu/donation.htm).

Enormous amounts of research remain to be started and completed. This must include, but not be limited to: systematic surveys (all species, wide geographic ranges); detailed descriptive taxonomy (quantitative, qualitative, type specimens, etc.), life cycle studies (all endogenous stages, cross-transmission), veterinary investigations (pathology, immunology), ecological and epidemiological studies (especially in habitats where multiple species ranges overlap), and molecular sequencing and analyses (multiple genes including nuclear, mitochondrial, etc.) need to be done sooner rather than later, before habitat loss and pollution eliminate at-risk vertebrate species and their parasites from the Earth forever. It would be gratifying to learn that this synopsis of what is *not* known will stimulate both American and Australian parasitologists and mammalogists along with those from every other country and continent to work together.

MOLECULAR TOOLS

The Apicomplexan order Eucoccidiorida is taxonomically the most diverse and the phylogenetic relationships between its many families, genera, and species are unclear, at best. Species identifications have primarily been based on analyzing qualitative features and quantifying oocyst characteristics, and to a lesser extent, on host specificity, pathology, and geographic distribution data (Duszynski and Wilber, 1997). However, some *Eimeria*, and most *Sarcocystis* and *Cryptosporidium* oocysts, are morphologically similar and occur in several hosts. These factors compromise species identification (Zhao and Duszynski, 2001a; Power et al., 2009). As alluded to in several chapters, and as can be seen in Chapter 10, many taxonomic studies on coccidian exogenous stages have inadequate descriptions based on the morphology of oocysts recovered from feces. What is truly lacking in our discipline is information on the biology, life cycles (experimental infections), host specificity (cross-transmission), and analysis of multiple gene sequences to help understand phylogenetic relationships. However, undertaking efforts to monitor the developmental history in controlled experimental infections, and determining host specificity at the level of species and genera via cross-transmission studies, can be time consuming, labor intensive, and expensive. On the other hand, the development and continued refinement of molecular techniques now offer reasonably quick, highly sensitive, accurate, and inexpensive alternatives to conventional diagnosis of the Apicomplexa. These tools provide information on genetic variability of various isolates of presumed "species" and can demonstrate that a single species is not genetically uniform, but consists of several distinct genotypes or cryptic species. Genetic studies can now use parasite-specific PCR primers to overcome the problem of oocysts recovered from fecal specimens that have many contaminants. In the past, various tissue extraction kits (e.g., QIAGEN) required up to 500 or more oocysts of a single species before one could confidently isolate DNA from that species. However, simplified DNA extraction techniques are developing rapidly; Zhao et al. (2001a), using chemical lysis and bead beating, could isolate and amplify coccidia DNA from about 50 oocysts and, recently, Gerhold et al. (2015) developed a novel, and simple technique to extract and amplify DNA from 20 or fewer oocysts using a freeze–thaw and heat denaturation technique.

PCR applications include isolating DNA fragments by selective amplification of a specific region of the target DNA to produce copies of a piece of DNA and generate multiple copies of a particular sequence. Analysis of each sequence examines all bases at a particular locus and this has become the "gold standard" of genotyping studies (Fayer et al., 2000). To gain more phylogenetically significant comparisons between various genotype sequences from oocysts or tissue stages, one should attempt to include sequences of several genes, if possible, because molecular analysis of a single gene may not be adequate to uncover the full genetic diversity within one coccidian species. Examples of sequences currently being determined in a variety of species include small subunit ribosomal (SSU rRNA), 70 kDa heat shock protein (hsp70), actin, *Cryptosporidium* oocyst wall protein, and 60 kDa glycoprotein (gp60) loci, and others (Hill et al., 2012; Power et al., 2009). The outstanding benefit of PCR amplification is its use to analyze extremely small amounts of a sample. Once DNA pieces have been cloned and sequenced, DNA phylogenies can be constructed if similar gene regions are known from other related species, genera, or even families.

Other molecular tools include sodium dodecyl sulfate-polyacrylamide gel electrophoresis, immunofluorescent assay, slide agglutination test, SnSAG-specific ELISA RAPD, PCR-based restriction fragment length polymorphism, amplified fragment length polymorphism finger printing, and sequence analysis of surface protein genes, ribosomal genes, microsatellite alleles, and other molecular markers (Elsheikha and Mansfield, 2007). For those (mostly) North Americans working to distinguish between *Sarcocystis* species (Chapter 7), and their (mostly) Australians colleagues working to distinguish between *Cryptosporidium* species (Chapter 9), these techniques have proved to be invaluable in their work on these two difficult genera. Thus, molecular approaches are increasingly used to characterize the identity of various coccidians and to compliment earlier morphological descriptions (Power et al., 2009). Genetic information derived from these techniques not only contributes to a more stable taxonomy of coccidia genera and their species, but it also places each parasite in an evolutionary context, which may help enhance the resolution of the host clade in which it and its are found (Hill et al., 2012; Power et al., 2009).

REVISIONARY TRENDS

Since 1998, my colleagues and I have been doing revisionary monographic work on the coccidia of a widely divergent group of vertebrate hosts that have included marmotine squirrels (Wilber et al., 1998), primates and tree shrews (Duszynski et al., 1999), insectivores (Duszynski and Upton, 2000), *Eimeria* and *Cryptosporidium* in wild mammals (Duszynski and Upton, 2001), bats (Duszynski, 2002), amphibians (Duszynski et al., 2007), snakes (Duszynski and Upton, 2010), rabbits (Duszynski and Couch, 2013), turtles (Duszynski and Morrow, 2014); and this treatise on coccidians known from marsupials. The unifying theme in this body of work is that we have attempted to consolidate the world's literature, for each vertebrate lineage, regarding their coccidians that shed a resistant propagule (oocyst) into the environment, and then to look at all of the species identifications to try to evaluate their validity. Our earlier studies concentrated almost exclusively on intestinal coccidians (*Eimeria*, *Isospora*, *Caryospora*, *Cryptosporidium*), while some of the later treatises expanded their scope to include species with more complex life cycles (*Besnoitia*, *Klossiella*, *Sarcocystis*). Two constants in these works are: (1) Only a very small percentage of the total numbers of species in each vertebrate lineage have ever been examined for coccidian parasites; and (2) The families and genera of the apicomplexan species found to date differ from lineage to lineage.

Biodiversity Vacuum

In the **poikiotherms**, only 65/>5500 (<1%) known amphibian species (Jirků et al., 2009), 208/3108 (6.5%) known snake species (Duszynski and Upton, 2009), and 64/328 (19.5%) turtle species have been examined for intestinal coccidians. In mammalian species, we have learned that 86/925 (9%) bat species, 35/428 (9%) insectivore species, 4/19 (21) tree shrew (Scandentia) species, 18/233 (8%) primate species, 23/91 (25%) rabbit species, and 85/331 (26%) marsupial species have been examined for intestinal coccidians. Thus, in these nine distinct vertebrate lineages studied to date, only 588 of 10,963 (5%) extant species have been examined for coccidia.

Discoveries to Date

From these nine vertebrate lineages the following species and forms of coccidia have been discovered.

Amphibia. 38 *Eimeria*, 11 *Isospora*, two *Goussia*, and one *Hyaloklossia* species, and 10 *species inquirendae* (*Coccidium-*, *Eimeria-*, *Goussia-*, and *Isospora*-type forms) have been named.

Snakes. 52 *Caryospora*, two *Cryptosporidium*, four *Cyclospora*, 66 *Eimeria*, seven *Isospora*, 22 *Sarcocystis*, two *Tyzzeria*, and one *Wenyonella* species, and 106 *species inquirendae* (*Caryospora-*, *Cryptosporidium-*, *Dorisiella-*, *Eimeria-*, *Globidium-*, *Isospora-*, *Sarcocystis-*, *Toxoplasma-*, and *Tyzzeria*-type forms) have been named.

Turtles. 66 *Eimeria*, three *Isospora*, one *Caryospora*, and one *Sarcocystis* species, and 28 *species inquirendae* (*Caryospora-*, *Coccidium-*, *Cryptosporidium-*, *Eimeria-*, *Mantonella-* and *Sarcocystis*-type forms) have been named.

Bats. 31 *Eimeria* species and eight *species inquirendae* (*Coccidium-*, *Eimeria-*, and *Isospora*-type forms) have been named.

Insectivores. 48 *Eimeria*, 22 *Isospora*, five *Cyclospora* species, and 45 *species inquirendae* (*Coccidium-*, *Cyclospora-*, *Eimeria-*, *Isospora*-type forms) have been named.

Tree shrews. Four *Eimeria* species have been named.

Primates. One *Cyclospora*, seven *Eimeria*, seven *Isospora* species, and four *species inquirendae* (*Eimeria*-, *Isospora*-type forms) have been named.

Rabbits. Three *Besnoitia*, three *Cryptosporidium*, 73 *Eimeria*, two *Isospora*, five *Sarcocystis*, and one *Toxoplasma* species, and 33 *species inquirendae* (*Besnoitia*-, *Cryptosporidium*-, *Eimeria*-, *Sarcocystis*-type forms) have been named.

Marsupials. One *Besnoitia*, six *Cryptosporidium*, 56 *Eimeria*, one *Isospora*, 11 *Klossiella*, 10 *Sarcocystis*, one *Toxoplasma* species, and 68 *species inquirendae* (*Besnoitia*-, *Coccidium*-, *Cryptosporidium*-, *Eimeria*-, *Isospora*-, *Klossiella*-, *Sarcocystis*-, *Toxoplasma*- and *Tyzzeria*-type forms) have been named.

In all, 576 coccidian species in 13 genera (*Besnoitia*—4; *Caryospora*—53; *Cryptosporidium*—11; *Cyclospora*—10; *Eimeria*—389; *Goussia*—2; *Hyaloklossia*—1; *Isospora*—53; *Klossiella*—11; *Sarcocystis*—38; *Toxoplasma*—1; *Tyzzeria*—2; *Wenyonella*—1) have been reasonably well-enough described to be considered valid species, and another 302 coccidian forms in 15 genera (*Besnoitia*-, *Caryospora*-, *Coccidium*-, *Cryptosporidium*-, *Cyclospora*-, *Dorisiella*-, *Eimeria*-, *Globidium*-, *Goussia*-, *Isospora*-, *Klossiella*-, *Mantonella*-, *Sarcocystis*-, *Toxoplasma*-, and *Tyzzeria* types) have been identified at some level. All of this biodiversity of apicomplexan species and forms is found in only the 5% of the vertebrate species that have been examined for them in these nine evolutionary lineages. If we extrapolate that 576 real species are found in 5% of the individuals in these groups, then we might expect almost another 11,000 apicomplexans to be discovered in the other 95% of these species that have yet to be examined...from only these nine vertebrate groups. Using current estimates, there are about 84,000 extant vertebrate species (Chapman, 2009) remaining on Earth, so our modest efforts to date have examined the coccidian literature on only about 13% of all vertebrates. Just try to imagine the numbers and variety of species and forms still to be discovered!

FUTURE OF TAXONOMY OF APICOMPLEXANS

Given the daunting tasks noted above, what are the prospects that any significant portion of this work will ever be completed? From my viewpoint, the future looks bleak because there are two modern-day trends working against us. The first is the rate of loss of the biodiversity of extant vertebrates that seems to be accelerating around the world, and the second is the rate of loss of taxonomists/systematists, who are not being trained any longer in universities.

The loss of species, the communities they form, and their genetic heritage is accelerating in many parts of the world due mainly to the increase in human populations and all that such increases portend: loss of habitat, and the pollution of air, land, and groundwaters via industrial waste, pesticides, and fertilizers. Such population increases diminish our ability to be good stewards of Earth, restricts our ability to manage our environment, and imperils our ability to conserve our natural and biological resources. Accompanying the lack of focus on the importance of taxonomic training in universities is the loss of rudimentary knowledge along with the necessary expertise for identifying and inventorying the biota of Earth, including their parasites. Shifts in attitudes about organismal and evolutionary biology change the way we recruit new teachers/scholars, and reductions in the training of graduate students in these areas means that retiring taxonomists are not and cannot be replaced. Taxonomic expertise is needed to identify and classify the world's biological resources and to organize this knowledge in accessible databases in order to ensure stewardship and rational use. Unless such trends can be slowed or stopped, the rate of extinction of professional taxonomists and museum curators may exceed that of the taxons and the myriad of organisms they harbor.

TABLE 11.1   ALPHABETICAL LIST OF ALL APICOMPLEXAN PARASITES COVERED IN THIS BOOK AND THE MARSUPIAL HOSTS FROM WHICH THEY HAVE BEEN REPORTED

Besnoitia darlingi

　Caluromys derbianus, Brown-eared Woolly Opossum (experimental)

　Didelphis aurita, Big-eared Opossum

　Didelphis marsupialis, Common Opossum

　Didelphis virginiana, Virginia Opossum

　Philander opossum, Gray Four-eyed Opossum (experimental)

Besnoitia sp. of Conti-Diaz et al., 1970 (*species inquirenda*)

　Didelphis virginiana, Virginia Opossum

Besnoitia sp. of Stabler and Welch, 1961 (*species inquirenda*)

　Didelphis marsupialis, Common Opossum

Coccidium sp. of Johnston, 1910a (*species inquirenda*)

　Macropus eugenii, Tammar Wallaby

Coccidium sp. of Johnston, 1910b (*species inquirenda*)

　Macropus giganteus Eastern Grey Kangaroo

Cryptosporidium fayeri

　Macropus fuliginosus, Western Grey Kangaroo

　Macropus giganteus, Eastern Grey Kangaroo

　Macropus rufus, Red Kangaroo

　Perameles bougainville, Western Barred Bandicoot

　Petrogale xanthopus, Yellow-footed Rock Wallaby

　Phascolarctos cinereus, Koala

　Wallabia bicolor, Swamp Wallaby

Cryptosporidium hominis

　Macropus giganteus, Eastern Grey Kangaroo

Cryptosporidium macropodum

　Macropus fuliginosus, Western Grey Kangaroo

　Macropus giganteus, Eastern Grey Kangaroo

　Macropus rufus, Red Kangaroo

　Perameles bougainville, Western Barred Bandicoot

　Petrogale xanthopus, Yellow-footed Rock Wallaby

　Phascolarctos cinereus, Koala

　Wallabia bicolor, Swamp Wallaby

TABLE 11.1—cont'd

Cryptosporidium muris

Macrotis lagotis, Greater Bilby

Cryptosporidium parvum

Didelphis virginiana, Virginia Opossum (experimental)

Isoodon obesulus, Southern Brown Bandicoot

Macropus giganteus, Eastern Grey Kangaroo

Trichosurus vulpecula, Common Brushtail

Wallabia sp.

***Cryptosporidium parvum/hominis*-like of Ryan and Power, 2012 (*species inquirenda*)**

Isoodon obesulus, Southern Brown Bandicoot

Macropus giganteus, Eastern Grey Kangaroo

Perameles nasuta, Long-nosed Bandicoot

Trichosurus vulpecula, Common Brushtail

Cryptosporidium xiaoi

Macropus fuliginosus, Western Grey Kangaroo

***Cryptosporidium* sp., Burshtail possum genotype I of Ryan and Power, 2012 (*species inquirenda*)**

Trichosurus vulpecula, Common Brushtail

***Cryptosporidium* sp., kangaroo genotype I of Yang et al., 2011 (*species inquirenda*)**

Macropus fuliginosus, Western Grey Kangaroo

***Cryptosporidium* sp. of Barker et al., 1978 (*species inquirenda*)**

Antechinus stuartii, Brown Antechinus

***Cryptosporidium* sp. of Obendorf, unpub. observ. (in Ryan et al., 2008) (*species inquirenda*)**

Thylogale billardierii, Tasmanian Pademelon

***Cryptosporidium* sp. of O'Donoghue, 1985 (*species inquirenda*)**

Antechinus sp.

***Cryptosporidium* sp. of O'Donoghue, unpub. observ. (in Ryan et al., 2008) (*species inquirenda*)**

Macropus rufus, Red Kangaroo

***Cryptosporidium* sp. of Phillips et al., unpub. observ. (in Ryan et al., 2008) (*species inquirenda*)**

Phascolarctos cinereus, Koala

***Cryptosporidium* sp. of Power et al. 2003 (*species inquirenda*)**

Macropus eugenii, Tammar Wallaby

Continued

TABLE 11.1—cont'd

Cryptosporidium **sp. of Zanette et al., 2008 (*species inquirenda*)**

Didelphis albiventris, White-eared Opossum

Eimeria aepyprymni

Aepyprymnus rufescens, Rufous Rat Kangaroo

Eimeria arundeli

Vombatus ursinus, Common Wombat

Eimeria auritanensis

Didelphis aurita, Big-eared Opossum

Eimeria bicolor

Wallabia bicolor, Swamp Wallaby

Eimeria boonderooensis

Petrogale assimilis, Allied Rock Wallaby

Petrogale inorata, Unadorned Rock Wallaby

Eimeria caluromydis

Caluromys philander philander, Bare-tailed Wooly Opossum

Eimeria cochabambensis

Marmosops dorothea Thomas, 1911, Mouse Opossum

Monodelphis domestica, Short-tailed Opossum

Thylamys venustus, Mouse Opossum

Eimeria dendrolagi

Dendrolagus lumholtzi, Lumholtz's Tree Kangaroo

Eimeria desmaresti

Macropus rufogriseus, Red-necked Wallaby

Eimeria didelphidis

Didelphis aurita, Big-eared Opossum

Eimeria flindersi

Macropus antilopinus, Antilopine Kangaroo

Macropus eugenii, Tammar Wallaby

Macropus rufogriseus, Red-necked Wallaby

Eimeria gaimardi

Bettongia gaimardi, Eastern Bettong

TABLE 11.1—cont'd

Eimeria gambai

  Didelphis aurita, Big-eared Opossum

Eimeria godmani

  Petrogale assimilis, Allied Rock Wallaby

  Petrogale godmani, Godman's Rock Wallaby

  Petrogale inorata, Unadorned Rock Wallaby

  Petrogale lateralis pearsoni, Black-flanked Rock Wallaby

Eimeria gungahlinensis

  Macropus fuliginosus, Western Grey Kangaroo

  Macropus giganteus, Eastern Grey Kangaroo

Eimeria haberfeldi

  Caluromys philander, Bare-tailed Wooly Opossum

Eimeria hestermani

  Macropus dorsalis, Black-striped Wallaby

  Macropus eugenii, Tammar Wallaby

  Macropus fuliginosus, Western Grey Kangaroo

  Macropus giganteus, Eastern Grey Kangaroo

  Macropus rufogriseus, Red-necked Wallaby

Eimeria hypsiprymnodontis

  Hypsiprymnodon moschatus, Musky Rat Kangaroo

Eimeria indianensis

  Didelphis virginiana, Virginia Opossum

Eimeria inornata

  Petrogale inorata, Unadorned Rock Wallaby

  Petrogale lateralis pearsoni, Black-flanked Rock Wallaby

  Petrogale penicillata, Brush-tailed Rock Wallaby

Eimeria kairiensis

  Hypsiprymnodon moschatus, Musky Rat Kangaroo

Eimeria kanyana

  Permeles bougainville, Western Barred Bandicoot

Continued

TABLE 11.1—cont'd

***Eimeria kogoni* of Mykytowycz, 1964 (*species inquirenda*)**

Macropus giganteus, Eastern Grey Kangaroo

Eimeria lagorchestis

Lagorchestes conspicillatus, Spectacled Hare Wallaby

Eimeria lumholtzi

Dendrolagus lumholtzi, Lumholtz's Tree Kangaroo

Eimeria macropodis

Macropus dorsalis, Black-striped Wallaby

Macropus eugenii, Tammar Wallaby

Macropus fuliginosus, Western Grey Kangaroo

Macropus giganteus, Eastern Grey Kangaroo

Macropus irma, Western Brush Wallaby

Macropus parma Waterhouse, Parma Wallaby

Macropus parryi, Pretty-faced Wallaby

Macropus rufogriseus, Red-necked Wallaby

Macropus rufus, Red Kangaroo

Eimeria marmosopos

Didelphis marsupialis, Common Opossum

Marmosops dorothea, Mouse Opossum

Eimeria marsupialium

Macropus fuliginosus, Western Grey Kangaroo

Macropus giganteus, Eastern Grey Kangaroo

Eimeria micouri

Micoureus constantiae constantiae, Mouse Opossum

Eimeria mundayi

Potorous tridactylus, Long-nosed Potoroo

Eimeria mykytowyczi

Macropus agilis, Agile Wallaby

Macropus antilopinus, Antilopine Kangaroo

Macropus parryi, Pretty-faced Wallaby

Eimeria obendorfi

Thylogale billardierii, Tasmanian Pademelon

TABLE 11.1—cont'd

Eimeria occidentalis

Petrogale brachyotis, Short-eared Rock Wallaby

Petrogale lateralis, Black-flanked Rock Wallaby

Petrogale rothschildi, Rothschild's Rock Wallaby

Eimeria parma

Macropus parma Waterhouse, Parma Wallaby

Eimeria parryi

Macropus parryi, Pretty-faced Wallaby

Eimeria petrogale

Petrogale assimilis, Allied Rock Wallaby

Petrogale godmani, Godman's Rock Wallaby

Petrogale inornata, Unadorned Rock Wallaby

Petrogale lateralis, Black-flanked Rock Wallaby

Petrogale penicillata, Brush-tailed Rock Wallaby

Petrogale persephone, Proserpine Rock Wallaby

Eimeria philanderi

Philander opossum opossum, Gray Four-eyed Opossum

Eimeria potoroi

Potorous tridactylus, Long-nosed Potoroo

Eimeria prionotemni

Macropus agilis, Agile Wallaby

Macropus dorsalis, Black-striped Wallaby

Macropus eugenii, Tammar Wallaby

Macropus parryi, Pretty-faced Wallaby

Macropus rufogriseus, Red-necked Wallaby

Eimeria quokka

Setonix brachyurus, Quokka

Eimeria quenda

Isoodon obesulus urita, Southern Brown Bandicoot

Eimeria ringaroomaensis

Thylogale billardierii, Tasmanian Pademelon

Continued

TABLE 11.1—cont'd

Eimeria rufusi of **Prasad, 1960** (*species inquirenda*)

   Macropus rufus, Red Kangaroo

Eimeria setonicis

   Setonix brachyurus, Quokka

Eimeria sharmani

   Petrogale assimilis, Allied Rock Wallaby

   Petrogale godmani, Godman's Rock Wallaby

   Petrogale inornata, Unadorned Rock Wallaby

   Petrogale lateralis, Black-flanked Rock Wallaby

   Petrogale penicillata, Brush-tailed Rock Wallaby

   Petrogale persephone, Proserpine Rock Wallaby

   Petrogale rothschildi, Rothschild's Rock Wallaby

Eimeria spearei

   Hypsiprymnodon moschatus, Musky Rat Kangaroo

Eimeria **sp. of Barker et al., 1963** (*species inquirenda*)

   Macropus giganteus, Eastern Grey Kangaroo

Eimeria **sp. of Barker et al., 1988b** (*species inquirenda*)

   Lagorchestes conspicillatus, Spectacled Hare Wallaby

Eimeria **sp. of Barker et al., 1988c** (*species inquirenda*)

   Petrogale penicillata, Brush-tailed Rock Wallaby

Eimeria **sp. of Mackerras, 1958** (*species inquirenda*)

   Isoodon macrourus, Northern Brown Bandicoot

Eimeria **sp. of Obendorf and Munday, 1990** (*species inquirenda*)

   Perameles gunnii, Western Barred Bandicoot

Eimeria **sp. of O'Callaghan and Moore, 1986** (*species inquirenda*)

   Trichosurus vulpecula, Common Brushtail

Eimeria **sp. of O'Donoghue, 1997** (*species inquirenda*)

   Pseudocheirus peregrinus, Common Ringtail

Eimeria **sp. of O'Donoghue, 1997** (*species inquirenda*)

   Macropus rufus, Red Kangaroo

Eimeria **sp. of O'Donoghue and Adlard, 2000** (*species inquirenda*)

   Macropus agilis, Agile Wallaby

TABLE 11.1—cont'd

***Eimeria* sp. of O'Donoghue and Adlard, 2000 (*species inquirenda*)**

Macropus parryi, Pretty-faced Wallaby

***Eimeria* sp. of Speare et al., 1984 (*species inquirenda*)**

Hemibelideus lemuroides, Lemuroid Ringtail Possum

***Eimeria* sp. of Speare et al., 1984 (*species inquirenda*)**

Pseudochirops (syn. *Pseudocheirus*) *archeri*, Green Ringtail Possum

***Eimeria* sp. of Speare et al., 1989 (*species inquirenda*)**

Macropus dorsalis, Black-striped Wallaby

***Eimeria* sp. of Winter, 1959 (*species inquirenda*)**

Macropus giganteus, Eastern Grey Kangaroo

***Eimeria* spp. 1 & 2 of Bennett and Hobbs, 2011 (*species inquirenda*)**

Isoodon obesulus, Southern Brown Bandicoot

***Eimeria* spp. of Speare et al., 1984 (*species inquirenda*)**

Pseudochirulus herbertensis, Herbert River Ringtail

"*Eimeriina*" sp. of Yamada et al., 1981 (*species inquirenda*)

Macropus fuliginosis, Western Grey Kangaroo

Eimeria spratti

Hypsiprymnodon moschatus, Musky Rat Kangaroo

Eimeria thylogale

Thylogale billardierii, Tasmanian Pademelon

Eimeria tinarooensis

Hypsiprymnodon moschatus, Musky Rat Kangaroo

Eimeria toganmainensis

Macropus eugenii, Tammar Wallaby

Macropus fuliginosus, Western Grey Kangaroo

Macropus giganteus, Eastern Grey Kangaroo

Macropus rufogriseus, Red-necked Wallaby

Macropus rufus, Red Kangaroo

Eimeria trichosuri

Trichosurus caninus, Short-eared Possum

Trichosurus cunninghami, Mountain Brushtail Possum

Trichosurus vulpecula, Common Brushtail Possum

Continued

TABLE 11.1—cont'd

Eimeria ursini

  Lasiorhinus latifrons, Southern Hairy-nosed Wombat

Eimeria volckertzooni

  Setonix brachyurus, Quokka

Eimeria wallabiae

  Wallabia bicolor, Swamp Wallaby

Eimeria wilcanniensis

  Macropus fuliginosus, Western Grey Kangaroo

  Macropus giganteus, Eastern Grey Kangaroo

  Macropus robustus, Wallaroo

  Macropus rufogriseus, Red-necked Wallaby

  Macropus rufus, Red Kangaroo

Eimeria wombati

  Lasiorhinus latifrons, Southern Hairy-nosed Wombat

Eimeria xanthopus

  Petrogale xanthopus, Yellow-footed Rock Wallaby

Eimeria yathongensis

  Macropus fuliginosus, Western Grey Kangaroo

  Macropus giganteus, Eastern Grey Kangaroo

Isospora arctopitheci

  Didelphis marsupialis, Common Opossum

Isospora sp. of Ernst et al., 1969 (*species inquirenda*)

  Didelphis virginiana, Virginia Opossum

Isospora sp. of Joseph, 1974 (*species inquirenda*)

  Didelphis virginiana, Virginia Opossum

Isospora sp. of Lainson and Shaw, 1989 (*species inquirenda*)

  Philander opossum opossum, Gray Four-eyed Opossum

***Klossiella bettongiae* (*species inquirenda*)**

  Bettongia gaimardi, Tasmanian or Eastern Bettong

Klossiella beveridgei

  Lagorchestes conspicillatus, Spectacled Hare Wallaby

TABLE 11.1—cont'd

Klossiella callitris

Macropus fuliginosus melanops, Western Grey Kangaroo

Klossiella convolutor

Pseudocheirus peregrinus, Common Ringtail

Klossiella quimrensis

Isoodon obesulus, Southern Brown Bandicoot

Perameles bougainville, Western Barred Bandicoot

Perameles gunnii, Eastern Barred Bandicoot

Klossiella rufi

Macropus rufus, Red Kangaroo

Klossiella rufogrisei

Macropus rufogriseus, Red-necked or Bennett's Wallaby

Klossiella schoinobatis

Petauroides volans, Greater Glider

Klossiella serendipensis

Wallabia bicolor, Swamp Wallaby

***Klossiella* sp. of Barker et al., 1975 (*species inquirenda*)**

Potorous tridactylus, Long-nosed or Southern Potoroo

***Klossiella* sp. of Mackerras, 1958 (*species inquirenda*)**

Perameles nasuta, Long-nosed Bandicoot

***Klossiella* sp. of Munday et al., 1988 (*species inquirenda*)**

Macropus rufus, Red Kangaroo

***Klossiella* sp. of Speare et al., 1984 (*species inquirenda*)**

Pseudochirops (syn. *Pseudocheirus*) *archeri*, Green Ringtail Possum

***Klossiella* spp. of Speare et al., 1984 (*species inquirenda*)**

Pseudochirulus herbertensis, Herbert River Ringtail Possum

Klossiella tejerai

Didelphis aurita, Big-eared Opossum

Didelphis marsupialis, Common Opossum

Marmosa murina, Linnaeus's Mouse Opossum

Continued

TABLE 11.1—cont'd

Klossiella thylogale

   Thylogale billardierii, Red-bellied or Tasmanian Pademelon

Sarcocystis bettongiae **Bourne, 1934 (***species inquirenda***)**

   Bettongia lesueur grayii, Boodie or Short-nosed "Rat" Kangaroo (intermediate host)

Sarcocystis didelphidis

   Didelphis marsupialis, Common Opossum (intermediate host)

Sarcocystis falcatula

   Didelphis albiventris, White-eared Opossum (definitive host)

   Didelphis aurita, Big-eared Opossum (definitive host)

   Didelphis marsupialis, Common Opossum (definitive host)

   Didelphis virginiana, Virginia Opossum (definitive host)

Sarcocystis garnhami

   Didelphis marsupialis, Common Opossum (intermediate host)

   Philander mcihennyi, McIlhenny's Four-eyed Opossum (intermediate host)

Sarcocystis greineri

   Didelphis virginiana, Virginia Opossum (intermediate host)

Sarcocystis inghami

   Didelphis virginiana, Virginia Opossum (intermediate host)

Sarcocystis lindsayi

   Didelphis albiventris, White-eared Opossum (definitive host)

   Didelphis aurita, Big-eared Opossum (definitive host)

Sarcocystis marmosae

   Marmosa murina, Linnaeus's Mouse Opossum (intermediate host)

Sarcocystis mucosa

   Macropus rufogriseus, Red-necked or Bennett's Wallaby (intermediate host)

   Petrogale assimilis, Allied Rock Wallaby (intermediate host)

   Petrogale inorata, Unadorned Rock Wallaby (intermediate host)

   Petrogale penicillata, Brush-tailed Rock Wallaby (intermediate host)

   Thylogale billardierii, Tasmanian Pademelon (intermediate host)

Sarcocystis neurona

   Didelphis albiventris, White-eared Opossum (definitive host)

   Didelphis marsupialis, Common Opossum (definitive host)

   Didelphis virginiana, Virginia Opossum (definitive host)

TABLE 11.1—cont'd

Sarcocystis speeri

   Didelphis albiventris, White-eared Opossum (definitive host)

   Didelphis marsupialis, Common Opossum (definitive host)

   Didelphis virginiana, Virginia Opossum (definitive host)

"Sarcocystidae" sp. of Merino et al., 2008 (*species inquirenda*)

   Thylamys elegans, Elegant Fat-tailed Mouse Opossum (intermediate host?)

"Sarcocystidae" sp. of Merino et al., 2009 (*species inquirenda*)

   Dromiciops gliroides, Monito del Monte (intermediate host?)

"Sarcocystidae" sp. of Zhu et al., 2009 (*species inquirenda*)

   Petaurus australis, Yellow-bellied Glider (intermediate host?)

Sarcocystis **sp. of Carini, 1939 (*species inquirenda*)**

   Lutreolina crassicaudata, Lutrine Opossum (intermediate host?)

Sarcocystis **sp. of Dubey et al., 2001b (*species inquirenda*)**

   Didelphis virginiana, Virginia Opossum (?) (definitive host)

Sarcocystis **sp. of Duszynski and Box, 1978 (*species inquirenda*)**

   Didelphis virginiana, Virginia Opossum (definitive host)

Sarcocystis **sp. of Mackerras, 1958 (*species inquirenda*)**

   Dasyurus (syn. *Satanellus*) *hallucatus,* Northern Quoll (intermediate host)

Sarcocystis **sp. of Mackerras et al., 1953 (*species inquirenda*)**

   Isoodon obesulus, Southern Brown Bandicoot (intermediate host)

Sarcocystis **sp. of Munday, 1978 (*species inquirenda*)**

   Petrogale penicillata, Brush-tailed Rock wallaby (intermediate host)

Sarcocystis **sp. of Speare et al., 1989 (*species inquirenda*)**

   Dendrolagus lumholtzi, Lumholtz's Tree kangaroo (intermediate host)

Sarcocystis **sp. 1 of Munday et al., 1978 (*species inquirenda*)**

   Antechinus stuartii Macleay, Brown Antechinus (intermediate host)

   Antechinus swainsonii, Dusky Antechinus (intermediate host)

Sarcocystis **sp. 2 of Munday et al., 1978 (*species inquirenda*)**

   Dasyurus maculatus, Tiger Quoll or Tiger Cat (intermediate host)

Sarcocystis **sp. 3 of Munday et al., 1978 (*species inquirenda*)**

   Isoodon macrourus, Northern Brown Bandicoot (intermediate host)

Continued

TABLE 11.1—cont'd

Sarcocystis **spp. 4 A & B of Munday et al., 1978 (***species inquirenda***)**

  Macropus rufus, Red Kangaroo (intermediate host)

Sarcocystis **sp. (spp.?) 5 of Munday et al., 1978 (***species inquirenda***)**

  Macropus agilis, Agile Wallaby (intermediate host)

  Macropus giganteus, Eastern Grey Kangaroo (intermediate host)

  Macropus rufogriseus, Red-necked Wallaby (intermediate host)

  Thylogale billardierii, Tasmanian Pademelon (intermediate host)

  Wallabia bicolor, Swamp Wallaby (intermediate host)

Sarcocystis **sp. 6 of Munday et al., 1978 (***species inquirenda***)**

  Petrogale brachyotis (syn. *P. venustula*), Short-eared Rock wallaby (intermediate host)

  Petrogale (syn. *Peradorcas*) *concinna*, Nabarlek or Little-rock Wallaby (intermediate host)

Sarcocystis **sp. 7 of Munday et al., 1978 (***species inquirenda***)**

  Parmeles gunnii, Eastern Barred Bandicoot (intermediate host)

  Perameles nasuta, Long-nosed Bandicoot (intermediate host)

Sarcocystis **sp. 8 of Munday et al., 1978 (***species inquirenda***)**

  Pseudochirops (syn. *Pseudocheirus*) *archeri*, Green Ringtail (intermediate host)

Sarcocystis **sp. 9 of Munday et al., 1978 (***species inquirenda***)**

  Sarcophilus harrisii, Tasmanian Devil (intermediate host)

Sarcocystis **sp. 10 of Munday et al., 1978 (***species inquirenda***)**

  Sarcophilus harrisii, Tasmanian Devil (intermediate host)

Sarcocystis **sp (spp.?) 11 of Munday et al., 1978 (***species inquirenda***)**

  Trichosurus caninus, Short-eared Possum (intermediate host)

  Trichosurus vulpecula, Common Brushtail (intermediate host)

Sarcocystis **sp. of Seneviratna et al., 1975 (***species inquirenda***)**

  Didelphis virginiana, Virginia Opossum (intermediate host)

Sarcocystis **sp. of Scholtyseck et al., 1982 (***species inquirenda***)**

  Didelphis virginiana, Virginia Opossum (intermediate host)

Sarcocystis **sp. of Speare et al., 1989 (***species inquirenda***)**

  Dendrolagus lumholtzi Lumholtz's Tree Kangaroo (intermediate host)

Sarcocystis **sp. of Triffitt, 1927 (***species inquirenda***)**

  Macropus rufogriseus (syn. *Macropus bennetti*), Red-necked Wallaby (intermediate host)

Toxoplasma gondii

  Antechinomys laniger, Kultarr

TABLE 11.1—cont'd

Dasycercus cristicauda, Mulgara

Dasyuroides byrnei, Kowari

Dendrolagus lumholtzi, Lumholtz's Tree Kangaroo

Didelphis albiventris, White-eared Opossum

Didelphis aurita, Big-eared Opossum

Didelphis marsupialis, Common Opossum

Isoodon obesulus, Southern Brown Bandicoot

Lasiorhinus latifrons, Southern Hairy-nosed Wombat

Macropus agilis, Agile Wallaby

Macropus eugenii, Tammar Wallaby

Macropus fuliginosus, Western Grey Kangaroo

Macropus giganteus, Eastern Grey Kangaroo

Macropus parma, Waterhouse, Parma Wallaby

Macropus robustus, Wallaroo

Macropus rufogriseus, Red-necked Wallaby

Macropus rufus, Red Kangaroo

Macrotis lagotis, Greater Bilby

Marmosa murina, Linnaeus's Mouse Opossum

Metachirus nudicaudatus, Brown Four-eyed Opossum

Micoureus demerarae, Woolly Opossum

Monodelphis domestica, Gray Short-tailed Opossum

Myrmecobius fasciatus, Numbat

Parantechinus apicalis, Southern Dibbler

Perameles gunnii, Eastern Barred Bandicoot

Perameles nasuta, Long-nosed Bandicoot

Petrogale xanthopus, Yellow-footed Rock Wallaby

Phascolarctos cinereus, Koala

Potorous tridactylus, Long-nosed or Southern Potoroo

Pseudantechinus macdonnellensis, Fat-tailed False Antechinus

Setonix brachyurus, Quokka

Sminthopsis crassicaudata, Fat-tailed Dunnart

Sminthopsis leucopus, White-footed Dunnart

Continued

TABLE 11.1—cont'd

Sminthopsis macroura, Striped-faced Dunnart

Thylogale billardierii, Tasmanian Pademelon

Thylogale thetis, Red-necked Pademelon

Trichosurus vulpecula, Common Brushtail

Vombatus ursinus, Common Wombat

Wallabia bicolor, Swamp Wallaby

Toxoplasma sp. of Munday et al., 1978 (*species iquirenda*)

Perameles gunnii, Eastern Barred Bandicoot

Perameles nasuta, Long-nosed Bandicoot

Toxoplasma sp. of O'Donoghue and Adlard, 2000 (*species iquirenda*)

Antechinus minimus, Swamp Antechinus

Antechinus swainsonii, Dusky Antechinus

Dasyurus viverrinus, Eastern Quoll

Phascogale tapoatafa, Brush-tailed Phascogale

Tyzzeria sp. of Barker et al., 1988c (*species iquirenda*)

Thylogale thetis, Red-necked Pademelon

TABLE 11.2 ALPHABETICAL LIST OF ALL MARSUPIAL ORDERS, FAMILIES, GENERA, AND SPECIES COVERED IN THIS BOOK, AND THE APICOMPLEXA PARASITES WHICH HAVE BEEN REPORTED FROM THEM

ORDER DASYUROMORPHIA

Family Dasyuridae

Antechinomys laniger, **Kultarr**

　Toxoplasma gondii

Antechinus minimus, **Swamp Antechinus**

　Toxoplasma sp. of O'Donoghue and Adlard, 2000 (*species inquirenda*)

Antechinus stuartii, **Brown Antechinus**

　Cryptosporidium sp. of Barker et al., 1978 (*species inquirenda*)

　Sarcocystis sp. 1 of Munday et al., 1978 (*species inquirenda*) (intermediate host)

Antechinus swainsonii, **Dusky Antechinus**

　Sarcocystis sp. 1 of Munday et al., 1978 (*species inquirenda*) (intermediate host)

　Toxoplasma sp. of O'Donoghue and Adlard, 2000 (*species inquirenda*)

Antechinus **sp.**

　Cryptosporidium sp. of O'Donoghue, 1985 (*species inquirenda*)

Dasycercus cristicauda, **Mulgara**

　Toxoplasma gondii

Dasyuroides byrnei, **Kowari**

　Klossiella sp. of O'Donoghue and Adlard, 2000 (*species inquirenda*) (intermediate host)

　Toxoplasma gondii

Dasyurus (syn. *Satanellus*) *hallucatus*, **Northern Quoll**

　Sarcocystis sp. of Mackerras, 1958 (*species inquirenda*) (intermediate host)

Dasyurus maculatus, **Tiger Quoll or Tiger Cat**

　Sarcocystis sp. 2 of Munday et al., 1978 (*species inquirenda*) (intermediate host)

Dasyurus viverrinus, **Eastern Quoll**

　Toxoplasma sp. of O'Donoghue and Adlard, 2000 (*species inquirenda*)

Parantechinus apicalis, **Southern Dibbler**

　Toxoplasma gondii

Phascogale tapoatafa, **Brush-tailed Phascogale**

　Toxoplasma sp. of O'Donoghue and Adlard, 2000 (*species inquirenda*)

Pseudantechinus macdonnellensis, **Fat-tailed False Antechinus**

　Toxoplasma gondii

Continued

TABLE 11.2—cont'd

Sarcophilus harrisii, **Tasmanian Devil**

  Sarcocystis sp. 9 of Munday et al., 1978 (*species inquirenda*) (intermediate host)

  Sarcocystis sp. 10 of Munday et al., 1978 (*species inquirenda*) (intermediate host)

Sminthopsis crassicaudata, **Fat-tailed Dunnart**

  Toxoplasma gondii

Sminthopsis leucopus, **White-footed Dunnart**

  Toxoplasma gondii

Sminthopsis macroura, **Striped-faced Dunnart**

  Toxoplasma gondii

Family Myrmecobiidae

Myrmecobius fasciatus, **Numbat**

  Toxoplasma gondii

ORDER DIDELPHIMORPHIA

Family Didelphidae

Caluromys philander, **Bare-tailed Wooly Opossum**

  Eimeria caluromydis

  Eimeria haberfeldi

Didelphis albiventris, **White-eared Opossum**

  Cryptosporidium sp. of Zanette et al., 2008 (*species inquirenda*)

  Sarcocystis falcatula (definitive host)

  Sarcocystis lindsayi (definitive host)

  Sarcocystis neurona (definitive host)

  Sarcocystis speeri (definitive host)

  Toxoplasma gondii

Didelphis aurita, **Big-eared Opossum**

  Eimeria auritanensis

  Eimeria didelphidis

  Eimeria gambai

  Klossiella tejerai

  Sarcocystis falcatula (definitive host)

  Sarcocystis lindsayi (definitive host)

  Toxoplasma gondii

TABLE 11.2—cont'd

Didelphis marsupialis, Common Opossum

Besnoitia sp. of Stabler and Welch, 1961 (*species inquirenda*)

Eimeria marmosopos

Isospora arctopitheci

Klossiella tejerai

Sarcocystis didelphidis (intermediate host)

Sarcocystis falcatula (definitive host)

Sarcocystis garnhami (intermediate host)

Sarcocystis neurona (definitive host)

Sarcocystis speeri (definitive host)

Toxoplasma gondii

Didelphis virginiana, Virginia Opossum

Besnoitia sp. of Conti-Diaz et al., 1970 (*species inquirenda*)

Cryptosporidium parvum (experimental)

Eimeria indianensis

Isospora sp. of Ernst, Cooper, and Chobotar, 1969 (*species inquirenda*)

Isospora sp. of Joseph, 1974 (*species inquirenda*)

Sarcocystis falcatula (definitive host)

Sarcocystis greineri (intermediate host)

Sarcocystis inghami (intermediate host)

Sarcocystis neurona (definitive host)

Sarcocystis speeri (definitive host)

Sarcocystis sp. of Dubey et al., 2001b (*species inquirenda*) (definitive host?)

Sarcocystis sp. of Duszynski and Box, 1978 (*species inquirenda*) (definitive host)

Sarcocystis sp. of Seneviratna et al., 1975 (*species inquirenda*) (intermediate host)

Sarcocystis sp. of Scholtyseck et al., 1982 (*species inquirenda*) (intermediate host)

Lutreolina crassicaudata, Lutrine Opossum

Sarcocystis sp. of Carini, 1939 (*species inquirenda*) (definitive host)

Marmosa murina, Linnaeus's Mouse Opossum

Klossiella tejerai

Sarcocystis marmosae (intermediate host)

Toxoplasma gondii

Continued

TABLE 11.2—cont'd

Marmosops dorothea, **Mouse Opossum**

   Eimeria cochabambensis

   Eimeria marmosopos

Metachirus nudicaudatus, **Brown Four-eyed Opossum**

   Toxoplasma gondii

Micoureus constantiae, **Mouse Opossum**

   Eimeria micouri

Micoureus demerarae, **Woolly Opossum**

   Toxoplasma gondii

Monodelphis domestica, **Short-tailed Opossum**

   Eimeria cochabambensis

Philander mcihennyi, **McIlhenny's Four-eyed Opossum**

   Sarcocystis garnhami (intermediate host)

Philander opossum, **Gray Four-eyed Opossum**

   Eimeria philanderi

   Isospora sp. of Lainson and Shaw, 1989 (*species inquirenda*)

Thylamys elegans, **Elegant Fat-tailed Mouse Opossum**

   "Sarcocystidae" sp. of Merino et al., 2008 (*species inquirenda*) (intermediate host?)

Thylamys venustus, **Mouse Opossum**

   Eimeria cochabambensis

ORDER DIPROTODONTIA

Family Hypsiprymnodontidae

Hypsiprymnodon moschatus, **Musky Rat Kangaroo**

   Eimeria hypsiprymnodontis

   Eimeria kairiensis

   Eimeria spearei

   Eimeria spratti

   Eimeria tinarooensis

Family Macropodidae

Dendrolagus lumholtzi, **Lumholtz's Tree kangaroo**

   Eimeria dendrolagi

   Eimeria lumholtzi

TABLE 11.2—cont'd

Sarcocystis sp. of Speare et al., 1989 (*species inquirenda*) (intermediate host)

Toxoplasma gondii

Lagorchestes conspicillatus, Spectacled Hare-wallaby

Eimeria lagorchestis

Eimeria sp. of Barker et al., 1988b (*species inquirenda*)

Klossiella beveridgei

Macropus agilis, Agile Wallaby

Eimeria mykytowyczi

Eimeria prionotemni

Eimeria sp. of O'Donoghue and Adlard, 2000 (*species inquirenda*)

Sarcocystis sp. (spp.?) 5 of Munday et al., 1978 (*species inquirenda*) (intermediate host)

Toxoplasma gondii

Macropus antilopinus, Antilopine Kangaroo

Eimeria flindersi

Eimeria mykytowyczi

Macropus dorsalis, Black-striped Wallaby

Eimeria hestermani

Eimeria macropodis

Eimeria prionotemni

Eimeria sp. of Speare et al., 1989 (*species inquirenda*)

Macropus eugenii, Tammar Wallaby

Coccidium sp. of Johnston, 1910a (*species inquirenda*)

Cryptosporidium sp. of Power et al., 2003 (*species inquirenda*)

Eimeria flindersi

Eimeria hestermani

Eimeria macropodis

Eimeria prionotemni

Eimeria toganmainensis

Toxoplasma gondii

Macropus fuliginosus, Western Grey Kangaroo

Cryptosporidium fayeri

Cryptosporidium macropodum

Continued

TABLE 11.2—cont'd

Cryptosporidium sp., kangaroo genotype I of Yang et al., 2011 (*species inquirenda*)

Cryptosporidium xiaoi

Eimeria gungahlinensis

Eimeria hestermani

Eimeria macropodis

Eimeria marsupialium

Eimeria toganmainensis

Eimeria wilcanniensis

Eimeria yathongensis

"*Eimeriina*" of Yamada et al., 1981 (*species inquirenda*)

Klossiella callitris

Toxoplasma gondii

Macropus giganteus Eastern Grey Kangaroo

Coccidium sp. of Johnston, 1910b (*species inquirenda*)

Cryptosporidium fayeri

Cryptosporidium hominis

Cryptosporidium macropodum

Cryptosporidium parvum

Cryptosporidium parvum/hominis-like of Ryan and Power, 2012 (*species inquirenda*)

Eimeria gungahlinensis

Eimeria hestermani

Eimeria kogoni of Mykytowycz, 1964 (*species inquirenda*)

Eimeria macropodis

Eimeria marsupialium

Eimeria sp. of Barker et al., 1963 (*species inquirenda*)

Eimeria sp. of Winter, 1959 (*species inquirenda*)

Eimeria toganmainensis

Eimeria wilcanniensis

Eimeria yathongensis

Sarcocystis sp. (spp.?) 5 of Munday et al., 1978 (*species inquirenda*) (intermediate host)

Toxoplasma gondii

TABLE 11.2—cont'd

***Macropus irma*, Western Brush Wallaby**

   Eimeria macropodis

***Macropus parma* Waterhouse, Parma Wallaby**

   Eimeria macropodis

   Eimeria parma

   Toxoplasma gondii

***Macropus parryi*, Pretty-faced Wallaby**

   Eimeria macropodis

   Eimeria mykytowyczi

   Eimeria parryi

   Eimeria prionotemni

   Eimeria sp. of O'Donoghue and Adlard, 2000 (*species inquirenda*)

***Macropus robustus*, Wallaroo**

   Eimeria wilcanniensis

   Toxoplasma gondii

***Macropus rufogriseus*, Red-necked or Bennett's Wallaby**

   Eimeria desmaresti

   Eimeria flindersi

   Eimeria hestermani

   Eimeria macropodis

   Eimeria prionotemni

   Eimeria toganmainensis

   Eimeria wilcanniensis

   Klossiella rufogrisei

   Sarcocystis mucosa (intermediate host)

   Sarcocystis sp. (spp.?) 5 of Munday et al., 1978 (*species inquirenda*) (intermediate host)

   Sarcocystis sp. of Triffitt, 1927 (*species inquirenda*) (intermediate host)

   Toxoplasma gondii

***Macropus rufus*, Red Kangaroo**

   Cryptosporidium fayeri

   Cryptosporidium sp. of O'Donoghue, unpub. observ. (In Ryan et al., 2008) (*species inquirenda*)

Continued

TABLE 11.2—cont'd

Eimeria macropodis

Eimeria rufusi of Prasad, 1960 (*species inquirenda*)

Eimeria toganmainensis

Eimeria wilcanniensis

Eimeria sp. of O'Donoghue, 1997 (*species inquirenda*)

Klossiella rufi

Klossiella sp. of Munday, 1988 (*species inquirenda*)

Sarcocystis spp. (?) 4 A and B of Munday et al., 1978 (*species inquirenda*) (intermediate host)

Sarcocystis sp. (spp.?) 6 of Munday et al., 1978 (*species inquirenda*) (intermediate host)

Toxoplasma gondii

Petrogale assimilis, Allied Rock Wallaby

Cryptosporidium macropodum

Eimeria boonderooensis

Eimeria godmani

Eimeria petrogale

Eimeria sharmani

Sarcocystis mucosa (intermediate host)

Petrogale brachyotis (syn. *P. venustula*), Short-eared Rock-wallaby

Eimeria occidentalis

Sarcocystis sp. 6 of Munday et al., 1978 (*species inquirenda*) (intermediate host)

Petrogale (syn. *Peradorcas*) concinna, Nabarlek or Little-rock Wallaby

Sarcocystis sp. 6 of Munday et al., 1978 (*species inquirenda*) (intermediate host)

Petrogale godmani, Godman's Rock wallaby

Eimeria godmani

Eimeria petrogale

Eimeria sharmani

Petrogale inorata, Unadorned Rock Wallaby

Eimeria boonderooensis

Eimeria godmani

Eimeria inornata

Eimeria petrogale

Eimeria sharmani

Sarcocystis mucosa

TABLE 11.2—cont'd

***Petrogale lateralis*, Black-flanked Rock Wallaby**

Eimeria godmani

Eimeria inornata

Eimeria occidentalis

Eimeria petrogale

Eimeria sharmani

***Petrogale penicillata*, Brush-tailed Rock Wallaby**

Eimeria inornata

Eimeria petrogale

Eimeria sharmani

Eimeria sp. of Barker et al., 1988c (*species inquirenda*)

Sarcocystis mucosa (intermediate host)

Sarcocystis sp. of Munday, 1978 (*species inquirenda*) (intermediate host)

***Petrogale persephone*, Proserpine Rock Wallaby**

Eimeria petrogale

Eimeria sharmani

***Petrogale rothschildi*, Rothschild's Rock Wallaby**

Eimeria occidentalis

Eimeria sharmani

***Petrogale xanthopus*, Yellow-footed Rock Wallaby**

Cryptosporidium fayeri

Cryptosporidium macropodum

Eimeria xanthopus

Toxoplasma gondii

***Setonix brachyurus*, Quokka**

Eimeria quokka

Eimeria setonicis

Eimeria volckertzooni

Toxoplasma gondii

***Thylogale billardierii*, Tasmanian Padmelon**

Cryptosporidium sp. of Obendorf, unpub. observ. (in Ryan et al., 2008) (*species inquirenda*)

Eimeria obendorfi

Continued

TABLE 11.2—cont'd

Eimeria ringaroomaensis

Eimeria thylogale

Klossiella thylogale

Sarcocystis mucosa (intermediate host)

Sarcocystis sp. (spp.?) 5 of Munday et al., 1978 (*species inquirenda*) (intermediate host)

Toxoplasma gondii

Thylogale thetis, Red-necked Pademelon

Toxoplasma gondii

Tyzzeria sp. of Barker et al., 1988c (*species inquirenda*)

Wallabia bicolor, Swamp Wallaby

Cryptosporidium fayeri

Cryptosporidium macropodum

Eimeria bicolor

Eimeria wallabiae

Klossiella serendipensis

Sarcocystis sp. (spp.?) 5 of Munday et al., 1978 (*species inquirenda*) (intermediate host)

Toxoplasma gondii

Wallabia sp.

Cryptosporidium parvum

Family Petauridae

Petaurus australis, Yellow-bellied Glider

"Sarcocystidae" sp. of Zhu et al., 2009 (*species inquirenda*) (intermediate host)

Family Phalangeridae

Trichosurus caninus, Short-eared Possum

Eimeria trichosuri

Sarcocystis sp (spp.?) 11 of Munday et al., 1978 (*species inquirenda*) (intermediate host)

Trichosurus cunninghami, Mountain Brushtail Possum

Eimeria trichosuri

Trichosurus vulpecula, Common Brushtail

Cryptosporidium parvum

Cryptosporidium parvum/hominis-like of Ryan and Power, 2012 (*species inquirenda*)

Cryptosporidium sp., Brushtail possum genotype I of Ryan and Power, 2012 (*species inquirenda*)

TABLE 11.2—cont'd

Eimeria sp. of O'Callaghan and Moore, 1986 (*species inquirenda*)

Eimeria trichosuri

Sarcocystis sp (spp.?) 11 of Munday et al., 1978 (*species inquirenda*) (intermediate host)

Toxoplasma gondii

Family Phascolarctidae

***Phascolarctos cinereus*, Koala**

Cryptosporidium fayeri

Cryptosporidium macropodum

Cryptosporidium sp. of Phillips et al., unpub. observ. (in Ryan et al., 2008) (*species inquirenda*)

Toxoplasma gondii

Family Potoridae

***Aepyprymnus rufescens*, Rufous Rat Kangaroo**

Eimeria aepyprymni

***Bettongia gaimardi*, Eastern Bettong**

Eimeria gaimardi

Klossiella bettongiae

***Bettongia lesueur grayii*, Boodie or Short-nosed "Rat" Kangaroo**

Sarcocystis bettongiae of Bourne, 1934 (*species inquirenda*) (intermediate host)

***Potorous tridactylus*, Long-nosed or Southern Potoroo**

Eimeria mundayi

Eimeria potoroi

Klossiella sp. of Barker et al., 1975 (*species inquirenda*)

Toxoplasma gondii

Family Pseudocheiridae

***Hemibelideus lemuroides*, Lemuroid Ringtail**

Eimeria sp. of Speare et al., 1984 (*species inquirenda*)

Klossiella sp. (*species inquirenda*)

***Petauroides volans*, Greater Glider**

Klossiella schoinobatis

***Pseudocheirus peregrinus*, Common Ringtail**

Eimeria sp. of O'Donoghue, 1997 (*species inquirenda*)

Klossiella convolutor

Continued

TABLE 11.2—cont'd

Pseudochirops (syn. *Pseudocheirus*) *archeri*, **Green Ringtail**

Eimeria sp. of Speare et al., 1984 (*species inquirenda*)

Klossiella sp. of Speare et al., 1984 (*species inquirenda*)

Sarcocystis sp. 8 of Munday et al., 1978 (*species inquirenda*) (intermediate host)

Pseudochirulus herbertansis, **Herbert River Ringtail**

Eimeria spp. of Speare et al., 1984 (*species inquirenda*)

Klossiella sp. of Speare et al., 1984 (*species inquirenda*)

Family Vombatidae

Lasiorhinus latifrons, **Southern Hairy-nosed Wombat**

Eimeria ursini

Eimeria wombati

Toxoplasma gondii

Vombatus ursinus, **Common Wombat**

Eimeria arundeli

Toxoplasma gondii

ORDER MICROBIOTHERIA

Family Microbiotheriidae

Dromiciops gliroides, **Monito del Monte**

"Sarcocystidae" sp. of Merino et al., 2009 (*species inquirenda*) (intermediate host?)

ORDER PERAMELEMORPHIA

Family Thylacomyidae

Macrotis lagotis, **Greater Bilby**

Cryptosporidium muris

Toxoplasma gondii

Family Peramelidae

Isoodon macrourus, **Northern Brown Bandicoot**

Eimeria sp. of Mackerras, 1958 (*species inquirenda*)

Sarcocystis sp. 3 of Munday et al., 1978 (*species inquirenda*) (intermediate host)

Isoodon obesulus, **Southern Brown Bandicoot**

Cryptosporidium parvum (?)

Cryptosporidium parvum/hominis-like of Ryan and Power, 2012 (*species inquirenda*)

Eimeria quenda

TABLE 11.2—cont'd

Eimeria spp. 1 and 2 of Bennett and Hobbs, 2011 (*species inquirenda*)

Klossiella quimrensis

Sarcocystis sp. of Mackerras et al., 1953 (*species inquirenda*) (intermediate host)

Toxoplasma gondii

Perameles bougainville, Western Barred Bandicoot

Cryptosporidium fayeri

Cryptosporidium macropodum

Eimeria kanyana

Klossiella quimrensis

Parmeles gunnii, Eastern Barred Bandicoot

Eimeria sp. of Obendorf and Munday, 1990 (*species inquirenda*)

Klossiella quimrensis

Sarcocystis sp. 7 of Munday et al., 1978 (*species inquirenda*) (intermediate host)

Toxoplasma gondii

Toxoplasma sp. of Munday et al., 1978 (*species inquirenda*)

Perameles nasuta, Long-nosed Bandicoot

Cryptosporidium parvum/hominis-like of Ryan and Power, 2012 (*species inquirenda*)

Klossiella sp. of Mackerras, 1958 (*species inquirenda*)

Sarcocystis sp. 7 of Munday et al., 1978 (*species inquirenda*) (intermediate host)

Toxoplasma gondii

Toxoplasma sp. of Munday et al., 1978 (*species inquirenda*)

TABLE 11.3 A LIST OF ALL *EIMERIA* SPECIES COVERED IN CHAPTERS 3, 4, 5 OF THIS BOOK, TO DETERMINE IF THERE MAY BE ANY UNIFYING PATTERNS OF OOCYST AND/OR SPOROCYST MORPHOLOGY THAT COULD INDICATE A PHYLOGENETIC RELATIONSHIP WITHIN OR BETWEEN A MARSUPIAL GENUS/FAMILY/ORDER

Marsupial Super Order/ Order/Family/*Genus*/*E.* sp.	Oocyst[a]			Sporocyst[a]		
	L × W	M	OR	L × W	SB/SSB	SR
AMERIDELPHIA						
O. DIDELPHIMORPHIA						
DIDELPHIDAE						
CALUROMYDIS						
caluromydis	32 × 31	–	–	15 × 10	+/+	+
haberfeldi	30 × 20	–	–	13 × 8	+/–	+
DIDELPHIS						
auritanensis	32 × 30	–	–	13 × 10	+/–	+
cochabambensis	22 × 20	–	–	11 × 7	+/–	+
didelphidis	16 × 16	–	–	10 × 6	+/–	+
gambai	26 × 25	–	–	12 × 10	+/–	+
marmosopos	22 × 20	–	–	11 × 7	+/+	+
micouri	25 × 18	–	–	11 × 7	+/–	+
indianensis	18 × 16	–	–	9 × 6	+/–	+
philanderi	23 × 22	–	–	11 × 8	+/–	+
AUSTRALIDELPHIA						
O. DIPROTODONTIA						
HYPSIPRYMNODONTIDAE						
HYPSIPRYMNODON						
hypsiprymnodontis	29 × 23	–	–	17 × 8	+/+	+
kairiensis	13 × 13	–	–	8 × 5	+/–	+
spearei	17 × 16	–	–	10 × 6	+/+	+
spratti	21 × 19	–	–	13 × 8	+/+	+
tinarooensis	26 × 24	–	–	12 × 8	+/+	+
MACROPODIDAE						
DENDROLAGUS						
dendrolagi	34 × 18	+/–	–	14 × 9	+/+	+
lumholtzi	22 × 11	–	–	9 × 5	+/–	+

TABLE 11.3—cont'd

| Marsupial Super Order/ | Oocyst[a] | | | Sporocyst[a] | | |
Order/Family/*Genus*/E. sp.	L × W	M	OR	L × W	SB/SSB	SR
LAGORCHESTES						
lagorchestis	48 × 27	+	−	19 × 11	+/+	+
MACROPUS						
desmaresti	17 × 10	−	−	8 × 4	+/−	+
flindersi	44 × 29	+	−	18 × 11	+/+	+
gungahlinensis	18 × 17	−	−	9 × 6	+/−	+
hestermani	65 × 45	+	−	25 × 13	+/+	+
macropodis	26 × 13	+	−	9 × 6	+/−	+
marsupialium	23 × 16	−	−	11 × 7	+/−	+
mykytowyczi	31 × 17	+/−	−	11 × 8	+/−	+
parma	21 × 12	−	−	12 × 5	+/−	+
parryi	29 × 13	−	−	12 × 6	+/−	+
prionotemni	37 × 22	−	+	16 × 10	+/+	+
toganmainensis	41 × 26	+	−	16 × 10	+/+	+
wilcanniensis	32 × 20	+/−	−	13 × 10	+/−	+
yathongensis	21 × 14	−	−	11 × 6	+/−	+
PETROGALE						
boonderooensis	27 × 16	−	−	11 × 7	+/−	+
godmani	30 × 17	+	−	12 × 8	−(?)/−	+
inornata	35 × 20	−	−	13 × 8	+/+	+
occidentalis	23 × 18	−	−	11 × 6	+/−	+
petrogale	23 × 14	−	−	9 × 5	+/−	+
sharmani	28 × 17	−	−(?)	13 × 6	+/−	+
xanthopus	25 × 17	+/−(?)	+	10 × 7	+/−	+
SETONIX						
quokka	18 × 11	−	−	8 × 5	+/−	+
setonicis	30 × 18	−	−	12 × 8	+/+	+
volckertzooni	22 × 13	−	−(?)	13 × 5	+/−	+
THYLOGALE						
obendorfi	30 × 16	−	−	11 × 8	+/−	+
ringaroomaensis	28 × 18	−	−	12 × 8	+/+	+

Continued

TABLE 11.3—cont'd

Marsupial Super Order/ Order/Family/*Genus*/*E*. sp.	Oocyst[a]			Sporocyst[a]		
	L × W	M	OR	L × W	SB/SSB	SR
thylogale	32 × 21	–	+	15 × 8	+/+	+
WALLABIA						
bicolor	23 × 13	–	–	8 × 6	+/–	+
wallabiae	39 × 20	–	–	13 × 8	+/+	+
PHALANGERIDAE						
TRICHOSURUS						
trichosuri	41 × 23	+	+	16 × 10	+/+	+
POTORIDAE						
AEPYPRYMNUS						
aepyprymni	37 × 22	–	+/–	16 × 9	+/+	+
BETTONGIA						
gaimardi	35 × 24	–	–	15 × 10	+/+	+
POTOROUS						
mundayi	17 × 16	–	–	10 × 6	+/+	+
potoroi	26 × 18	+	+	12 × 8	+/+	+
VOMBATIDAE						
LASIORHINUS						
ursini	24 × 20	–	–	10 × 7	+/–	+
wombati	75 × 57	–	–	25 × 17	+/–	+
VOMBATUS						
arundeli	64 × 43	+	+	26 × 14	+/–	+
O. PERAMELEMORPHIA						
PERAMELIDAE						
ISOODON						
quenda	25 × 24	–	–	13 × 9	–/–	+
PERAMELES						
kanyana	19 × 18	–	–	9 × 7	+/–	+

Abbreviations: M = micropyle; OR = oocyst residuum; SB/SSB = stieda body/substieda body; SR = sporocyst residuum.

[a] *Approximate mean measurements for oocyst and sporocyst L/Ws.*

References

Adkesson, M.J., Gorman, M.E., Hsiao, V., Whittington, J.K., Langan, J.N., 2007. *Toxoplasma gondii* inclusions in peripheral blood leukocytes of a red-necked wallaby (*Macropus rufogriseus*). Veterinary Clinical Pathology 36, 97–100.

Alexeieff, A.G., 1913. Recherches sur les sarcosporidies. 1. Etude morphologique. Archives de Zoologie Expérimentale et Gènerale 51, 543–551.

Alves, M., Matos, O., Antunes, F., 2001. Multilocus PCR-RFLP analysis of *Cryptosporidium* isolates from HIV-infected patients from Portugal. Annals of Tropical Medicine and Parasitolory 95, 627–632.

Amrine-Madsen, H., Scally, M., Westerman, M., Stanhope, M.J., Krajewski, C., Springer, M.S., 2003. Nuclear gene sequences provide evidence for the monophyly of australidelphian marsupials. Molecular Phylogenetic Evolution 28, 186–196.

Anderson, B.C., 1988. Gastric cryptosporidiosis of feeder cattle, beef cows, and dairy cows. Bovine Practitioner 23, 99–101.

Anderson, B.C., 1991. Experimental infection in mice of *Cryptosporidium muris* isolated from a camel. Journal of Protozoology 38, 16s–17s.

Andrews, J.M., 1927. Host–parasite specificity in the coccidia of mammals. Journal of Parasitology 13, 183–194.

Angus, K.W., 1987. Cryptosporidiosis in domestic animals and humans. Practice 9, 47–49.

Arcay-de-Peraza, L., 1967. Coccidiosis en monos y su comparacion con la isosporosis humana, con descripcion de una nueva especie de *Isospora* en *Cacajao rubicundus* (Uakari monkey o mono chucuto). Acta Biologia Venezuelica 5, 203–222.

Arrowood, M.J., 1997. Diagnosis. In: Fayer, R. (Ed.), *Cryptosporidium* and Cryptosporidiosis. CRC Press, Boca Raton, FL, pp. 43–64.

Arundel, J.H., Barker, I., Beveridge, I., 1977. Diseases of marsupials. In: Stonehouse, B., Gilmore, D. (Eds.), The Biology of Marsupials. Macmillan Press Ltd, Melbourne, pp. 141–154.

Attwood, H.D., Woolley, P.A., 1973a. Toxoplasmosis in dasyurid marsupials. Pathology 2, 77–78.

Attwood, H.D., Woolley, P.A., 1973b. Spontaneous malignant neoplasms in dasyurid marsupials. Journal of Comparative Pathology 83, 569–581.

Attwood, H.D., Woolley, P.A., Rickard, M.D., 1975. Toxoplasmosis in dasyurid marsupials. Journal of Wildlife Diseases 11, 543–551.

Ayala, S.C., D'Alessandro, A., Mackenzie, R., Angel, D., 1973. Hemoparasite infections in 830 wild animals from eastern Llanos of Columbia. Journal of Parasitology 59, 52–59.

Aydin, Y., 1991. Experimental cryptosporidiosis in laboratory animals: pathological findings and cross-transmission studies. Ankara Üniversitesi Veteriner Fakültesi Dergisi 38, 465–482.

Babudieri, B., 1932. I sarcosporidi e le sarcosporidiosi. (Studio monografico). Archiv für Protistenkunde 76, 421–580.

Baird, K.L., Cheadle, M.A., Greiner, E.C., 2002. Prevalence and site specificity of *Sarcocystis greineri* sarcocysts in Virginia opossum (*Didelphis virginiana*) in Florida. Journal of Parasitology 88, 624–625.

Baker, A.M., Mutton, T.Y., Mason, E.D., Gray, E.L., 2015. A taxonomic assessment of the Australian dusky *Antechinus* complex: a new species, the Tasman Peninsula dusky antechinus (*Antechinus vandycki* sp. nov.) and an elevation to species of the mainland dusky antechinus (*Antechinus swainsonii mimetes* (Thomas)). Memoirs of the Queensland Museum – Nature 59, 75–126.

Barker, I.K., Beveridge, I., Bradley, A.J., Lee, A.K., 1978. Observations on spontaneous stress-related mortality among males of the dasyurid marsupial *Antechinus stuartii* Macleay. Australian Journal of Zoology 26, 435–447.

Barker, I.K., Calaby, J.H., Sharman, G.B., 1963. Diseases of Australian laboratory marsupials. Veterinary Bulletin 33, 539–544.

Barker, I.K., Harrigan, K.E., Dempster, J.K., 1972. Coccidiosis in wild gray kangaroos. International Journal for Parasitology 2, 187–192.

Barker, I.K., Munday, B.L., Harrigan, K.E., 1975. *Klossiella* spp. in the kidneys of peramelid, petaurid, and macropodid marsupials. Zeitschrift für Parasitenkunde 46, 35–41.

Barker, I.K., Munday, B.L., Hartley, W.J., 1985. *Klossiella* (Apicomplexa: Klossiellidae) in petaurid and macropodid marsupials in Australia. Journal of Protozoology 32, 520–522.

Barker, I.K., Munday, B.L., Presidente, P.J.F., 1979. Coccidia of wombats: correction of host–parasite relationships. *Eimeria wombati* (Gilruth and Bull, 1912) comb. nov. and *Eimeria ursini* Supperer, 1957 from the hairy-nosed wombat and *Eimeria arundeli* sp. n. from the common wombat. Journal of Parasitology 65, 451–456.

Barker, I.K., O'Callaghan, M.G., Beveridge, I., 1988a. *Eimeria* spp. (Apicomplexa: Eimeriidae) parasitic in the rat-kangaroos *Hypsiprymnodon moschatus*, *Potorous tridactylus*, *Aepyprymnus rufescens* and *Bettongia gaimardi* (Marsupialia: Potoroidae). International Journal for Parasitology 18, 947–953.

Barker, I.K., O'Callaghan, M.G., Beveridge, I., 1988b. *Eimeria* spp. (Apicomplexa: Eimeriidae) parasitic wallabies and kangaroos of the genera *Setonix*, *Thylogale*, *Wallabia*, *Lagorchestes* and *Dendrolagus* (Marsupialia: Macropododidae). International Journal for Parasitology 18, 955–962.

Barker, I.K., O'Callaghan, M.G., Beveridge, I., 1989. Host-parasite associations of *Eimeria* spp. (Apicomplexa: Eimeriidae) in kangaroos and wallabies of the genus *Macropus* (Marsupialia: Macropodidae). International Journal for Parasitology 19, 241–263.

Barker, I.K., O'Callaghan, M.G., Beveridge, I., Close, R.L., 1988c. Host–parasite associations of *Eimeria* spp. (Apicomplexa: Eimeriidae) in rock wallabies, *Petrogale* spp. (Marsupialia: Macropodidae). International Journal for Parasitology 18, 353–363.

Barretto, M.P., 1940. Contribuição au estudo dos Sarcosporidia Bütschli, 1882, com a descrição de uma nova especie: *S. jacarinae* n. sp. parasita do "tiziu" (*Volantina jacarina* L.). Arquivos de Zoologia (São Paulo) 1, 339–368.

Barta, J.R., 2000. Suborder Adeleorina Léger, 1911. In: Lee, J.J., Leedale, G.F., Bradbury, P. (Eds.), An Illustrated Guide to the Protozoa, second ed. Society of Protozoologists, P.O. Box 368, Lawrence, Kansas, vol. 1. pp. 305–318.

Barta, J.R., Schrenzel, M.D., Carreno, R., Rideout, B.A., 2005. The genus *Atoxoplasma* (Garnham 1950) as a junior objective synonym of the genus *Isospora* (Schneider 1881) species infecting birds and resurrection of *Cystoisospora* (Frenkel 1977) as the correct genus for *Isospora* infecting mammals. Critical comment. Journal of Parasitology 91, 726–727.

Basso, W., Venturini, M.C., Moré, G., Quiroga, A., Bacigalupe, D., Unzaga, J.M., Larsen, A., Laplace, R., Venturini, L., 2007. Toxoplasmosis in captive Bennett's wallabies (*Macropus rufogriseus*) in Argentina. Veterinary Parasitology 144, 157–161.

Beck, R.M.D., 2008. A dated phylogeny or marsupials using a molecular supermatrix and multiple fossil constraints. Journal of Mammalogy 89, 175–189.

Beech, J., 1974. Equine protozoan encephalomyelitis. Veterinary Medicine/Small Animal Clinician 69, 1562–1566.

Beech, J., Dodd, D.C., 1974. *Toxoplasma*-like encephalitis in the horse. Veterinary Pathology 11, 87–96.

Begg, M., Beveridge, I., Chilton, N.B., Johnson, P.M., O'Callaghan, M.G., 1995. Parasites of the Proserpine rock-wallaby, *Petrogale persephone* (Marsupialia: Macropodidae). Australian Mammalogy 18, 45–53.

Bennett, M.D., Hobbs, R.P., 2011. A new *Eimeria* species parasitic in *Isoodon obesulus* (Marsupialia: Peramelidae) in Western Australia. Journal of Parasitology 97, 1129–1131.

Bennett, M.D., Woolford, L., O'Hara, A.J., Nicholls, P.K., Warren, K., Hobbs, R.P., 2006. A new *Eimeria* species parasitic in western barred bandicoots, *Perameles bougainville* (Marsupialia; Permelidae), in Western Australia. Journal of Parasitology 93, 1292–1294.

Bennett, M.D., Woolford, L., O'Hara, A.J., Nicholls, P.K., Warren, K.S., Friend, J.Q., Swan, R.A., 2007. *Klossiella quimrensis* (Apicomplexa: Klossiellidae) causes renal coccidiosis in western barred bandicoots *Perameles bougainville* (Marsupiala: Peramelidae) in western Australia. Journal of Parasitology 93, 89–92.

Bettoil, S.S., Obendorf, D.L., Nowarkowski, M., Goldsmid, J.M., 2000a. Pathology of experimental toxoplasmosis in eastern barred bandicoots in Tasmania. Journal of Wildlife Diseases 36, 141–144.

Bettoil, S.S., Obendorf, D.L., Nowarkowski, M., Milstein, T., Goldsmid, J.M., 2000b. Earthworms as paratenic hosts of toxoplasmosis in eastern barred bandicoots in Tasmania. Journal of Wildlife Diseases 36, 145–148.

Black, A., Orr, M., 1996. Review of veterinary diagnostic cases—July to September 1996. Surveillance 23, 3–5.

Blanchard, R., 1885a. Note sur les Sarcosporidies et sur un essai de classification de ces Sporozoaires. Bulletin de la Societe Zoologique de France 10, 244–276.

Blanchard, R., 1885b. Sur un nouveau type de Sarcosporidies. Comptes Rendus de l'Academie des Sciences 100, 1599–1601.

Bolon, B., Greiner, E.C., Calderwood Mays, M.B., 1989. Microscopic features of *Sarcocystis falcatula* in skeletal muscle from a Patagonian conure. Veterinary Pathology 26, 282–284.

Boorman, G.A., Kollias, G.V., Taylor, R.F., 1977. An outbreak of toxoplasmosis in wallaroos (*Macropus robustus*) in a California zoo. Journal of Wildlife Diseases 13, 64–68.

Boulard, Y., 1975. Étude morphologique des coccidies (Adeleidae) *Klossiella killicki* n. sp. chez des microchiroptères africains et *Klossiella tejerai* Scorza, 1957, chez un marsupial sud- américain. Bulletin du Muséum National d'Histoire Naturelle 284, 83–89.

Bourne, G., 1934. Sarcosporidia. Journal of the Royal Society of Western Australia 19, 1–8.

Box, E.D., Duszynski, D.W., 1977. Survey for *Sarcocystis* in brown-headed cowbirds (*Molothrus ater*): a comparison of macroscopic, microscopic and digestion techniques. Journal of Wildlife Diseases 13, 356–359.

Box, E.D., Duszynski, D.W., 1978. Experimental transmission of *Sarcocystis* from icterid birds to sparrows and canaries by sporocysts from the opossum. Journal of Parasitology 64, 682–688.

Box, E.D., Duszynski, D.W., 1980. *Sarcocystis* of passerine birds: sexual stages in the opossum (*Didelphis virginiana*). Journal of Wildlife Diseases 16, 209–215.

Box, E.D., Smith, J.H., 1982. The intermediate host spectrum in a *Sarcocystis* species of birds. Journal of Parasitology 68, 668–673.

Box, E.D., Marchiondo, A.A., Duszynski, D.W., Davis, C.P., 1980. Ultrastructure of *Sarcocystis* from passerine birds and opossums: comments on classification of the genus *Isospora*. Journal of Parasitology 66, 68–74.

Box, E.D., Meier, J.L., Smith, J.H., 1984. Description of *Sarcocystis falcatula* Stiles, 1893, a parasite of birds and opossums. Journal of Protozoology 31, 521–524.

Brown, C.C., 1988. Endogenous lipid pneumonia in opossums from Louisiana. Journal of Wildlife Diseases 24, 214–219.

Brumpt, E., 1913. Précis de Parasitologie, second ed. Masson, Paris. 1011 p.

Burbridge, A.A., Eldridge, M.D.B., Groves, C., Harrison, P.L., Jackson, S.M., Reardon, T.B., Westerman, M., Woinarski, J.C.Z., 2014. 2. A list of native Australian mammal species and subspecies. In: Woinarski, J.C.Z., Burbridge, A.A., Harrison, P.L. (Eds.), The Action Plan for Australian Mammals 2012. CSIRO Publishing, Collingwood, Victoria, Australia, pp. 16–32.

Burridge, M.J., Bigler, W.J., Forrester, D.J., Hennemann, J.M., 1979. Serologic survey for *Toxoplasma gondii* in wild animals in Florida. Journal of the American Veterinary Medical Association 175, 964–967.

Cabrera, A., 1919. Genera Mammalium: Monotremata, Marsupialia, vol. 1. Museo Nacional de Ciencias Naturales, Madrid.

Cabrera, A., 1958 (1957). Catálogo de los mamíferos de América del Sur. Part 1. Revista del Museo Argentino de Ciencias Naturales "Bernardino Rivadavia" (Ciencias Zoológicas) 4 (i–iv), 1–307.

Canfield, P.J., Hartley, W.J., Dubey, J.P., 1990. Lesions of toxoplasmosis in Australian marsupials. Journal of Comparative Pathology 103, 159–167.

Carini, A., 1936. *Eimeria didelphydis* n. sp. dell'intestino del *Didelphys aurita*. Archivio Italiano di Scienze Medicina Tropical e di Parassitologia (Colon) 17 (n.s.2), 332–333.

Carini, A., 1937a. Sur une nouvelle *Eimeria*, parasite de l'intestin du *Caluromys philander*. Annales de Parasitologie, Humaine et Comparee 15, 453–455.

Carini, A., 1938 (1937). Mais uma *Eimeria*, parasita do intestino do *Didelphys aurita*. Archivos de Biologia (São Paulo) 22, 61–62.

Carini, A., 1939. Sobre uma nova *Isospora* do intestino da *Lutreolina crassicaudata*. Archivos de Biologia (São Paulo) 23, 5–6.

Carreno, R.A., Barta, J.R., 1999. An Eimeriid origin of isosporid coccidia with Stieda bodies as shown by phylogenetic analysis of small subunit ribosomal RNA gene sequences. Journal of Parasitology 85, 77–83.

Casemore, D.P., 1991. The epidemiology of human cryptosporidiosis and the water route of infection. Water Science Technology 24, 157–164.

Casemore, D.P., Wright, J.T., Coop, R.L., 1997. Cryptosporidiosis—human and animal epidemiology. In: Fayer, R. (Ed.), Cryptosporidium and Cryptosporidiosis. CRC Press, Boca Raton, FL, pp. 65–92.

Chalmers, R.M., Sturdee, A.P., Casemore, D.P., Curry, A., Miller, A., Parker, N.D., Richmond, T.M., 1994. *Cryptosporidium muris* in wild house mice (*Mus musculus*): first report in the UK. European Journal of Protistology 30, 151–155.

Chapman, A.D., 2009. Numbers of Living Species in Australia and the World, second ed. Australian Biological Resources Study, Canberra, Australia, 80 p. ISBN: 978-0-642-56861-8. (also available online in PDF version).

Cheadle, M.A., 2001. *Sarcocystis greineri* n. sp. (Protozoa: Sarcocystidae) in the Virginia opossum (*Didelphis virginiana*). Journal of Parasitology 87, 1085–1089.

Cheadle, M.A., Dame, J.B., Greiner, E.C., 2001a. Sporocyst size of isolates of *Sarcocystis* shed by the Virginia opossum (*Didelphis virginiana*). Veterinary Parasitology 95, 305–311.

Cheadle, M.A., Tanhauser, S.M., Dame, J.B., Sellon, D.C., Hines, M., Ginn, P.E., MacKay, R.J., Griener, E.C., 2001b. The nine-banded armadillo (*Dasypus novemcinctus*) is an intermediate host for *Sarcocystis neurona*. International Journal for Parasitology 31, 330–335.

Chatton, E., 1912. Sur quelques genres d'amibes libres et parasites. Synonymies, homonymie, impropriété. Bulletin de la Societe Zoologique de France-Evolution et Zoologie 37, 109–115, 168.

Chilvers, B.L., Cowan, P.E., Waddington, D.C., Kelly, P.J., Brown, T.J., 1998. The prevalence of infection of *Giardia* spp. and *Cryptosporidium* spp. in wild animals on farmland, southeastern North Island, New Zealand. International Journal of Environmental Health Research 8, 59–64.

Chinchilla, M., Valerio, I., Duszynski, D.W., 2015. Endogenous life cycle of *Eimeria marmosops* (Apicomplexa: Eimeriidae) from the opossum *Didelphis marsupialis* (Didelphimorphia: Didelphidae). Journal of Parasitology 101, 436–444.

Clark, E.G., Townsend, H.G.G., McKenzie, N.T., 1981. Equine protozoal myeloencephalitis: a report of 2 cases from Western Canada. Canadian Veterinary Journal 22, 140–144.

Clarke, J.J., 1895. Memoirs: a study of coccidia met with in mice. Quarterly Journal of Microscopical Science 2 (147), 277–283.

Clemens, W.A., 1968. Origin and early evolution of marsupials. Evolution 22, 1–18.

Clubb, S.L., Frenkel, J.K., 1992. *Sarcocystis falcatula* of opossums: transmission by cockroaches with fatal pulmonary disease in psittacine birds. Journal of Parasitology 78, 116–124.

Clubb, S.L., Frenkel, J.K., Gardiner, C.H., Graham, D.L., 1988. An acute fatal illness in Old World Psittacine birds associated with *Sarcocystis falcatula* of opossums. In: Annual Proceedings of the Association of Avian Veterinarians, September 27 to October 1, Houston, TX, pp. 139–149.

Conti-Diaz, I.A., Turner, C., Tweeddale, D.T., Furcolow, M.L., 1970. Besnoitiasis in the opossum (*Didelphis marsupialis*). Journal of Parasitology 56, 457–460.

Cook, I., Pope, J.H., 1959. *Toxoplasma* in Queensland, III. A preliminary survey of animal hosts. Australian Journal of Experimental Biology and Medical Science 37, 253–262.

Coutelen, F., 1932. Existence d'une encephalite toxoplasmique spontanee chez les wombats. Un toxoplasme nouveau. Comptes Rendus des Seances Socété de Biologia (Paris) 110, 1245–1247.

Coutelen, F., 1933. Sur la position systématique de *Globidium mucosa* (R. Blanchard, 1885), parasite du kangourou des rouchers *Macropus* (*Petrogale*) *penicillatus*. Annales de Parasitologie, Humaine et Comparee 11, 1–6.

Cusick, P.K., Sells, D.M., Hamilton, D.P., Hardenbrook, H.J., 1974. Toxoplasmosis in two horses. Journal of the American Veterinary Medical Association 164, 77–80.

Dame, J.B., MacKay, R.J., Yowell, C.A., Cutler, T.J., Marsh, A., Greiner, E.C., 1995. *Sarcocystis falcatula* from passerine and psittacine birds: synonymy with *Sarcocystis neurona*, agent of equine protozoal myeloencephalitis. Journal of Parasitology 81, 930–935.

da Silva Stabenow, C., Ederli, N.B., Lopes, C.W.G., de Oliveira, F.C.R., 2012. *Didelphis aurita* (Marsupialia: Didelphidae): a new host for *Sarcocystis lindsayi* (Apicomplexa: Sarcocystidae). Journal of Parasitology 98, 1262–1265.

Darling, S.T., 1910. Sarcosporidiosis in the opossum and its experimental production in the guinea pig by the intramuscular injection of sporozoites. Bulletin de la Societe de Pathologie Exotique 3, 513–518.

Daszak, P., Cunningham, A.A., Hyatt, A.D., 2000. Emerging infectious disease of wildlife—threats to biodiversity and human health. Science 287, 443–449.

de Thoisy, B., Michel, J.-C., Vogel, I., Vie, J.-C., 2000. A survey of hemoparasite infections in free-ranging mammals and reptiles in French Guiana. Journal of Parasitology 86, 1035–1040.

Deane, L.M., Deane, M.P., 1961. Sobre dois hemocitozoários encontrados em mamíferos silvestres da Região Amazónica. Revista do Instituto de Medicina Tropical de São Paulo 3, 107–110.

Dickens, R.K., 1978. The Koala in Health and Disease. Post-Graduate Committee in Veterinary Science, vol. 36. University of Sydney, pp. 105–118.

Dobos-Kovacs, M., Meszaros, J., Pellérdy, L.P., Balsai, A., 1974a. Studies on source of *Toxoplasma* infections in captive kangaroos. Acta Veterinaria Academiae Scientiarum Hungaricae, Tomus 24, 293–301.

Dobos-Kovacs, M., Meszaros, J., Pellérdy, L.P., Balsai, A., 1974b. Toxoplasmose bei Kanguruhs (*Thylogale eugenii*) verursacht durch *Toxoplasma* oozysten entheltendes Futter. Parasitologica Hungarica 7, 85–89.

Doube, L.J., 1981. Diseases of wombats. In: Wildlife Diseases of the Pacific Basin and Other Countries. Proceedings of the 4th International Conference of the Wildlife Disease Association. Sydney, Australia, pp. 63–75.

Dubey, J.P., 2000. Prevalence of *Sarcocystis* species sporocysts in wild-caught opossums (*Didelphis virginiana*). Journal of Parasitology 86, 705–710.

Dubey, J.P., 2001. Migration and development of *Sarcocystis neurona* in tissues of interferon gamma knockout mice fed sporocysts from a naturally-infected opossums. Veterinary Parasitology 95, 341–351.

Dubey, J.P., 2004. Toxoplasmosis—A waterborne zoonosis. Veterinary Parasitology 126, 57–72.

Dubey, J.P., Beattie, C.P., 1988. Toxoplasmosis of Animals and Man. CRC Press, Boca Raton, FL. 220 p.

Dubey, J.P., Crutchley, C., 2008. Toxoplasmosis in wallabies (*Macropus rufogriseus* and *Macropus eugenii*): blindness, treatment with atovaquone, and isolation of *Toxoplasma gondii*. Journal of Parasitology 94, 929–933.

Dubey, J.P., Hamir, A.N., 2000. Immunohistochemical confirmation of *Sarcocystis neurona* infections in raccoons, mink, cat, skunk and pony. Journal of Parasitology 86, 1150–1152.

Dubey, J.P., Lindsay, D.S., 1998. Isolation in immunodeficient mice of *Sarcocystis neurona* from opossum (*Didelphis virginiana*) faeces and its differentiation from *Sarcocystis falcatula*. International Journal for Parasitology 28, 1823–1828.

Dubey, J.P., Lindsay, D.S., 1999. *Sarcocystis speeri* n. sp. (Protozoa: Sarcocystidae) from the opossum (*Didelphis virginiana*). Journal of Parasitology 85, 903–909.

Dubey, J.P., Miller, S., 1986. Equine protozoal myeloencephalitis in a pony. Journal of the American Veterinary Medical Association 188, 1311–1313.

Dubey, J.P., Odening, K., 2001. Toxoplasmosis and related infections. In: Samuel, W.M., Pybus, M.J., Kocan, A.A. (Eds.), Parasitic Diseases of Wild Mammals, second ed. Iowa State University Press, Ames, IA, pp. 478–519.

Dubey, J.P., Black, S.S., Rickard, L.G., Rosenthal, B.M., Lindsay, D.S., Shen, S.K., Kwok, O.C.H., Hurst, G., Rashmir-Raven, A., 2001a. Prevalence of *Sarcocystis neurona* sporocysts in opossums (*Didelphis virginiana*) from rural Mississippi. Veterinary Parasitology 95, 283–293.

Dubey, J.P., Calero-Bernal, R., Speer, C.A., Rosenthal, B.M., Fayer, R., 2015. Sarcocystosis of Animals and Man. CRC Press, Boca Raton, FL. ISBN: 978-1-49-871012-1, in press.

Dubey, J.P., Davis, G.W., Koestner, A., Kiryu, K., 1974. Equine encephalomyelitis due to a protozoan parasite resembling *Toxoplasma gondii*. Journal of the American Veterinary Medical Association 165, 249–255.

Dubey, J.P., Davis, S.W., Speer, C.A., Bowman, D.D., de Lahunta, A., Granstrom, D.E., Topper, M.J., Hamir, A.N., Cummings, J.F., Suter, M.M., 1991a. *Sarcocystis neurona* n. sp. (Protozoa: Apicomplexa), the etiologic agent of equine protozoal myeloencephalitis. Journal of Parasitology 77, 212–218.

Dubey, J.P., Garner, M.M., Stetter, M.D., Marsh, A.E., Barr, B.C., 2001b. Acute *Sarcocystis falcatula*-like infection in a carmine bee-eater (*Merops nubicus*) and immunohistochemical cross reactivity between *Sarcocystis falcatula* and *Sarcocystis neurona*. Journal of Parasitology 87, 824–832.

Dubey, J.P., Hamir, A.N., Niezgoda, M., Rupprecht, C.E., 1996. A *Sarcocystis neurona*-like organism associated with encephalitis in a striped skunk (*Mephitis mephitis*). Journal of Parasitology 82, 172–174.

Dubey, J.P., Hedstrom, O., Machado, C.R., Osborn, K.G., 1991b. Disseminated toxoplasmosis in a captive koala (*Phascolarctos cinereus*). Journal of Zoo and Wildlife Medicine 22, 348–350.

Dubey, J.P., Johnson, G.C., Bermudez, A., Suedmeyer, K.W., Fritz, D.L., 2001c. Neural sarcocystosis in a straw-necked ibis (*Carphibis spinicollis*) associated with a *Sarcocystis neurona*-like organism and description of muscular sarcocysts of an unidentified *Sarcocystis* species. Journal of Parasitology 87, 1317–1322.

Dubey, J.P., Kerber, C.E., Lindsay, D.S., Kasai, N., Pena, H.F.J., 2000a. The South American opossum, *Didelphis marsupialis*, from Brazil as another definitive host for *Sarcocystis speeri* Dubey and Lindsay, 1999. Parasitology 121, 589–594.

Dubey, J.P., Lindsay, D.S., Kerber, C.E., Kasai, N., Pena, H.F.J., Gennari, S.M., Kwok, O.C.H., Shen, S.K., Rosenthal, B.M., 2001d. First isolation of *Sarcocystis neurona* from the South American opossum, *Didelphis albiventris*, from Brazil. Veterinary Parasitology 95, 295–304.

Dubey, J.P., Lindsay, D.S., Rezende, P.C.B., Costa, A.J., 2000b. Characterization of an unidentified *Sarcocystis falculata*-like parasite from the South American oppoum, *Didelphis albiventris* from Brazil. Journal of Eukaryotic Microbiology 47, 538–544.

Dubey, J.P., Lindsay, D.S., Rosenthal, B.M., Kerber, C.E., Kasai, N., Pena, H.F.J., Kwok, O.C.H., Shen, S.K., Gennari, S.M., 2001e. Isolates of *Sarcocystis falcatula*-like organisms from South American opossums *Didelphis marsupialis* and *Didelphis albiventris* from São Paulo, Brazil. Journal of Parasitology 87, 1449–1453.

Dubey, J.P., Lindsay, D.S., Saville, W.J.A., Reed, S.M., Granstrom, D.E., Speer, C.A., 2001f. A review of *Sarcocystis neurona* and equine protozoal myeloencephatitis (EPM). Veterinary Parasitology 95, 89–131.

Dubey, J.P., Lindsay, D.S., Venturini, L., Venturini, C., 2000c. Characterization of *Sarcocystis falcatula* isolates from Argentinian opossum, *Didelphis albiventris*. Journal of Eukaryotic Microbiology 47, 260–263.

Dubey, J.P., Ott-Joslin, J., Torgerson, R.W., Topper, J.J., Sundberg, J.P., 1988. Toxoplasmosis in black-faced kangaroos (*Macropus fuliginosus melanops*). Veterinary Parasitology 30, 97–105.

Dubey, J.P., Rosenthal, B.M., Speer, C.A., 2001g. *Sarcocystis lindsayi* n. sp. (Protozoa: Sarcocystidae) from the South American opossum, *Didelphis albiventris* from Brazil. Journal of Eukaryotic Microbiology 48, 595–603.

Dubey, J.P., Rosypal, A.C., Rosenthal, B.M., Thomas, N.J., Lindsay, D.S., Stanek, J.F., Reed, S.M., Saville, W.J.A., 2001h. *Sarcocystis neurona* infections in sea otter (*Enhydra lutris*): evidence for natural infections with sarcocysts and transmission of infection to opossums (*Didelphis virginiana*). Journal of Parasitology 87, 1387–1393.

Dubey, J.P., Saville, W.J.A., Lindsay, D.S., Sitch, R.W., Stanek, J.F., Speer, C.A., Rosenthal, B.M., Njoku, C.J., Kwok, O.C.H., Shen, S.K., Reed, S.M., 2000d. Completion of the life cycle of *Sarcocystis neurona*. Journal of Parasitology 86, 1276–1280.

Dubey, J.P., Saville, W.J.A., Stanek, J.F., Lindsay, D.S., Rosenthal, B.M., Oglesbee, M.J., Rosypal, A.C., Njoku, C.J., Stich, R.W., Kwok, O.C.H., Shen, S.K., Hamir, A.N., Reed, S.M., 2001i. *Sarcocystis neurona* infections in raccoons (*Procyon lotor*): evidence for natural infection with sarcocysts, transmission of infection to opossums (*Didelphis virginiana*), and experimental induction of neurologic disease in raccoons. Veterinary Parasitology 100, 117–129.

Dubey, J.P., Speer, C.A., Bowman, D.D., Horton, K.M., Venturini, C., Venturini, L., 2000e. Experimental transmission of *Sarcocystis speeri* Dubey and Lindsay, 1999 from the South American opossum (*Didelphis albiventris*) to the North American opossum (*Didelphis virginiana*). Journal of Parasitology 86, 624–627.

Dubey, J.P., Speer, C.A., Fayer, R., 1989. Sarcocystosis of Animals and Man. CRC Press, Boca Raton, FL. 215 p.

Dubey, J.P., Speer, C.A., Lindsay, D.S., 1998. Isolation of a third species of Sarcocystis in immunodeficient mice fed feces from opossums (*Didelphis virginiana*) and its differentiation from *Sarcosystis falcatula* and *Sarcocystis neurona*. Journal of Parasitology 84, 1158–1164.

Dubey, J.P., Speer, C.A., Lindsay, D.S., 2000f. In vitro cultivation of schizonts of *Sarcocystis speeri* Dubey and Lindsay, 1999. Journal of Parasitology 86, 671–678.

Dubey, J.P., Venturini, L., Venturini, C., Basso, W., Unzaga, J., 1990. Isolation of *Sarcocystis falcatula* from the South American opossum (*Didelphis albiventris*) from Argentinian. Veterinary Parasitology 86, 239–244.

Dubey, J.P., Venturini, L., Venturini, M.C., Speer, C.A., 2000g. Isolation of *Sarcocystis speeri* Dubey and Lindsay, 1999 from the South American opossum (*Didelphis albiventris*) from Argentina. Journal of Parasitology 86, 160–163.

Duszynski, D.W., 2002. Coccidia (Apicomplexa: Eimeriidae) of the mammalian order Chiroptera. Special Publication of the Museum of Southwestern Biology, No. 5. First Impressions, Inc, Albuquerque, New Mexico, USA, 45p.

Duszynski, D.W., Box, E.D., 1978. The opossum (*Didelphis virginiana*) as a host for *Sarcocystis debonei* from cowbirds (*Molothrus ater*) and grackles (*Cassidix mexicanus, Quiscalus quiscula*). Journal of Parasitology 64, 326–329.

Duszynski, D.W., Bolek, M.G., Upton, S.J., 2007. Coccidia (Apicomplexa: Eimeriidae) of amphibians of the world. (Zootaxa 1667). Magnolia Press, Auckland, New Zealand, pp.1–77.

Duszynski, D.W., Couch, L., 2013. The Biology and Identification of the Coccidia (Apicomplexa) of Rabbits of the World. Academic Press, Amsterdam, 340 p. ISBN: 978-0-12-397899-8.

Duszynski, D.W., Morrow, J.J., 2014. The Biology and Identification of the Coccidia (Apicomplexa) of Turtles of the World. Academic Press, Amsterdam, 210 p. ISBN: 978-0-12-801367-0.

Duszynski, D.W., Upton, S.J., 2000. Coccidia (Apicomplexa: Eimeriidae) of the mammalian order Insectivora. Special publication of the Museum of Southwestern Biology. No. 4. University of New Mexico Printing Services, Albuquerque, New Mexico, USA, 67p.

Duszynski, D.W., Upton, S.J., 2001. *Cyclospora, Eimeria, Isopora* and *Cryptosporidium* spp. In: Samuel, W.M., Pybus, M.J., Kocan, A.A. (Eds.), Parasitic Diseases of Wild Mammals, second ed. Iowa State University Press, Ames, IA, pp. 416–459.

Duszynski, D.W., Upton, S.J., 2010. The Biology of the Coccidia (Apicomplexa) of Snakes of the World. A Scholarly Handbook for Identification and Treatment. CreateSpace, 422 p. ISBN: 10: 1448617995. https://www.CreateSpace.com/3388533.

Duszynski, D.W., Wilber, P.G., 1997. A guideline for the preparation of species descriptions in the Eimeriidae. Invited critical comment. Journal of Parasitology 83, 333–336.

Duszynski, D.W., Wilson, W.D., Upton, S.J., Levine, N.D., 1999. Coccidia (Apicomplexa: Eimeriidae) in the Primates and Scandentia. International Journal of Primatology 20, 761–797.

d'Utra e.Silva, O., Arantes, J.B., 1916. Sobres uma hemogregarina da gambá, *Hemogregarina didelphydis* n. sp. Memorias do Instituto Oswaldo Cruz, Rio de Janeiro 8, 61–64.

Eden, R., 1555. The Decades of the newe worlde or west India, conteynyng the navigations and conquests of the Spanyardes, with the particular description of the moste ryche and large landes and Ilandes lately founde in the west Ocean perteynyng to the inheritaunce of the kinges of Spayne [etc.]. Londini: In aedibus Guilhelmi Powell. In: Arber, E. (Ed.), The First Three English Books on America. Turnbull, and Spears, Edinburgh (1885).

Edgcomb, J.H., Walker, D.H., Johnson, C.M., 1976. *Klossiella* in the opossum. Veterinary Pathology 13, 315–318.

Elsheikha, H.M., Mansfield, L.S., 2007. Molecular typing of *Sarcocystis neurona*: current status and future trends. Veterinary Parasitology 149, 43–55.

Elsheikha, H.M., Fitzgerald, S.D., Mansfield, L.S., Mahdi Saeed, A., 2003. *Sarcocystis inghami* n. sp. (Sporozoa: Sarcocystidae) from the skeletal muscles of the Virginia opossum *Didelphis virginiana* in Michigan. Systematic Parasitology 56, 77–84.

Elsheikha, H.M., Fitzgerald, S.D., Rosenthal, B.M., Mansfield, L.S., 2004a. Concurrent presence of *Sarcocystis neurona* sporocysts, *Besnoitia darlingi* tissue cysts, and *Sarcocystis inghami* sarcocysts in naturally infected opossums (*Didelphis virginiana*). Journal of Veterinary Diagnostic Investigation 16, 352–356.

Elsheikha, H.M., Murphy, A.J., Mansfield, L.S., 2004b. Prevalence of *Sarcocystis* species sporocysts in Northern Virginia opossums (*Didelphis virginiana*). Parasitology Research 93, 427–431.

Enders, R.K., 1937. *Panniculus carnosus* and formation of the pouch in didelphids. Journal of Morphology 61, 1–26.

Ernst, J.V., Cooper Jr., C., Chobotar, B., 1969. *Isospora boughtoni* Volk, 1938 and *Isospora* sp. (Protozoa: Eimeriidae) from an opossum *Didelphis marsupialis*. Bulletin of the Wildlife Disease Association 5, 406–409.

Ernst, J.V., Todd, K.S., Barnard, W.P., 1977. Endogenous stages of *Eimeria sigmodontis* (Protozoa: Eimeriidae) in the cotton rat, *Sigmodon hispidus*. Journal of Parasitology 7, 373–381.

Esteban, E., Anderson, B.C., 1995. *Cryptosporidium muris*: prevalence, persistency, and detrimental effect on milk production in a dry lot dairy. Journal of Dairy Science 78, 1068–1072.

Eymann, J., Herbert, C.A., Cooper, D.W., Dubey, J.P., 2006. Serologic survey for *Toxoplasma gondii* and *Neospora caninum* in the common brushtail possum (*Trichosurus vulpecula*) from urban Sydney, Australia. Journal of Parasitology 92, 267–272.

Fayer, R., 2010. Taxonomy and species delimitation in *Cryptosporidium*. Experimental Parasitology 124, 90–97.

Fayer, R., Smith, M., 2009. *Cryptosporidium xiaoi* n. sp. (Apicomplexa: Cryptosporidiidae) in sheep (*Ovis aries*). Veterinary Parasitology 164, 192–200.

Fayer, R., Morgan, U., Upton, S.J., 2000. Epidemiology of *Cryptosporidium*: transmission, detection and identification. International Journal for Parasitology 30, 1305–1322.

Fayer, R., Phillips, L., Anderson, B.C., Bush, M., 1991. Chronic cryptosporidiosis in a bactrian camel (*Camelus bactrianus*). Journal of Zoo and Wildlife Medicine 22, 228–232.

Feng, Y., Ortega, Y., He, G., Das, P., Xu, M., Zhang, X., Fayer, R., Gatei, W., Cama, V., Xiao, L., 2007. Wide geographic distribution of *Cryptosporidium bovis* and the deer-like genotype in bovines. Veterinary Parasitology 144, 1–9.

Fenger, C.K., Granstrom, D.E., Langemeier, J.L., Gajadhar, A., Cothran, G., Tramontin, R.R., Stamper, S., Dubey, J.P., 1994. Phylogenetic relationship of *Sarcocystis neurona* to other members of the family Sarcocystidae based on the sequence of the small ribosomal subunit gene. Journal of Parasitology 79, 966–975.

Fenger, C.K., Granstrom, D.E., Langemeier, J.L., Stamper, S., Donahue, J.M., Patterson, J.S., Gajadhar, A.A., Marteniuk, J.V., Xiaomin, Z., Dubey, J.P., 1995. Identification of opossums (*Didelphis virginiana*) as the putative definitive host of *Sarcocystis neurona*. Journal of Parasitology 81, 916–919.

Flatt, R.E., Nelson, L.R., Patton, N.M., 1971. *Besnoitia darlingi* in the opossum (*Didelphis marsupialis*). Laboratory Animal Science 2, 106–109.

Frenkel, J.K., 1955 (1953). Infections with organisms resembling *Toxoplasma*, together with the description of a new organism: *Besnoitia jellisoni*. Atti del VI Congresso Internazionale di Microbiologia, Roma 5, 426–434.

Frens, K., 2011. Peramelemorphia (on-line) Animal Diversity Web. Accessed February 11, 2015 at: http://animaldiversity.org/accounts/Peramelemorphia/.

Frey, J.K., Yates, T.L., Duszynski, D.W., Gannon, W.L., Gardner, S.L., 1992. Designation and curatorial management of type host specimens (symbiotypes) for new parasite species. Journal of Parasitology 78, 930–932.

Gardner, A.L., 2005a. Order Didelphimorphia. In: Wilson, D.E., Reeder, D.M. (Eds.), Mammal Species of the World: a Taxonomic and Geographic Reference, third ed., vol. 1. The Johns Hopkins University Press, Baltimore, MD, pp. 3–18.

Gardner, A.L., 2005b. Order Microbiotheria. In: Wilson, D.E., Reeder, D.A. (Eds.), Mammal Species of the World: a Taxonomic and Geographic Reference, third ed., vol. 1. The Johns Hopkins University Press, Baltimore, MD, p. 21.

Gardner, A.L. (Ed.), 2008 (2007). Mammals of South America. vol. 1. Marsupials, Xenarthrans, Shrews, and Bats. Chicago University Press, Chicago, p. 669.

Gardner, S.L., Duszynski, D.W., 1990. Polymorphism of eimerian oocysts can be a problem in naturally infected hosts: an example from subterranean rodents in Bolivia. Journal of Parasitology 76, 805–811.

Garner, M.M., Gardiner, C.H., Wellehan, J.F.X., Johnson, A.J., McNamara, T., Linn, M., Terrell, S.P., Childress, A., Jacobson, E.R., 2006. Intranuclear coccidiosis in tortoises: nine cases. Veterinary Pathology 43, 311–320.

Garnham, P.C.C., 1964. Discovery of Besnoitia in the basilisk lizard. Transactions of the Royal Society of Tropical Medicine and Hygiene 58, 286.

Garnham, P.C.C., 1965. Besnoitia in Lizards. Progress in Protozoology. Abstracts of papers read at the Second International Conference of Protozoology, London, UK, 29 July–5 August, 1965, International Congress Series No. 91, Excerpta Medica Foundation, Amsterdam, Abstract No. 126: 124.

Garnham, P.C.C., 1966. Besnoitia (Protozoa: Toxoplasmea) in lizards. Parasitology 56, 329–334.

Garnham, P.C.C., Lewis, D.J., 1958. Demonstration. Some parasites from British Honduras. Transactions of the Royal Society of Tropical Medicine and Hygiene 52, 295–296.

Gerhold, R.W., McDougald, L.R., Beckstead, R.B., 2015. A novel, simplified technique to amplify Eimeria (Coccidia: Apicomplexa) DNA from oocysts. Journal of Parasitology 101, 102–103.

Gibb, D.G., Kakulas, B.A., Perret, D.J., Jenkyn, D.J., 1966. Toxoplasmosis in the Rottnest Quokka (Setonix brachyurus). Australian Journal of Experimental Biology and Medical Science 44, 665–672.

Giles, M., Chalmers, R., Pritchard, G., Elwin, K., Mueller-Dolbies, D., Clifton-Hadley, F., 2009. Cryptosporidium parvum in a goat and a sheep in the UK. Veterinary Record 164, 24–25.

Gilruth, J.A., Bull, L.B., 1912. Article XXVIII. Enteritis, associated with infection of the intestinal wall by cyst-forming protozoa (Neosporidia), occurring in certain native animals (wallaby, kangaroo, and wombat). Proceedings of the Royal Society of Victoria, NSW 24 (Part II), 432–450.

Granstrom, D.E., MacPherson, J.M., Gajadhar, A.A., Dubey, J.P., Tramontin, R., Stamper, S., 1994. Differentiation of Sarcocystis neurona from eight related coccidia by random amplified polymorphic DNA assay. Molecular and Cellular Probes 8, 353–356.

Groves, C.P., 2005a. Order Dasyuromorphia. In: Wilson, D.E., Reeder, D.M. (Eds.), Mammal Species of the World: a Taxonomic and Geographic Reference, third ed., vol. 1. The Johns Hopkins University Press, Baltimore, MD, pp. 23–37.

Groves, C.P., 2005b. Order Peramelemorphia. In: Wilson, D.E., Reeder, D.M. (Eds.), Mammal Species of the World: a Taxonomic and Geographic Reference, third ed., vol. 1. The Johns Hopkins University Press, Baltimore, MD, pp. 38–42.

Grünberg, W., 1959. Toxoplasmose beim Bennett-Känguruh (Makropus bennetti Gould) und einem Klippschilefer (Hydrax syriacus Schreb). Wiener Tierärztliche Monatsschrift 46, 586–593.

Guyot, K., Follet-Dumoulin, A., Lelievre, E., Sarfati, C., Rabodonirina, M., Nevez, G., Cailliez, J.C., Camus, D., Dei-Cas, E., 2001. Molecular characterization of Cryptosporidium isolates obtained from humans in France. Journal of Clinical Microbiology 39, 3472–3480.

Hackel, D.B., Kinney, T.D., Wendt, W., 1953. Pathologic lesions in captive wild animals. III. Toxoplasmosis in a kangaroo. Laboratory Investigations 2, 154–163.

Harding, H.R., 1987. Interrelationships of the families of the Diprotodontia—a view based on spermatozoan ultrastructure. In: Archer, M. (Ed.), Possums and Opossums: Studies in Evolution. Surrey Beatty and Sons, Chipping Norton, New South Wales, Australia, pp. 195–216.

Hartley, M., English, A., 2005. A seroprevalence survey of Toxoplasma gondii in common wombats (Vombatus ursinus). European Journal of Wildlife Research 51, 65–67.

Hartley, W.J., Dubey, J.P., Spielman, D.S., 1990. Fatal toxoplasmosis in koalas (Phascolarctos cinereus). Journal of Parasitology 76, 271–272.

Heckscher, S.K., Wickersberg, B.A., Duszynski, D.W., Gardner, S.L., 1999. Three new species of Eimeria from Bolivian marsupials. International Journal for Parasitology 29, 275–284.

Henry, A., Masson, G., 1932. Considérations sur le genre Globidium, Globidium cameli n. sp., parasite du dromedaire. Annales de Parasitologie, Humaine et Comparee 10, 385–401.

Hendricks, L.D., 1974. A redescription of Isospora artopitheci Rodhain, 1933 (Protozoa: Eimeriidae) from primates of Panama. Proceedings of the Helminthological Society of Washington 41, 229–233.

Hendricks, L.D., 1977. Host range characteristics of the primate coccidian Isospora arctopitheci Rodhain 1933 (Protozoa: Eimeriidae). Journal of Parasitology 63, 32–35.

Hendricks, L.D., Walton, B.C., 1974. Vertebrate intermediate hosts in the life cycle of an isosporan from a non-human primate. Proceedings of the International Congress of Parasitology 1, 96–97.

Herskhovitz, P., 1999. Dromiciops gliroides Thomas, 1894, last of the Microbiotheria (Marsupialia) with a review of the family Microbiotheriidae. Fieldiana Zoology 93, 1–60.

Hilgenfeld, M., 1965. Enzootic outbreak of toxoplasmosis in kangaroos. In: Progress in Protozoology. Proceedings of the 2nd International Conference of Protozoology, 29 July–5 August, London, United Kingdom. Excerpta Medica Foundation, New York, p. 184. Abstract No. 211.

Hill, N.J., Deane, E.M., Power, M.L., 2008. Prevalence and genetic characterization of *Cryptosporidium* isolates from common brushtail possums (*Trichosurus vulpecula*) adapted to urban settings. Applied and Environmental Microbiology 74, 5549–5555.

Hill, N.J., Richter, C., Power, M.L., 2012. Pinning down a polymorphic parasite: new genetic and morphological descriptions of *E. macropodis* from the tammar wallaby (*Macropus eugenii*). Parasitology International 61, 461–465.

Hillyer, E.V., Anderson, M.P., Greiner, E., Atkinson, C.T., Frenkel, J.K., 1991. An outbreak of *Sarcocystis* in a collection of psittacines. Journal of Zoo and Wildlife Medicine 22, 434–445.

Hnida, J.A., Duszynski, D.W., 1999a. Taxonomy and systematics of some *Eimeria* species of murid rodents as determined by the ITS1 region of the ribosomal gene complex. Parasitology 199, 349–357.

Hnida, J.A., Duszynski, D.W., 1999b. Taxonomy and phylogeny of some *Eimeria* (Apicomplexa: Eimeriidae) species of rodents as determined by polymerase chain reaction/restriction-fragment-length polymorphism analysis of 18s rDNA. Parasitology Research 85, 887–894.

Hoberg, E.P., Phillips, A.J., 2014. Transfer of the U.S. National parasite collection. Comparative Parasitology 81, 300–301 and Syst Parasitol 89:1–2.

Horovitz, L., Sánchez-Villagra, M.R., 2003. A morphological analysis of marsupial mammal higher-level phylogenetic relationships. Cladistics 19, 181–212.

Houk, A.E., Goodwin, D.G., Zajac, A.M., Barr, S.C., Dubey, J.P., Lindsay, D.S., 2010. Prevalence of antibodies to *Trypanosoma cruzi*, *Toxoplasma gondii*, *Encephalitozoon cuniculi*, *Sarcosystis neurona*, *Besnoitia darlingi*, and *Neospora caninum* in North American opossums, *Didelphis virginiana*, from Southern Louisiana. Journal of Parasitology 96, 1119–1122.

Hum, S., Barton, N.J., Obendorf, D., Barker, I.K., 1991. Coccidiosis in common wombats (*Vombatus ursinus*). Journal of Wildlife Diseases 27, 697–700.

Hutton, J.B., 1979. Some diseases of possums. In: Goldsmith, M. (Ed.), Opossum Field Day. Ministry of Agriculture and Fisheries, Rangiora, pp. 22–25.

Iseki, M., 1979. *Cryptosporidium felis* sp. n. (Protozoa, Eimeriorina) from the domestic cat. Japanese Journal of Parasitology 22, 285–307.

Iseki, M., 1986. Two species of *Cryptosporidium* naturally infecting house rats, *Rattus norvegicus*. Japanese Journal of Parasitology 35, 521–526.

Iseki, M., Maekawa, T., Moriya, K., Uni, S., Takada, S., 1989. Infectivity of *Cryptosporidium muris* (strain RN 66) in various laboratory animals. Parasitology Research 75, 218–222.

Jakes, K.A., 1998. *Sarcocystis mucosa* in Bennett's wallabies and pademelons from Tasmania. Journal of Wildlife Diseases 34, 594–599.

Jensen, J.M., Patton, S., Wright, B.G., Loeffler, D.G., 1985. Toxoplasmosis in marsupials in a zoological collection. Journal of Zoo Animal Medicine 16, 129–131.

Jirků, M., Kirků, M., Oborník, M., Lukeš, J., Modrý, D., 2009. A model for taxonomic work on homoxenous coccidia: redescription, host specificity, and molecular phylogeny of *Eimeria ranae* Dobell, 1909, with a review of anuran-host *Eimeria* (Apicomplexa: Eimeriorina). Journal of Eukaryotic Microbiology 56, 39–51.

Johnson, A.M., Roberts, H., Munday, B.L., 1988. Prevalence of *Toxoplasma gondii* antibody in wild macropods. Australian Veterinary Journal 65, 199–201.

Johnson, A.M., Roberts, H., Statham, P., Munday, B.L., 1989. Serodiagnosis of acute toxoplasmosis in macropods. Veterinary Parasitology 34, 25–33.

Johnston, T.H., 1910a. Exhibition of a *Coccidium* sp. from the intestinal walls of *M. thetidis* hosts. Proceedings of the Linnean Society of New South Wales 44, 523–524.

Johnston, T.H., 1910b. Exhibition of a portion of the small intestine of a kangaroo, *Macropus giganteus* Zimm., showing the presence of a *Coccidium* sp. Proceedings of the Linnean Society of New South Wales 44, 804.

Jolly, S.E., 1993. Biological control of possums. New Zealand Journal of Zoology 20, 335–339.

Joseph, T., 1974. *Eimeria indianensis* sp. n. and an *Isospora* sp. from the opossum *Didelphis virginiana* (Kerr). Journal of Protozoology 21, 12–15.

Kalyakin, V.N., Zasukhin, D.N., 1975. Distribution of *Sarcocystis* (Protozoa: Sporozoa) in vertebrates. Folia Parasitologica 22, 289–307.

Karanis, P., Plutzer, J., Halim, N.A., Igori, K., Nagasawa, H., Ongerth, J., Liqing, M., 2007. Molecular characterization of *Cryptosporidium* from animal sources in Qinghai province of China. Parasitology Research 101, 1575–1580.

Kirsch, J.A.W., 1977. The comparative serology of Marsupialia and a classification of marsupials. Australian Journal of Zoology Supplemental Series 52, 1–152.

Kirsch, J.A.W., Palma, R.E., 1995. DNA/DNA hybridization studies of carnivorous marsupials. V. A further estimate of relationships among opossums (Marsupialia: Didelphidae). Mammalia 59, 403–425.

Kirsch, J.A.W., Poole, W.E., 1972. Taxonomy and distribution of the grey kangaroos, *Macropus giganteus* Shaw and *Macropus fuliginosus* (Desmarest), and their subspecies (Marsupialia: Macropodidae). Australian Journal of Zoology 20, 315–339.

Kirsch, J.A.W., Lapointe, F.-J., Springer, M.S., 1997. DNA-hybridization studies of marsupials and their implications for metatherian classification. Australian Journal of Zoology 45, 211–280.

Krieg, H., 1924. Beobachtungen an argentinischen Beutelratten. Zeitschrift für Morphologie und Ökologie der Tiere 1, 637–659.

Kriegs, J.O., Churakov, G., Kiefmann, M., Jordan, U., Brosius, J., Schmitz, J., 2006. Retroposed elements as archives for the evolutionary history of placental mammals. PLoS Biology 4 (4), e91.

Kullberg, M., Hallström, B., Arnason, U., Janke, A., 2008. Expressed sequence tags from the platypus reject the Marsupionata and acknowledge the Theria hypothesis. Zoologica Scripta 37, 115–127.

Kvičerova, J., Pakandl, M., Hypša, V., 2008. Phylogenetic relationships among Eimeria spp. (Apicomplexa, Eimeriidae) infecting rabbits: evolutionary significance of biological and morphological features. Parasitology 135, 443–452.

Lainson, R., Shaw, J.J., 1989. Two new species of Eimeria and three new species of Isospora (Apicomplexa: Eimeriidae) from Brazilian mammals and birds. Bulletin du Muséum National d'Histoire Naturelle (Paris) Ser. 4 Sect. A 11, 349–365.

Lapointe, J.M., Duignan, P.J., Marsh, A.E., Gulland, F.M., Barr, B.C., Naydan, D.K., King, D.P., Farman, C.A., Huntingdon, K.A.B., Lowenstine, L.J., 1998. Meningoencephalitis due to a Sarcocystis neurona-like protozoan in Pacific harbor seals (Phoca vitulina richardsi). Journal of Parasitology 84, 1184–1189.

Lee, J.J., Leedale, G.F., Bradbury, P. (Eds.), 2000. An Illustrated Guide to the Protozoa, second ed. Society of Protozoologists, P.O. Box 368, Lawrence, KS, vol. 1. p. 689.

Leighton, F.A., Gajadhar, A.A., 2001. Besnoitia spp. and besnoitiosis. In: Samuel, W.M., Pybus, M.J., Kocan, A.A. (Eds.), Parasitic Diseases of Wild Mammals, second ed. Iowa State University Press, Ames, IA, pp. 468–478.

Levine, N.D., 1973. Protozoan Parasites of Domestic Animals and of Man, second ed. Burgess, Minneapolis, MN. 406 p.

Levine, N.D., 1977. Taxonomy of Toxoplasma. Journal of Protozoology 24, 36–41.

Levine, N.D., 1979. What is 'Sarcocystis' mucosa? Annals of Tropical Medicine and Parasitolory 73, 91–92.

Levine, N.D., 1982. Taxonomy and life cycles of coccidia. In: Long, P.L. (Ed.), The Biology of the Coccidia, second ed. University Park Press Inc., Baltimore, MD, USA, pp. 1–33.

Levine, N.D., 1986. The taxonomy of Sarcocystis (Protozoa, Apicomplexa) species. Journal of Parasitology 72, 372–382.

Levine, N.D., 1988. The coccidia: Adeleinorina. The Protozoan Phylum Apicomplexa, vol. I. CRC Press, Boca Raton, FL, pp. 133–134.

Levine, N.D., Ivens, V., 1965. The Coccidian Parasites (Protozoa, Apicomplexa) of Rodents. Illinois Biological Monograph No. 33. University of Illinois Press, Urbana, IL, 356 p.

Levine, N.D., Ivens, V., 1981. The Coccidian Parasites (Protozoa, Apicomplexa) of Carnivores. Illinois Biological Monograph No. 51. University of Illinois Press, Urbana, IL, 248 p.

Lindsay, D.S., Dubey, J.P., Horton, K.M., Bowman, D.D., 1999. Development of Sarcocystis falcatula in cell cultures demonstrates that it is different from Sarcocystis neurona. Parasitology 118, 227–233.

Lindsay, D.S., Hendricks, C.M., Blagburn, B.L., 1988. Experimental Cryptosporidium parvum infections in opossums (Didelphis virginiana). Journal of Wildlife Diseases 24, 157–159.

Lindsay, D.S., Thomas, N.J., Dubey, J.P., 2000. Biological characterization of Sarcocystis neurona isolated from a southern sea otter (Enhydra lutris nereis). International Journal for Parasitology 30, 617–624.

Linnaeus, C., 1758. Systema naturae per regna tria naturae, secundum classes, ordines, genera, species, cum characteribus, differentiis, synonymis, locis, tenth ed., vol. 1. Laurentii Salvii, Stockholm.

Lobos, G., Charrier, A., Carrasco, G., Palma, R.E., 2005. Presence of Dromiciops gliroides (Microbiotheria: Microbiotheriidae) in the deciduous forests of central Chile. Mammalian Biology 70, 376–380.

Lou, Z., Ji, Q., Wible, J.R., Yuan, C.-X., 2003. An early Cretaceous tribosphenic mammal and metatherian evolution. Science 302, 1934–1940.

Lujan, N.K., Page, L.M., February 27, 2015. Libraries of Life. Op-ed Contribution. New York Times.

Lynch, M.J., Obendorf, D.L., Statham, P., Reddacliff, G.L., 1993. An evaluation of a live Toxoplasma gondii vaccine in Tammar wallabies (Macropus eugenii). Australian Veterinary Journal 70, 352–353.

Mackerras, I.M., Mackerras, M.J., 1960. Taxonomy of the common short-nosed marsupial bandicoot in eastern Queensland. Australian Journal of Science 23, 51–52.

Mackerras, I.M., Mackerras, M.J., Sandars, D.F., 1953. Parasites of the bandicoot, Isoodon obesulus. Proceedings of the Royal Society of Queensland (for 1951) 63, 61–63.

Mackerras, M.J., 1958. Catalogue of Australian mammals and their recorded internal parasites. Part I. Monotremes and marsupials. Proceedings of the Linnean Society of New South Wales 83, 101–160.

Mandelli, G., Cerioli, G., Hahn, E.E.A., Strozzi, F., 1966. Osservazioni anatomohistologiche e parassitologiche su di un episocio de toxoplasmosi nel canguro di Bennett (Macropis bennetti Gould). Bollettino del Istituto Sieroterapico Milanese 45, 177–192.

Mandour, A.M., 1965. Sarcocystis garnhami n. sp. in the skeletal muscle of an opossum, Didelphis marsupialis. Journal of Protozoology 12, 606–609.

Marsh, A.E., Barr, B.C., Tell, L., Koski, M., Greiner, E., Dame, J., Conrad, P.A., 1997. In vitro cultivation and experimental inoculation of Sarcocystis falcatula and Sarcocystis neurona merozoites into budgerigars (Melopsittacus undulatus). Journal of Parasitology 83, 1189–1192.

Marsh, A.E., Barr, B.C., Tell, L., Bowman, D.D., Conrad, P., Ketcherside, C., Green, T., 1999. Comparison of the internal transcribed spacer, ITS-1, from Sarcocystis falcatula isolates and Sarcocystis neurona. Journal of Parasitology 85, 750–757.

Martinez, F.A., 1990. *Sarcocystis* spp. (Protozoa: Toxoplasmatinae) in *Didelphis albiventris*. Veterinaria Argentina 7, 389–392.

Matschie, P., 1916. Bemerkungen über die Gattung *Didelphis* L. Sitzungsber. Ges. Naturforsch. Freunde Berlin 1916, 259–272.

Mayhew, I.G., Dellers, R.W., Timoney, J.F., Kemen, M.J., Fayer, R., Lunde, M.N., 1978. Microbiology and serology, (Chapter 7). In: Mayhew, I.G., de Lahunta, A., Whitlock, R.H., Krook, L., Tusker, J.B. (Eds.), Spinal Cord Disease in the Horse, pp. 148–160.

McCarthy, S., Ng, J., Gordon, C., Miller, R., Wyber, A., Ryan, U.M., 2008. Prevalence of *Cryptosproidium* and *Giardia* species in animals in irrigation catchments in the southwest of Australia. Experimental Parasitology 118, 596–599.

McKenna, M.C., Bell, S.K., 1997. Classification of Mammals above the Species Level. Columbia University Press, New York City, New York. 637 p.

McKenna, P.B., 1998. Checklist of protozoan and closely related parasites of terrestrial mammals in New Zealand. New Zealand Journal of Zoology 25, 213–221.

McLauchlin, J., Amar, C., Pedraza-Diaz, S., Nichols, G.L., 2000. Molecular epidemiological analysis of *Cryptosporidium* spp. in the United Kingdom: results of genotyping *Cryptosporidium* spp. in 1,705 faecal samples from humans and 105 faecal samples from livestock animals. Journal of Clinical Microbiology 38, 3984–3990.

McLauchlin, J., Pedraza-Diaz, S., Amar-Hoetzeneder, C., Nichols, G.L., 1999. Genetic characterization of *Cryptosporidium* strains from 218 patients with diarrhea diagnosed as having sporadic cryptosporidiosis. Journal of Clinical Microbiology 37, 3153–3158.

Meredith, R.W., Westerman, M., Case, J.A., Springer, M.S., 2008a. A phylogeny and timescale for marsupial evolution based on sequences for five nuclear genes. Journal of Mammalian Evolution 15, 1–36.

Meredith, R.W., Westerman, M., Springer, M.S., 2008b. A timescale and phylogeny for "Bandicoots" (Peramelemorphia: Marsupialia) based on sequences for five nuclear genes. Molecular Phylogenetic Evolution 47, 1–20.

Meredith, R.A., Westerman, M., Springer, M.S., 2009. A phylogeny of Diprotodontia (Marsupialia) based on sequences for five nuclear genes. Molecular Phylogenetic Evolution 51, 554–571.

Merino, S., Martínez, J., Vásquez, R.A., Šlapeta, J., 2010. Monophyly of marsupial intraerythrocytic apicomplexan parasites from South America and Australia. Parasitology 137, 37–43.

Merino, S., Vásquez, R.A., Martínez, J., Celis-Diez, J.L., Martínez-de la Puente, J., Marín-Vial, P., Sánchez-Monsalvez, I., Peirce, M.A., 2008. A sarcocystid misidentified as *Hepatozoon didelphydis*: molecular data from a parasitic infection in the blood of the southern mouse opossum (*Thylamys elegans*) from Chile. Journal of Eukaryotic Microbiology 55, 536–540.

Merino, S., Vásquez, R.A., Martínez, J., Celis-Diez, J.L., Gutiérrez-Jiménez, L., Ippi, S., Sánchez-Monsalvez, I., Martínez-de la Puente, J., 2009. Molecular characterization of an ancient *Hepatozoon* species parasitizing the 'living fossil' marsupial 'monito del monte' *Dromiciops gliroides* from Chile. Biological Journal of the Linnean Society 98, 568–576.

Mikkelsen, T.S., Wakefield, M.J., Aken, B., Amemiya, C.T., Chang, J.L., Duke, S., Garber, M., Gentles, A.J., Goodstadt, L., Heger, A., et al., 2007. Genome of the marsupial *Monodelphis domestica* reveals innovation in non-coding sequences (+46 other co-authors) Nature 447, 167–177.

Miller, M.A., Ehlers, K., Dubey, J.P., van Steenbergh, K., 1992. Outbreak of toxoplasmosis in wallabies on an exotic animal farm. Journal of Veterinary Diagnostic Investigation 4, 480–483.

Minchin, E.A., 1903. Sporozoa. In: Lankester, E.R. (Ed.), Treatise on Zoology. A & C Black, London, United Kingdom, pp. 150–360.

Modrý, D., Slapeta, R.R., Jirkù, M., Oborník, M., Lukeš, J., Koudela, R., 2001. Phylogenetic position of a renal coccidium of the European green frogs, '*Isospora' lieberkuehni* Labbe, 1894 (Apicomplexa: Sarcocystidae) and its taxonomic implications. International Journal of Systematic and Evolutionary Microbiology 51, 767–772.

Monteiro, R.M., Keid, L.B., Richtzenhain, L.J., Valadas, S.Y., Muller, G., Soares, R.M., 2013. Extensively variable surface antigens of *Sarcocystis* spp. infecting Brazilian marsupials in the genus *Didelphis* occur in myriad allelic combinations, suggesting sexual recombination has aided their diversification. Veterinary Parasitology 196, 64–70.

Morgan, U.M., Constantine, C.C., Forbes, D.A., Thompson, R.C.A., 1997. Differentiation between human and animal isolates of *Cryptosporidium parvum* using rDNA sequencing and direct PCR analysis. Journal of Parasitology 83, 825–830.

Morgan, U.M., Morris, P.T., Fayer, R., Deplazes, P., Thompson, R.C.A., 1999a. Phylogenetic relationships among isolates of *Cryptosporidium*: evidence for several new species. Journal of Parasitology 85, 1126–1133.

Morgan, U.M., Deplazes, P., Forbes, D.A., Spano, F., Hertzberg, H., Sargent, K.D., Elliot, A., Thompson, R.C.A., 1999b. Sequence and PCR-RFLP analysis of the internal transcribed spacers of the rDNA repeat unit in isolates of *Cryptosporidium* from different hosts. Parasitology 118, 49–58.

Morgan, U.M., Pallant, L., Dwyer, B.W., Forbes, D.A., Rich, G., Thompson, R.C.A., 1998. Comparison of PCR and microscopy for detection of *Cryptosporidium* in human faecal samples: clinical trial. Journal of Clinical Microbiology 36, 995–998.

Morgan-Ryan, U.M., Fall, A., Ward, L.A., Hijjawi, N., Sulaiman, I., Fayer, R., Thompson, R.C.A., Olson, M., 2002. *Cryptosporidium hominis* n. sp. (Apicomplexa: Cryptosporidiidae) from *Homo sapiens*. Journal of Eukaryotic Microbiology 49, 433–440.

Munday, B.L., 1970. The Epidemiology of Toxoplasmosis with Particular Reference to the Tasmanian Environment (MVSc thesis). University of Melbourne. Published as a monograph by the Tasmanian Department of Agriculture.

Munday, B.L., 1988. Marsupial Diseases, vol. 104. ,Postgraduate Committee in Veterinary Science, University of Sydney. pp. 299–365.

Munday, B.L., Mason, R.W., Hartley, W.J., Presidente, P.J.A., Obendorf, D., 1978. Sarcocystis and related organisms in Australian wildlife. I. Survey findings in mammals. Journal of Wildlife Diseases 14, 417–433.

Munemasa, M., Nikaido, M., Donnellan, S., Austin, C.C., Okada, N., Hasegawa, M., 2006. Phylogenetic analysis of diprotodontian marsupials based on complete mitochondrial genomes. Genes and Genetic Systematics 81, 181–191.

Mykytowycz, R., 1964. Coccidia in wild populations of the red kangaroo Megaleia rufa (Desmarest). Parasitology 54, 105–115.

Naiff, R.D., Arias, J.R., 1983. Besnoitia (Protozoa: Toxoplasmatinae) isolado de mucuras Didelphis marsupialis na Região Amazônica, Brasil. Memorias do Instituto Oswaldo Cruz, Rio de Janeiro 78, 431–435.

Neill, P.J.G., Smith, J.H., Box, E.D., 1989. Pathogenesis of Sarcocystis falcatula (Apicomplexa: Sarcocystidae) in the budgerigar (Melopsittacus undulatus). IV. Ultrastructure of developing, mature and degenerating sarcocysts. Journal of Protozoology 36, 430–437.

Ng, J., Yang, R., Whiffin, V., Cox, P., Ryan, U., 2011. Identification of zoonotic Cryptosporidium and Giardia genotypes infecting animals in Sydney's water catchments. Experimental Parasitology 128, 138–144.

Nicolle, C., Manceaux, L., 1908. Sur une infection e corps de Leishman (ou organismes voisins) du gondi. Comptes Rendus de l'Academie des Sciences 147, 763–766.

Nicolle, C., Manceaux, L., 1909. Sur un protozoaire nouveau du gondi: Toxoplasma N. Gen. Masson, 1909. Comptes Rendus de l'Academie des Sciences 148, 369–372.

Nilsson, M.A., Arnason, U., Spencer, P.B.S., Janke, A., 2004. Marsupial relationships and a timeline for marsupial radiation in South Gondwana. Gene 340, 189–196.

Nilsson, M.A., Churakov, G., Sommer, M., Van Tran, N., Zemann, A., Brosius, J., Schmitz, J., 2010. Tracking marsupial evolution using archaic genomic retroposon insertions. PLoS Biology 8 (7), e100436 (9 pgs.).

Nilsson, M.A., Gullberg, A., Spotorno, A.E., Arnason, U., Janke, A., 2003. Radiation of extant marsupials after the K/T boundary: evidence from complete mitochondrial genomes. Journal of Molecular Evolution 57, S3–S12.

Nöller, W., 1920. Globidium (Gastrocystis, Besnoitia). In: Prowazek, S. (Ed.), Handbuch der Pathologenen Protozoen, II. Johann Ambrosius Barth Pub, Leipzig, pp. 919–933.

Nowak, R.M., 1991. fifth ed. Walker's Mammals of the World, vol. 1. ,Johns Hopkins University Press, Baltimore, Maryland. 642 p.

Oakwood, M., Pritchard, D., 1999. Little evidence of toxoplasmosis in a declining species, the northern quoll (Dasyurus hallucatus). Wildlife Research 26, 329–333.

Obendorf, D.L., 1983. Diseases of dasyurid marsupials. Journal of Wildlife Diseases 19, 132–137.

Obendorf, D.L., Munday, B.L., 1983. Toxoplasmosis in wild Tasmanian wallabies. Australian Veterinary Journal 60, 62.

Obendorf, D.L., Munday, B.L., 1990. Toxoplasmosis in wild eastern barred bandicoots, Perameles gunnii. In: Seebeck, J.H., Brown, P.R., Wallis, R.L., Kemper, C.M. (Eds.), Bandicoots and Bilbies. Surrey Beaty & Sons, Sidney, Australia, pp. 193–197.

Obendorf, D.L., Statham, P., Driessen, M., 1996. Detection of agglutinating antibodies to Toxoplasma gondii in sera from free-ranging eastern barred bandicoots (Perameles gunnii). Journal of Wildlife Diseases 32, 623–626.

Odening, K., 1998. The present state of species-systematics in Sarcocystis Lankester, 1882 (Protista, Sporozoa, Coccidia). Systematic Parasitology 41, 209–233.

O'Brien, E., McInnes, L., Ryan, U., 2008. Cryptosporidium GP60 genotypes from humans and domesticated animals in Australia, North America and Europe. Experimental Parasitology 118, 118–121.

O'Callaghan, M.G., Moore, E., 1986. Parasites and serological survey of the common brushtail possum (Trichosurus vulpecula) from Kangaroo Island, South Australia. Journal of Wildlife Diseases 22, 589–591.

O'Callaghan, M.G., O'Donoghue, P.J., 2001. A new species of Eimeria (Apicomplexa: Eimeriidae) from the brushtail possum, Trichosurus vulpecula (Diprotodontia: Phalangeridae). Transactions of the Royal Society of South Australia 125, 129–132.

O'Callaghan, M.G., Barker, I.K., Beveridge, I., Hornsby, P., 1998. Eimeria species in the Pearson Island rock wallaby, Petrogale lateralis pearsoni. International Journal for Parasitology 28, 1889–1892.

O'Donoghue, P.J., 1985. Cryptosporidium infection in man, animals, birds and fish. Australian Veterinary Journal 62, 253–258.

O'Donoghue, P.J., 1995. Cryptosporidium and cryptosporidiosis in man and animals. International Journal for Parasitology 25, 139–195.

O'Donoghue, P.J., 1997. Protozoan parasites of wildlife in south-east Queensland. In: Tribe, A. (Ed.), Proceedings of the 1997 Conference of the Australian Association of Veterinary Conservation Biologists. Australian Veterinary Association, Brisbane, pp. 119–136.

O'Donoghue, P.J., Adlard, R.D., 2000. Catalogue of protozoan parasites recorded in Australia. Memoirs of the Queensland Museum, Part I, Brisbane 45, 1–163.

O'Donoghue, P.J., Obendorf, D.L., O'Callaghan, M.G., Moore, E., Dixon, B.R., 1987. Sarcocystis mucosa (Blanchard 1885) Labbé 1889 in an unadorned rock wallabies (Petrogale assimilis) and Bennett's wallabies (Macropus rufogriseus). Parasitology Research 73, 113–120.

Ogedengbe, J.D., Hanner, R.H., Barta, J.R., 2011. DNA barcoding identifies *Eimeria* species and contributes to the phylogenetics of coccidian parasites (Eimeriorina, Apicomplexa, Alveolata). International Journal for Parasitology 41, 843–850.

Olcott, A.T., Speer, C.A., Hendricks, L.D., 1982. Endogenous development of *Isospora arctopitheci* Rodhain, 1933 in the marmoset *Sanguinus geoffroyi*. Proceedings of the Helminthological Society of Washington 49, 118–126.

Oliver, L.R., 1976. The management of yapoks (*Chironectes minimus*) at Jersey Zoo, with observations on their behavior. Jersey Wildlife Preservation Trust 13, 32–36.

Özkul, I.A., Aydin, Y., 1994. Natural *Cryptosporidium muris* infection of the stomach in laboratory mice. Veterinary Parasitology 55, 129–132.

Patton, S., Johnson, S.L., Loeffler, D.G., Wright, B.G., Jensen, J.M., 1986. Epizootic of toxoplasmosis in kangaroos, wallabies, and potaroos: Possible transmission via domestic cats. Journal of the American Veterinary Medical Association 189, 1166–1169.

Pavlásek, I., Lavička, M., 1995. The first finding of natural *Cryptosporidium* infection of stomach in desert hamsters (*Phodopus roborovskii* Satunin, 1903). Veterinarni Medicina-Czech 40, 261–263.

Pedraza-Diaz, S., Amar, C., Nichols, G.L., McLauchlin, J., 2001. Nested polymerase chain reaction for amplification of the *Cryptosporidium* oocyst wall protein gene. Emerging Infectious Diseases 7, 49–56.

Pellérdy, L.P., 1965. Coccidia and Coccidiosis. Akademia Kiado, Budapest, Hungary. 657 p.

Pellérdy, L.P., 1974. Coccidia and Coccidiosis, second ed. Verlag Paul Parey, Berlin and Hamburg, and Akademia Kiado, Budapest, Hungary. 959 p.

Perkins, F.O., Barta, J.R., Clopton, R.E., Peirce, M.A., Upton, S.J., 2000. Phylum Apicomplexa Levine, 1970. In: Lee, J.J., Leedale, G.F., Bradbury, P. (Eds.), An Illustrated Guide to the Protozoa, second ed. Society of Protozoologists, P.O. Box 368, Lawrence, Kansas, vol. 1. , pp. 190–369.

Phillips, M.J., McLenachan, P.A., Down, C., Gibb, G.C., Penny, D., 2006. Combined mitochondrial and nuclear DNA sequences resolve the interrelations of the major Australasian marsupial radiations. Systematic Biology 55, 122–137.

Phillips, P., 1986. Toxoplasmosis in yellow footed rock wallabies. Veterinary Pathology Report, Australian Registry Veterinary Pathology 11, 211–216.

Poelma, F.G., 1966. *Eimeria lemuris* n. sp., *E. galago* n. sp. and *E. otolicni* n. sp. from a Galago *Galago senegalensis*. Journal of Protozoology 13, 547–549.

Pope, J.H., Bicks, V.A., Cook, I., 1957a. Toxoplasmosis in Queensland. II. Natural infections in bandicoots and rats. Australian Journal of Experimental Biology and Medical Science 35, 481–490.

Pope, J.H., Derrick, E.H., Cook, I., 1957b. *Toxoplasma* in Queensland. I. Observations on a strain of *Toxoplasma gondii* isolated from a bandicoot, *Thylacis obesulus*. Australian Journal of Experimental Biology 35, 467–480.

Power, M.L., 2010. Biology of *Cryptosporidium* from marsupial hosts. Experimental Parasitology 124, 40–44.

Power, M.L., Ryan, U.M., 2008. A new species of *Cryptosporidium* (Apicomplexa: Cryptosporidiidae) from eastern grey kangaroos (*Macropus giganteus*). Journal of Parasitology 94, 1114–1117.

Power, M.L., Cheung-Kwok-Sang, C., Slade, M., Williamson, S., 2009a. *Cryptosporidium fayeri*: diversity within the GP60 locus of isolates from different marsupial hosts. Experimental Parasitology 121, 219–223.

Power, M.L., Richter, C., Emery, S., Hufschmid, J., Gillings, M.R., 2009b. *Eimeria trichosuri*: phylogenetic position of a marsupial coccidium based on 18S rDNA sequences. Experimental Parasitology 122, 165–168.

Power, M.L., Shanker, S.R., Sangster, N.C., Veal, D.A., 2003. Evaluation of a combined immunomagnetic separation/flow cytometry technique for epidemiological investigation of *Cryptosporidium* in domestic and Australian native animals. Veterinary Parasitology 112, 21–31.

Power, M.L., Sangster, N.C., Slade, M.B., Veal, D.A., 2005. Patterns of *Cryptosporidium* oocyst shedding by eastern grey kangaroos inhabiting an Australian watershed. Applied and Environmental Microbiology 71, 6159–6164.

Power, M.L., Slade, M.B., Sangster, N.C., Veal, D.A., 2004. Genetic characterization of *Cryptosporidium* from a wild population of eastern grey kangaroos *Macropus giganteus* inhabiting a water catchment. Infection Genetics and Evolution 4, 56–97.

Prasad, H., 1960. A new species of coccidia of the red kangaroo *Macropus rufus* Mamm. Zeitschrift für Parasitenkunde 20, 385–389.

Presidente, P.J.A., 1982. Common wombat *Vombatus ursinus*: maintenance in captivity, blood values, infectious and parasitic diseases. In: Evans, D.D. (Ed.), The Management of Australian Mammals in Captivity. The Zoological Board of Victoria, Melbourne, Australia, pp. 133–143.

Presidente, P.J.A., 1984. Parasites and diseases of brushtail possums (*Trichosurus* spp.): occurrence and significance. In: Smith, A.P., Hume, I.D. (Eds.), Possums and Gliders. Australian Mammal Society and Surrey Beatty and Sons Pty. Ltd, Chipping Norton, New South Wales, pp. 171–190.

Presidente, P.J.A., Barnett, J.L., How, R.A., Humphreys, W.F., 1982. Effects of habitat, host sex and age on the parasites of *Trichosurus caninus* (Marsupialia: Phalangeridae) in north- eastern New South Wales. Australian Journal of Zoology 30, 33–47.

Ratcliffe, H.L., Worth, C.B., 1951. Toxoplasmosis in captive wild birds and mammals. American Journal of Pathology 27, 655–667.

Ratnasingham, S., Hebert, P.D., 2007. BOLD: the barcode of life data system. Molecular Ecology Notes 7, 355–364. http://www.barcodinglife.org.

Reddacliff, G.L., Hartley, W.J., Dubey, J.P., Cooper, D.W., 1993. Pathology of experimentally- induced, acute toxoplasmosis in macropods. Australian Veterinary Journal 70, 4–6.

Reduker, D.W., Duszynski, D.W., Yates, T.L., 1987. Evolutionary relationships among *Eimeria* spp. (Apicomplexa) infecting cricitid rodents. Canadian Journal of Zoology 65, 722–735.

Regendanz, R., Kikuth, W., 1928. Sur les Hémogrégarines de "gamba" (*Haemogregarina didelphydis*) de la "quica" (*Haemogregarina metachiri* n. sp.). Comptes Rendus des Seances Socété de Biologia (Paris) 98, 565–567.

Reichenow, E., Carini, A., 1937. Über *Eimeria travassosi* und die Gattung *Globidium*. Archiv für Protistenkunde 88, 374–386.

Reig, O.A., Kirsch, J.A.W., Marshall, L.G., 1985. New conclusions on the relationships of the opossum-like marsupials, with an annotated classification of the Didelphimorphia. Ameghiniana 21, 335–343.

Reig, O.A., Kirsch, J.A.W., Marshall, L.G., 1987. Systematic relationships of the living and Neocenozoic American "opossum-like" marsupials (suborder Didelphimorphia), with comments on the classification of these and of the Cretaceous and Paleogene New World and European metatherians. In: Archer, M. (Ed.), Possums and opossums: studies in evolution, vol. 1. Surrey Beatty, Sydney, Australia, pp. 1–89.

Rejmanek, D., VanWormer, E., Miller, M.A., Mazet, J.A.K., Nichelason, A.E., Melli, A.C., Packham, A.E., Jessup, D.A., Conrad, P.A., 2009. Prevalence and risk factors associated with *Sarcocystis neurona* infections in opossums (*Didelphis virginiana*) from central California. Veterinary Parasitology 166, 8–14.

Rejmanek, D., Miller, M.A., Grigg, M.E., Crosbie, P.R., Conrad, P.A., 2010. Molecular characterization of *Sarcocystis neurona* strains from opossums (*Didelphis virginiana*) and intermediate hosts from Central California. Veterinary Parasitology 170, 20–29.

Rhee, J.K., Seu, Y.S., Park, B.K., 1991a. Isolation and identification of *Cryptosporidium* from various animals in Korea. I. Prevalence of *Cryptosporidium* in various animals. Korean Journal of Parasitology 29, 139–148.

Rhee, J.K., Seu, Y.S., Park, B.K., 1991b. Isolation and identification of *Cryptosporidium* from various animals in Korea. II. Identification of *Cryptosporidium muris* from mice. Korean Journal of Parasitology 29, 149–159.

Rhee, J.K., Wang, S.S., Kim, H.C., 1999. Age-dependent resistance to *Cryptosporidium muris* (strain MCR) infection in golden hamsters and mice. Korean Journal of Parasitology 37, 33–37.

Rhee, J.K., Yook, S.Y., Park, B.K., 1995. Oocyst production and immunogenicity of *Cryptosporidium muris* (strain MCR) in mice. Korean Journal of Parasitology 33, 377–383.

Rickard, L.G., Black, S.A., Rashmir-Raven, A., Hurst, G., Dubey, J.P., 2001. Risk factors associated with the presence of *Sarcocystis neurona* sporocysts in opossums (*Didelphis virginiana*). Veterinary Parasitology 102, 179–184.

Ride, W.D.L., Cogger, H.G., Dupuis, C., Kraus, O., Minelli, A., Thompson, F.C., Tubbs, P.K. (Eds.), 2000. International Code of Zoological Nomenclature, fourth ed. Published by The International Trust for Zoological Nomenclature, The Natural History Museum, London SW7 5BD, United Kingdom. 306 p. (In English and French).

Riemann, H.P., Behymer, D.E., Fowler, M.E., Schulz, T., Lock, A., Orthoefer, J.G., Silverman, S., Franti, C.E., 1974. Prevalence of antibodies to *Toxoplasma gondii* in captive exotic mammals. Journal of the American Veterinary Medical Association 165, 798–800.

Robinson, G., Chalmers, R.M., 2010. The European rabbit (*Oryctolagus cuniculus*) a source of zoonotic cryptosporidiosis. Zoonoses Public Health 57, 1–13.

Rodhain, J., 1933. On a coccidia from the intestine of a titi monkey. Comptes Rendus des Seances Socété de Biologia (Paris) 114, 1357–1358.

Rose, A.B., Pekelharing, C.J., Platt, K.H., Woolmore, C.B., 1993. Impact of invading brushtail possum populations on mixed beech-broadleaf forests, South Westland, New Zealand. New Zealand Journal of Ecology 17, 19–28.

Rosenthal, B.M., Lindsay, D.S., Dubey, J.P., 2001. Relationships among *Sarcocystis* species transmitted by New World Opossum (*Didelphis* spp.). Veterinary Parasitology 95, 133–142.

Rosonke, B.J., Brown, S.R., Tornquist, S.J., Snyder, S.P., Garner, M.M., Blythe, L.L., 1999. Encephalomyelitis associated with a *Sarcocystis neurona*-like organism in a sea otter. Journal of the American Veterinary Medical Association 215, 1839–1842.

Ryan, U.M., Power, M.L., 2012. *Cryptosporidium* species in Australian wildlife and domestic animals. Parasitology 139, 1673–1688.

Ryan, U.M., Power, M.L., Xiao, L., 2008. *Cryptosporidium fayeri* n. sp. (Apicomplexa: Cryptosporidiidae) from a red kangaroo (*Macropus rufus*). Journal of Eukaryotic Microbiology 55, 22–26.

Schneideer, C.R., 1965. *Besnoitia panamensis* sp. n. (Protozoa: Toxoplasmatidae) from Panamanian lizards. Journal of Parasitology 51, 340–344.

Schneideer, C.R., 1966. Experimental infection of short-tailed bats, *Carollia perspicillata*, with *Besnoitia panamensis* (Protozoa: Toxoplasmatidae). Journal of Parasitology 52, 703.

Schneideer, C.R., 1967a. *Besnoitia darlingi* (Brumpt, 1913) in Panama. Journal of Protozoology 14, 78–82.

Schneideer, C.R., 1967b. Cross-immunity evidence of the identity of *Besnoitia panamensis* from lizards and *B. darlingi* from opossums. Journal of Parasitology 53, 886.

Schneideer, C.R., 1967c. The distribution of lizard besnotiosis in Panama, and its transfer to mice. Journal of Protozoology 14, 674–678.

Schneideer, C.R., 1967d. Susceptibility of the marmoset, *Saguinus geoffroyi* Pucheran, to intraperitoneal and oral infections with *Besnoitia* (Protozoa: Toxoplasmea). Journal of Parasitology 53, 1135–1139.

Scholtyseck, E., Entzeroth, R., Chobotar, B., 1982. Light and electron microscopy of *Sarcocystis* sp. in the skeletal muscle of an opossum (*Didelphis virginiana*). Protistologica 18, 527–532.

Scorza, J.V., Torrealba, J.F., Dagert, C., 1957. *Klossiella tejerai* nov. sp. y *Sarcocystis didelphidis* nov. sp. parasitos de un *Didelphis marsupialis* de Venezuela. Acta Biologia Venezuelica 2, 97–108.

Seneviratna, P., Edward, A.G., DiGiusti, D.L., 1975. Frequency of *Sarcocystis* spp. in Detroit, metropolitan area, Michigan. American Journal of Veterinary Research 36, 337–339.

Shaw, J.J., Lainson, R., 1969. *Sarcocystis* of rodents and marsupials in Brazil. Parasitology 59, 233–244.

Shedlock, A., Okada, N., 2004. SINEs of speciation: tracking lineages with retroposons. Trends in Ecological Evolution 19, 545–553.

Siqueira, D.B., Aléssio, F.M., Mauffrey, J.F., Marvulo, M.F.V., Ribeiro, V.O., Oliveira, R.L., Pena, H.F.J., Gennari, S.M., Mota, R.A., Faustino, M.A.G., Alves, L.C., Dubey, J.P., Silva, J.C.R., 2013. Seroprevalence of *Toxoplasma gondii* in wild marsupials and rodents from the Atlantic Forest of Pernambuco State, Northeastern Region, Brazil. Journal of Parasitology 99, 1140–1143.

Skerratt, L.F., 1998. Diseases and parasites of the common wombat in the Healsville area of Victoria. In: Wells, R.T., Pridmore, P.A. (Eds.), Wombats. Surrey Beatty & Sons, Chipping Norton, New South Wales, Australia, pp. 317–328.

Skerratt, L.F., Phelan, J., McFarlane, R., Speare, R., 1997. Serodiagnosis of toxoplasmosis in a common wombat. Journal of Wildlife Diseases 33, 346–351.

Šlapeta, J., Modry, D., Votypka, J., Jirku, M., Lukes, J., Koudela, B., 2003. Evolutionary relationships among cyst-forming coccidia *Sarcocystis* spp. (Alveolata: Apicomplexa: Coccidea) in endemic African tree vipers and perspective for evolution of heteroxenous life cycle. Molecular Phylogenetic Evolution 27, 464–475.

Smith, D.D., Frenkel, J.K., 1977. *Besnoitia darlingi* (Protozoa: Toxoplasmatinae): cyclic transmission by cats. Journal of Parasitology 63, 1066–1071.

Smith, D.D., Frenkel, J.K., 1984. *Besnoitia darlingi* (Apicomplexa, Sarcocystidae, Toxoplasmatinae): transmission between opossums and cats. Journal of Parasitology 31, 584–587.

Smith, J.H., Meier, J.L., Neill, P.J.G., Box, E.D., 1987a. Pathology of *Sarcocystis falcatula* in the budgerigar. I. Early pulmonary schizogony. Laboratory Investigations 56, 60–71.

Smith, J.H., Meier, J.L., Neill, P.J.G., Box, E.D., 1987b. Pathology of *Sarcocystis falcatula* in the budgerigar. II. Pulmonary pathology. Laboratory Investigations 56, 72–84.

Smith, J.H., Neill, P.J.G., Box, E.D., 1989. Pathogenesis of *Sarcocystis falcatula* (Apicomplexa: Sarcocystidae) in the budgerigar (*Melopsittacus undulatus*). III. Pathologic and quantitative parasitologic analysis of extrapulmonary disease. Journal of Parasitology 75, 270–287.

Smith, J.H., Neill, P.J.G., Dillard III, E.A., Box, E.D., 1990a. Pathology of experimental *Sarcocystis falcatula* infections of canaries (*Serinus canarius*) and pigeons (*Columba livia*). Journal of Parasitology 76, 59–68.

Smith, J.H., Craig, T.M., Dillard III, E.A., Neill, J.G., Jones, L.P., 1990b. Naturally occurring apicomplexan acute interstitial pneumonitis in thick-billed parrots (*Rhynchopsitta pachyrhyncha*). Journal of Parasitology 76, 285–288.

Smith, T.G., 1996. The genus *Hepatozoon* (Apicomplexa: Adeleina). Journal of Parasitology 82, 565–585.

Speare, R., Haffenden, A.T., Daniels, P.W., Thomas, A.D., Seawright, C.D., 1984. Diseases of the Herbert River ringtail, *Pseudocheirus herbertensis*, and other north Queensland rainforest possums. In: Smith, A., Hume, I. (Eds.), Possums and Gliders. Surrey Beatty & Sons with the Australian Mammal Society, Sydney, Australia, pp. 283–302.

Speare, R., Donovan, J.A., Thomas, A.D., Speare, P.J., 1989. Diseases of free-ranging Macropodoidea. In: Grigg, G., Jarman, P., Hume, I. (Eds.), Kangaroos, Wallabies and Rat-kangaroos. Surrey Beatty and Sons, Sydney, pp. 705–734.

Speer, C.A., Dubey, J.P., 1999. Ultrastructure of schizonts and merozoites of *Sarcocystis falcatula* in the lungs of budgerigars *Melopsittacus undulatus*. Journal of Parasitology 85, 630–637.

Spitz dos Santos, C., Berto, B.P., Lopes, B., Do, B., Cordeiro, M.D., da Fonseca, A.H., Filho, W.L.T., Lopes, C.W.G., 2014. Coccidial dispersion across New World marsupials: *Klossiella tejerai* Scorza, Torrealba and Dagert, 1957 (Apicomplexa: Adeleorina) from the Brazilian common opossum *Didelphis aurita* (Wied-Neuwied) (Mammalia: Didelphimorphia). Systematic Parasitology 89, 83–89.

Springer, M.S., Kirsch, J.A.W., Case, J.A., 1997a. The chronicle of marsupial evolution. In: Givnish, T.J., Sytsma, K.J. (Eds.), Molecular Evolution and Adaptive Radiation. Cambridge University Press, New York, pp. 129–161.

Springer, M.S., Burk, A., Kavanagh, J.R., Waddell, V.G., Stanhope, M.J., 1997b. The interphotoreceptor retinoid binding protein gene in therian mammals: implications for higher level relationships and evidence for loss of function in the marsupial mole. Proceedings of the National Academy of Science, USA, 94, 13754–13759.

Stabenow, C.S., Ederli, N.B., Lopes, C.W.G., de Oliveira, F.C.R., 2012. *Didelphis aurita* (Marsupialia: Didelphidae): a new host for *Sarcocystis lindsayi* (Apicomplexa: Sarcocystidae). Journal of Parasitology 98, 1262–1265.

Stabler, R.M., Welch, K., 1961. *Besnoitia* from an opossum. Journal of Parasitology 47, 576.

Stankiewicz, M., Heath, D.D., Cowan, P.E., 1997a. Internal parasites of possums (*Trichosurus vulpecula*) from Kawau Island, Chatham Island and Stewart Island. New Zealand Veterinary Journal 45, 247–250.

Stankiewicz, M., Cowan, P.E., Heath, D.D., 1997b. Endoparasites of brushtail possums (*Trichosurus vulpecula*) from the South Island, New Zealand. New Zealand Veterinary Journal 45, 257–260.

Stankiewicz, M., Jowett, G.H., Roberts, M.G., Heath, D.D., Cowan, P., Clark, J.M., Jowett, J., Charleston, W.A.G., 1996. Internal and external parasites of possums (*Trichosurus vulpecula*) from forest and farmland, Wanganui, New Zealand. New Zealand Veterinary Journal of Zoology 23, 345–353.

Strahan, R. (Ed.), 1983. The Complete Book of Australian Mammals. Agnus and Robertson, Sydney, pp. 207–223.

Sulaiman, I.M., Morgan, U.M., Thompson, R.C.A., Lai, A.A., Xiao, L., 2000. Phylogenetic relationships of *Cryptosporidium* parasites based on the 70-kilodalton heat shock protein (HSP70) gene. Applied and Environmental Microbiology 66, 2385–2391.

Sulaiman, I.M., Xiao, L., Yang, C., Rscalante, L., Moore, A., Beard, C.B., Arrowood, M.J., Lal, A.A., 1998. Differentiating human and animal isolates of *Cryptosporidium parvum*. Emerging Infectious Diseases 4, 681–685.

Supperer, R., 1957. Zwei Coccidien, *Eimeria* (*Globidium*) *tasmaniae* n. sp. und *Eimeria* (*Eimeria*) *ursini* n. sp aus dem Wombat (*Phascolomys ursinus* Shaw). Zeitschrift für Parasitenkunde 17, 510–513.

Szalay, F.S., 1982. A new appraisal of marsupial phylogeny and classification. In: Archer, M. (Ed.), Carnivorous Marsupials. Royal Zoological Society of New South Wales, Sydney, Australia, pp. 621–640.

Tanhauser, S.M., Yowell, C.A., Cutler, T.J., Greiner, E.C., MacKay, R.J., Dame, J.B., 1999. Multiple DNA markers differentiate *Sarcocystis neurona* and *Sarcocystis falcatula*. Journal of Parasitology 85, 221–228.

Tanhauser, S.M., Cheadle, M.A., Massey, E.T., Mayer, B.A., Schrodeder, D.E., Dame, J.B., Griener, E.C., MacKay, R.J., 2001. The nine-banded-armadillo (*Dasypus novemcinctus*) is naturally infected with *Sarcocystis neurona*. International Journal for Parasitology 31, 325–329.

Teixeira, M., Rauta, P.R., Albuquerque, G.R., Lopes, C.W.G., 2007. *Eimeria auritanensis* n. sp. and *E. gambai* Carini, 1938 (Apicomplexa: Eimeriidae) from the opossum *Didelphis aurita* Wied-Newied, 1826 (Marsupialia: Didelphidae) from southeastern Brazil. Revista Brasileira de Parasitologia Veterinária 16, 83–86.

Tenter, A.M., Barta, J.R., Beveridge, I., Duszynski, D.W., Mehlhorn, H., Morrison, D.A., Thompson, R.C.A., Conrad, P.A., 2002. The conceptual basis for a new classification of the coccidia. International Journal for Parasitology 32, 595–616.

Thomas, O., 1888. Catalogue of the Marsupialia and Monotremata in the Collection of the British Museum (Natural History). Trustees of the British Museum (Natural History), London. 401 p. + 28 Plates (digitized by Google).

Thompson, J.D., 2007. *Cryptosporidium* and *Giardia* in Australian Marsupials (Honors Thesis). Veterinary and Biomedical Sciences, Murdoch, Perth, Australia. 141 p.

Thompson, S.W., Reed, T.H., 1957. Toxoplasmosis in a swamp wallaby. Journal of the American Veterinary Medical Association 131, 545–549.

Triffitt, M.J., 1926. Some sporozoan parasites found in the intestinal wall of Bennett's wallaby (*Macropus bennetti*). Protozoology 2, 31–46.

Triffitt, M.J., 1927. Note on the occurrence of a sarcocyst, parasitic in a wallaby. Protozoology 3, 75–76.

Tyson, E., 1698. Carigueya, seu marsupiale americanum. Or, the anatomy of an opossum, dissected at Gresham College by Edw. Tyson, M.D. Fellow of the College of Physicians, and of the Royal Society, and Reader of Anatomy at the Chyrurgeons-Hall in London. Philosophical Transactions 20, 105–164.

Tyzzer, E.E., 1907. A sporozoan found in the peptic glands of the common mouse. Proceedings of the Society for Experimental Biology and Medicine 5, 12–13.

Tyzzer, E.E., 1910. An extracellular coccidium, *Cryptosporidium muris* (gen. et sp. nov.), of the gastric glands of the common mouse. Journal of Medical Research 23, 487–509.

Tyzzer, E.E., 1912. *Cryptosporidium parvum* (sp. nov.), a coccidium found in the small intestine of the common mouse. Archiv für Protistenkunde 26, 394–418.

Upton, S.J., 2000. Suborder Eimeriorina Léger, 1911. In: Lee, J.J., Leedale, G.F., Bradbury, P. (Eds.), An Illustrated Guide to the Protozoa, second ed. Society of Protozoologists, P.O. Box 368, Lawrence, KN, vol. 1. pp. 318–339.

Upton, S.J., Current, W.L., 1985. The species of *Cryptosporidium* (Apicomplexa: Cryptosporidiidae) infecting mammals. Journal of Parasitology 71, 625–629.

Valerio-Campos, I., Chinchilla-Carmona, M., Duszynski, D.W., 2015. *Eimeria marmosopos* (Coccidia: Eimeriidae) from the opossum, *Didelphis marsupialis*, L., 1758 in Costa Rica. Comparative Parasitology 82, 148–150.

Viggers, K., Spratt, D., 1995. The parasites recorded from *Trichosurus* species (Marsupialia, Phalangeridae). Wildlife Research 22, 311–332.

Vogelsang, E.G., 1929. Beiträge zur Kenntnis der Parasitenfauna Uruguays. Sarkosporidian bei Vögeln. Zentralblatt für Bakteriologie. I. Abteilung Originale 113, 206–208.

Volk, J.J., 1938. *Isospora boughtoni* n. sp. from the American opossum, *Didelphis virginiana*. Journal of Parasitology 24, 547–548.

Voss, R.S., Jansa, S.A., 2009. Phylogenetic relationships and classification of dedelphid marsupials in extant radiation of New World metatherian mammals. Bulletin of the American Museum of Natural History 322, 1–177.

Waddell, P.J., Kishino, H., Ora, R., 2001. A phylogenetic foundation for comparative mammalian genomics. Genomic Information Service Workshop. Genome Information 12, 141–154.

Waldron, L.S., Cheung-Kwok-Sang, C., Power, M.L., 2010. Wildlife-associated *Cryptosporidium fayeri* in humans, Australia. Emerging Infectious Diseases 16, 2006–2007.

Walker, E.P., Warnick, F., Hamlet, S.E., Lang, K.I., Davis, M.A., Uible, H.E., Wright, P.F., 1975. (revised by Paradiso, J.L.) Mammals of the World, third ed., vols 2, Johns Hopkins University Press, Baltimore, MD, 1500 p.

Warren, K.S., Swan, R.A., Morgan-Ryan, U.M., Friend, J.A., Elliot, A., 2003. *Cryptosporidium muris* infection in bilbies (*Macrotis lagotis*). Australian Veterinary Journal 81, 739–741.

Warren, W.C., Hillier, L.W., Marshall Graves, J.A., Birney, E., Ponting, C.P., Grützner, F., Belov, K., Miller, W., Clarke, L., Chinwalla, A.T., et al., 2008. Genome analysis of the platypus reveals unique signatures of evolution (+92 other co-authors) Nature 453, 175–183.

Watson, A.D., Farrow, B.R., McDonald, P.J., 1982. Prevalence of *Toxoplasma gondii* antibodies in pet dogs and cats [letter]. Australian Veterinary Journal 58, 213–214.

Weiss, L.M., Kim, K. (Eds.), 2007. *Toxoplasma gondii*: The Model Apicomplexan: Perspectives and Methods. Elsevier/Academic Press, Amsterdam, p. 777.

Wenyon, C.M., 1926. Protozoology, vols 2. ,Wood, New York, 1563 p.

Wenyon, C.M., Scott, H.H., 1925. Exhibitions of sections of intestine of Bennett's wallaby (*Macropus bennetti*) containing various parasites. Transactions of the Royal Society of Tropical Medicine and Hygiene 19, 7–8.

Widmer, G., Akiyoshi, D., Buckholt, M.A., Feng, X., Rich, S.M., Deary, K.M., Bowman, C.A., Xu, P., Wang, Y., Wang, X., Buck, G.A., Tzipori, S., 2000. Animal propagation and genomic survey of a genotype 1 isolate of *Cryptosporidium parvum*. Molecular and Biochemical Parasitology 108, 187–197.

Wilber, P.G., Duszynski, D.W., Upton, S.J., Seville, R.S., Corliss, J.O., 1998. A revision of the taxonomy and nomenclature of the *Eimeria* (Apicomplexa: Eimeriidae) from rodents in the Tribe Marmotini (Sciuridae). Systematic Parasitology 39, 113–135.

Wilhelmsen, C.L., Montali, R.J., 1980. Toxoplasmosis in a parma wallaby. Annual Proceedings of the American Association of Zoo Veterinarians 141–143.

Wilson, D.E., Reeder, D.M. (Eds.), 1993. Mammal Species of the World, second ed. Smithsonian Institution Press, Washington, DC, p. 1207.

Wilson, D.E., Reeder, D.M. (Eds.), 2005. Mammal Species of the World, third ed. vol. 1. Johns Hopkins University Press, Baltimore, MD, p. 743.

Winter, H., 1959. Coccidiosis in kangaroos. Australian Veterinary Journal 35, 301–303.

Xiao, L.H., Bern, C., Limor, J., Sulaiman, I., Roberts, J., Checkley, W., Cabrera, L., Gilman, R.H., Lal, A.A., 2001d. Identification of 5 types of *Cryptosporidium* parasites in children in Lima, Peru. Journal of Infectious Diseases 183, 492–497.

Xiao, L., Fayer, R., Ryan, U., Upton, S.J., 2004. *Cryptosporidium* taxonomy: recent advances and implications for public health. Clinical Microbiology Reviews 17, 72–97.

Xiao, L., Limor, J.R., Li, L., Morgan, U., Thompson, R.C.A., Lal, A.A., 1999a. Presence of heterogeneous copies of the small subunit rRNA gene in *Cryptosporidium parvum* human and marsupial genotypes and *Cryptosporidium felis*. Journal of Eukaryotic Microbiology 46, 44S–45S.

Xiao, L., Limor, J., Morgan, U.M., Sulaiman, I.M., Thompson, R.C.A., Lal, A.A., 2000. Sequence differences in the diagnostic target region of the oocysts wall protein gene of *Cryptosporidium* parasites. Applied and Environmental Microbiology 66, 5499–5502.

Xiao, L., Morgan, U.M., Limor, J., Escalante, A., Arrowood, M., Shulaw, W., Thompson, R.C.A., Fayer, R., Lal, A.A., 1999c. Genetic diversity within *Cryptosporidium parvum* and related *Cryptosporidium* species. Applied and Environmental Microbiology 65, 3386–3391.

Xiao, L., Escalante, L., Yang, C.F., Sulaiman, I., Escalante, A.A., Montali, R.J., Fayer, R., Lal, A.A., 1999b. Phylogenetic analysis of *Cryptosporidium* parasites based on the small subunit ribosomal RNA gene locus. Applied and Environmental Microbiology 65, 1578–1583.

Xiao, L., Sulaiman, I.M., Ryan, U.M., Zhou, L., Atwill, E.R., Tischler, M.L., Zhang, X., Fayer, R., Lal, A.A., 2002. Host adaptation and host–parasite co-evolution in *Cryptosporidium*: implications for taxonomy and public health. International Journal for Parasitology 32, 1773–1785.

Yakimoff, W.L., Matschoulsky, S.N., 1936. Coccidiosis in the kangaroo. Journal of Parasitology 22, 514–515.

Yamada, M.-O., Takeuchi, H., Kamo, S., Inoki, S., 1981. A cyst-forming Eimeriina found in the kangaroo imported from Australia. Zentralblatt für Bakteriologie. I. Abteilung Originale A 250, 361–367.

Yang, R., Fenwick, S., Potter, A., Ng, J., Ryan, U., 2011. Identification of novel *Cryptosporidium* genotypes in kangaroos from Western Australia. Veterinary Parasitology 179, 22–27.

Yoshikawa, H., Iseki, M., 1992. Freeze-fracture study of the site of attachment of *Cryptosporidium muris* in gastric glands. Journal of Protozoology 39, 539–544.

Zanette, R.A., da Silvia, A.S., Aleksandrro, S., Lunardi, F., Santurio, J.M., Monteiro, S.G., 2008. Occurrence of gastrointestinal protozoa in *Didelphis albiventris* (opossum) in the central region of Rio Grande do Sul State. Parasitology International 57, 217–218.

Zhao, X., Duszynski, D.W., 2001a. Phylogenetic relationships among rodent *Eimeria* species determined by plastid ORF470 and nuclear 18S rDNA sequences. International Journal for Parasitology 31, 715–719.

Zhao, X., Duszynski, D.W., 2001b. Molecular phylogenies suggest the oocyst residuum can be used to distinguish two independent lineages of *Eimeria* spp. in rodents. Parasitology Research 87, 638–643.

Zhao, X., Duszynski, D.W., Loker, E.S., 2001a. A simple method of DNA extraction for *Eimeria* species. Journal of Microbiological Methods 44, 131–137.

Zhao, X., Duszynski, D.W., Loker, E.S., 2001b. Phylogenetic position of *Eimeria antrozoi*, a bat coccidium (Apicomplexa: Eimeriidae) and its relationship to morphologically similar *Eimeria* spp. from bats and rodents based on nuclear 18S and plastid 23S rDNA sequences. Journal of Parasitology 87, 1120–1123.

Zhu, B.Y., Hartigan, A., Reppas, G., Higgins, D.P., Canfield, P.J., Šlapeta, J., 2009. Looks can deceive: molecular identity of an intraerythrocytic apicomplexan parasite in Australian gliders. Veterinary Parasitology 159, 105–111.

Zhu, G., Keithly, J.S., Philippe, H., 2000. What is the phylogenetic position of *Cryptosporidium*? International Journal of Systematic and Evolutionary Microbiology 50, 1673–1681.

Zwart, P., Strik, W.J., 1964. Globidiosis in a Bennett's wallaby. Tijdschr Diergeneesk 89 (Suppl. 1), 138–143.

Glossary and Abbreviations

Allopatric A form of speciation that occurs when a vicariant event isolates two populations of the same species for an extensive period of time that interferes with gene flow between them. Also called geographic speciation.

Ameridelphia Refers to the American marsupial orders that include the Didelphimorphia, Microbiotheria, and Pacituberculata.

Anlagen An embryonic area capable of forming a structure; the primordium, germ, or bud.

Apomorphy A specialized, derived, or novel trait or character that is unique to a group or species and all of its descendants and that can be used as a defining character in a phylogenetic context.

Australidelphia Refers to the Australian marsupial orders that include the Dasyuromorphia, Diprotodontia, Notoryctemorphia, and Peramelemorphia.

Baculum A penis bone. This is a bone found in the penis of many placental mammals such as carnivores, rodents, bats, and some primates, but not in humans.

Bifid A unique feature of marsupial reproductive systems in which the reproductive structures of both males (penis) and females (vagina, uterus) are doubled.

Binomial nomenclature A formal system of naming species by giving each a name composed of two parts using Latin (or Greek, or other) grammatical forms. The first part of the name identifies the genus to which the species belongs and the second part identifies the species within that genus and, when correctly written, this scientific name is italicized (e.g., *Homo sapiens*). The application of such names—initiated in 1753 by the Swedish naturalist Carl Linnaeus—is now governed by internationally agreed upon codes, which, for animals, is the *International Code of Zoological Nomenclature*.

Bradyzoites Slowly dividing zoites that reproduce asexually by endodyogeny within the tissue cysts of members of the Sarcocystidae (*Besnoitia, Sarcocystis, Toxoplasma*).

CLAJP Continuous lower ankle joint pattern, an anatomical distinction used at one time to separate the Australidelphia from the Ameridelphia. The former, along with the Microbiotheria, are characterized by CLAJP.

Comparative genomics The use of sequences from multiple genomes and comparing and analyzing them to understand evolutionary processes both within and between hypothesized clades.

Convergent evolution The independent evolution of a feature in species of different lineages. For example, wings have evolved many times independently (flies, birds, bats); and Australian koalas have fingerprints that are indistinguishable from those of humans.

Cytophaneres Species of *Sarcocystis* produce sarcocysts in their intermediate hosts. These sarcocysts have very characteristic cyst walls, some of which have radial spines composed of fibrils and coarse, electron-dense granules when viewed with the transmission electron microscope.

Diprotodonty The condition of having two front teeth, a dental condition that unifies the largest order of Australian marsupials, the Diprotodontia.

Endodyogeny A specialized form of asexual reproduction in which two progeny form within the parent parasite, consuming it in the process.

Endopolygeny Formation of daughter cells, each surrounded by its own membrane, while still in the mother cell.

Eutherian Mammals that have a placenta within which to nourish their young during gestation.

Extant Those species still living now versus those that are extinct.

Facultative Optional. In parasitology, establishing a relationship with a host only if an opportunity presents itself, but there is no physiological dependence to do so.

g gram.

Gamogony (gametogony) The process of gamete formation.

HCN An abbreviation used throughout this book to refer to the host cell nucleus.

Herbivore An animal that eats plants almost exclusively.

Heteroxenous Describes a parasite that lives with more than one host during its life cycle.

Homoxenous A parasite life cycle where only a single host species is involved.

Hypertrophic Enlargement, increase in volume, or overgrowth of a cell or body part.

Insectivore A plant or animal that eats insects almost exclusively.

Intraperitoneal (IP) Injection of a substance into the peritoneum or body cavity.

IUCN International Union for the Conservation of Nature.

Karyotype The number and appearance of chromosomes in the nucleus of a eukaryotic cell. Also, a picture of an organism's chromosomes that have been isolated from the nucleus of one of its cells, then fixed, put on slides, and stained.

kg Kilogram = 1000 g.

M An abbreviation used throughout this book to refer to the micropyle, usually a circular opening at one end of the oocyst, usually the more pointed end.

Marsupium (sing.)/Marsupia (pl.) A pouchlike enclosure found in marsupials for nursing their young.

Merogony The process of merozoite formation via asexual reproduction. Also called schizogony in the older literature.

Metatherian(s) Marsupials.

m_n An abbreviation used to refer to a merozoite of a particular asexual generation (first, second, etc.) during asexual reproduction (merogony) in a host.

M_n An abbreviation used to refer to the meront of a particular asexual generation (first, second, etc.) during asexual reproduction (merogony) in a host.

Molecular homoplasies Similar shared characteristics of organisms that lack a common ancestry; that is, those characteristics driven by mutational pressures from something like a vicariant event.

Monophyly/Monophyletic In cladistic usage, refers to a taxon or group that forms a clade consisting of an ancestral species and all of its known descendents.

Monotremes Egg-laying mammals such as spiny ant-eaters (echidnas) and the duck-billed platypus.

MYA Million years ago.

N An abbreviation used throughout this book to refer either to the nucleus (sing.) or nuclei (pl.) within various coccidian stages.

Nocturnal Active or occurring at night.

Omnivore/omnivorous An organism that eats food of both plant and animal origin.

OR An abbreviation used throughout this book to refer to the oocyst residuum, a structure often found within the oocyst.

Orthologous genes Two genes that diverged after a speciation event so that the history of the gene reflects the history of the species.

Parasitophorous vacuole (PV) A vacuolated space inside a host cell that surrounds a developing stage (e.g., meront, gamont) of an apicomplexan parasite.

Parous Females that are in the process of or have produced offspring.

PAS granules Periodic acid-Schiff (PAS) is a staining method used to detect polysaccharides (e.g., glycogen) and granules that take up this stain indicate the presence of various sugars.

Pelage Fur, hair, or wool of a mammal.

Per os Orally.

PG An abbreviation used throughout this book to refer to the polar granule, a small, usually refractile structure often found within the oocyst.

PI An abbreviation used throughout this book to refer to postinoculation, usually in days, meaning the time period between when a host is inoculated with a parasite and the day a particular stage of the parasite's life history is seen/discovered.

Placental(s) Those mammals possessing a placenta, an organ that connects the developing fetus to the uterine wall to allow gas exchange, nutrient uptake, and waste elimination.

Platypus A semiaquatic, egg-laying mammal endemic to eastern Australia.

Poikilotherms Organisms such as amphibians, fishes, and reptiles whose internal temperatures vary considerably with the ambient temperature.

Polyprotodontia Marsupials characterized by four or more pairs of upper incisor teeth in their jaw.

PSB An abbreviation used throughout this book to refer to the parastieda body, a structure of unknown composition that is found at the more rounded end of the sporocyst (SP), opposite the Stieda body (SB) that is located at its more pointed end.

Retroposed elements/retroposons Repetitive fragments of DNA that are inserted randomly into chromosomes after they have been reverse-transcribed from any RNA. Their presence or absence can provide a uniquely informative source of rare genomic changes that can be used in molecular systematics.

RG An abbreviation used throughout this book to refer to the refractile granule or globule, a spheroidal to subspheroidal structure or structures often, but not always, found inside sporozoites (SZ).

SB An abbreviation used throughout this book to refer to the Stieda body, a nipplelike structure found at the more pointed end of the sporocyst (SP).

Semifossorial An organism adapted for digging and spending some, but not all (fossorial) of its time underground (e.g., badgers).

SLAJP Separate lower ankle joint pattern, an anatomical distinction used at one time to separate the Australidelphia from the Ameridelphia. The latter group of orders, except for the Microbiotheria, are characterized by SLAJP.

SP An abbreviation used throughout this book to refer to the sporocyst, which encloses sporozoites (SZ).

Sporogony The formation of spores, or in the case of intestinal coccidia, it is the process by which sporocysts form and develop inside the oocyst, usually when it leaves the confines of the host gastrointestinal tract.

SR An abbreviation used throughout this book to refer to the sporocyst residuum, a structure often found within a sporocyst (SP).

SSB An abbreviation used throughout this book to refer to the substieda body, a structure that lies immediately under the Stieda body (SB) at the more pointed end of the sporocyst (SP).

Symbiotype host A single museum specimen of a host animal from which a new species of parasite has been described. This specimen is considered the type host for that parasite. The name comes from the Greek "*symbio*" meaning to live together.

Synapomorphy In cladistic analysis: A character state that is shared between two or more taxa and inferred to have been present in their most recent common ancestor.

Syndactyly A condition in the Peramelemorphia where the second and third toes on their hind foot are fused together (although they maintain separate claws); thought to be an adaptation for climbing.

Syngamy Fusion of gametes that are whole cells.

Syzygy The pairing of male and female gametes or the pairing of chromosomes in meiosis.

SZ An abbreviation used throughout this book to refer to the sporozoites that are enclosed within the sporocyst (SP).

Tachyzoites The rapidly multiplying stage of zoites in the Sarcocystidae that reproduce asexually by endodyogeny inside the body of the intermediate host. These are crescent-shaped forms, ~6×2, that actively enter host cells.

USNPC United States National Parasite Collection, now housed at the Smithsonian Institution, Washington, D.C., USA.

Vestigial A genetically determined structure (or trait) that has lost most or all of its ancestral function (e.g., appendix in humans).

Vibrissae Longer, thicker hairs of many mammals that have a tactile function with well-innervated hair follicles.

WFB An abbreviation for wall-forming bodies, globular structures found in fertilized macrogamonts that migrate to the periphery of the gamont to eventually coalesce and form the oocyst wall.

Zoonosis (sing.)/zoonoses (pl.) Disease agents of wild or domesticated animals that are transmissible to humans when they come in contact with each other.

Index

Printed in the United States
By Bookmasters